Making Choices: Ethics Issues for Health Care Professionals

Edited by Emily Friedman

AHA.

American Hospital Publishing, Inc.,
a wholly owned subsidiary of the
American Hospital Association

Library of Congress Cataloging-in-Publication Data
Main entry under title:

Making choices.

  Bibliography: p.
  "Catalog no. 025100"—T.p. verso.
  1. Medical ethics. 2. Hospital care—Moral and
ethical aspects. 3. Medicine—Decision making.
I. Friedman, Emily.
R724.M165   1986   174'.2   85-30681
ISBN 0-939450-77-1

Catalog no. 025100
©1986 by
American Hospital Publishing, Inc.,
a wholly owned subsidary of the
American Hospital Association

AHA is a service mark of American Hospital Association used under license by American Hospital
Publishing, Inc.
Printed in the U.S.A.
Text set in Baskerville
2.5M-4/86-0117

Audrey Young Kaufman, Editor
Peggy DuMais, Production Coordinator
Patrick J. Kane, Manager, Graphic Design
Melanie Campillo, Designer
Dorothy Saxner, Vice-President, Books

To the memory of

William Bartling, who helped establish
the right of patients to seek a high quality of death as
well as a high quality of life,

and

Donje McNair, a low-income Illinois child,
who died of liver disease in 1983 because funding
was not available for a liver transplant

Our heritage is composed of all the voices
that can answer our questions.
—Andre Malraux

About the Author

Emily Friedman, Chicago, is a contributing editor for *Hospitals* magazine and a contributing writer for *Medical World News, Medical Staff News, Health Progress, Healthcare Forum,* and other publications. She also serves as director of program analysis for Community Programs for Affordable Health Care, a Robert Wood Johnson Foundation project, cosponsored by the American Hospital Association and the Blue Cross and Blue Shield Association. Ms. Friedman lectures and teaches on health care ethics, the medically indigent, and American health services. She has written on health care ethics for *Hospitals, Trustee, The Hospital Medical Staff, Health Progress, Primary Care,* and *Society,* and is coauthor of a forthcoming book on the issues surrounding heart transplants.

Contents

Foreword

Aldous Huxley tells us that "All great truths began as heresy." Many people are asking both heretical and nonheretical questions about America's health care system. It is a time of great flux and change and challenge in the health care field. Our system is one of the most technologically advanced and ingenious. However, it is also one of the most expensive in the world, and it increasingly is being shown to have obvious flaws. The questions being asked of America's health care professionals are not only appropriate, they are overdue.

We are moving into a brave new world of medical science, in many ways as new as the world that Columbus discovered. We are on the threshold of the bionic man. Medical science explodes with ingenuity, yet the public's ability to fund this inventiveness is severely limited. America has a massive federal deficit and an economy that no longer can fully afford all the health care that medical science can bring us. Infinite needs have run into finite resources.

In my opinion, there is something fundamentally wrong in a society that no longer makes radios, black-and-white television sets, or video recorders (even though we invented all of them), but does have enough money to provide kidney dialysis on demand. We give smokers heart transplants, but we close our steel mills. We spend money to manufacture artificial hearts but not to repair our infrastructure, reform our school systems, or retool our economy. We are great at treating sick people, but we do little to treat our sick economy. In our search to be humane, we are uneconomic; our consciences may be clear, but our pockets are nearly empty. We are treating our illnesses at the expense of our livelihood.

America spends $1,500 per capita on health care. England spends $400, and Singapore spends $200. Yet the mortality and morbidity rates in all three nations are approximately the same. We spend far more, but for what result? If I had a department head who was spending four times as much as his counterpart in other states, I would fire him immediately. But not only do we not fire our health care system, we really have only begun to ask it some very hard questions.

We are told that "expense is no consideration when a life is at stake." This is patently absurd. I govern a state that loses many, many people every year in plane crashes in our mountains. Many times we cannot find the crash site immediately. Should I send massive search teams into our mountains every time because "a life is at stake," even if it means cannibalizing the money from our school system, our roads, and our prison system? If I did so, I would rightly be impeached. We have to make a value judgment as to how many resources we can correctly allocate to each search. We must make a hard decision every time.

The Greeks tell us that to know what to ask is to know half the answer. The value of this book is that it raises issues that will not go away and that must be solved. We can hide from these issues. We can wish they would go away. We can say, like Charlie Brown in *Peanuts,* "There is no issue so big that we can't run away from it." But ultimately society, and especially health care providers, must confront these issues.

I believe that by not asking these hard questions, we have started down a number of wrong roads:

- Humana's budget for the artificial heart is approximately the same amount of money that the world spent in eradicating smallpox. Does it make any sense for a society that doesn't provide prenatal care to many low-income women to be spending money on artificial hearts?

- Does it make any sense to give an organ transplant to an 85-year-old man, even if he is otherwise healthy? How much sense does it make to spend $5,000 to repair a car that has 200,000 miles on it?

- How do we allocate the limited number of donor organs that are available for transplant? Currently, we often seem to allocate them on the basis of who can get the most publicity. We treat the people we can point the television camera at; we turn our backs on those that we cannot see.

We can prevent far more heart disease than we can ever treat with transplants or artificial hearts, but, as others have pointed out, prevention affects statistics, whereas curative approaches affect individuals. This media-driven humanitarianism misallocates our health resources toward the dramatic. We do not care so much if people die; we just don't want to see them die on television. It is not the tragedy, but the knowledge, the witnessing of it, that we abhor.

Does it make any sense to spend half of all medical expenditures on 4 percent of the sick, with 40 percent being spent on 1 percent of them? Dramatic treatments often bring fame to doctors and hospitals, but can they be justified in a nation that needs to retool its economy, improve its infrastructure, and better educate its kids? And even within health care, does it make any sense to spend most of our resources on a few when we could, for the same money, achieve much better health for the American public as a whole through prevention and treatment of more common ailments?

I know how volatile these questions are. And when it comes to death and dying, they are not only volatile, but volcanic. Yet we must address this last taboo. Shakespeare observed, "We all owe God a death." In my opinion, many times we spend scarce societal resources keeping hopelessly ill people alive so that they can suffer for a couple of more days. If we all must die sometime, then we must make wise judgments as to whether certain procedures constitute treatment—or torture. I am all for spending money if it produces a medically happy outcome. However, if all we do is prolong dying, often extending patients' suffering as well, our moral ambivalence is not only causing pain but also costing society resources that are desperately needed elsewhere. A Catholic priest once likened much of our treatment of the terminally ill to "taping the leaves to the trees in the winter." It is not only fruitless, it is unseemly. And it is often cruel.

The process of policy development in the United States moves in fits and starts, and while it does so, these questions—which are the basis of theoretical debate for many—constitute a daily, practical burden for health care professionals. Hospital executives, managers, medical and nursing staffs, and trustees must decide how resources should be allocated. Those who care for the patient at the bedside must try to determine the appropriate level and duration of care while, it sometimes seems, attorneys, governments, third-party payers, churches, and the hospital itself are peering over their shoulders. The hospital, as a social institution, has to determine what is right, not only in the case of the individual patient within its walls, but in terms of the community it is committed to serve. It is probably unfair to ask hospitals and those who work within them to make frontline, life-or-death decisions every day while the policy debate moves at a snail-like pace. But it is their lot for now, and to some degree—no matter what decisions society does or does not ultimately make—it always will be.

In identifying issues and in trying to provide some wisdom for those who must resolve them, this book performs one of the ultimate public services—it forces us to confront reality and to consider what we are doing, whether we are policymakers, citizens, or health care professionals who end up making policy by default. *Making Choices* reminds us that the unthinkable must eventually meet the inevitable. In the end, it does not add to our comfort level, but it adds to the body of our wisdom.

Richard D. Lamm
Governor of Colorado
November 1985

Preface

Health care ethics today, as one of the preeminent people in the field has observed, is in danger of becoming a fad. It has all the ingredients: timeliness, intellectual challenge, news media attention, complexity, life-and-death stakes, and an aura of earth-shaking importance. With so much to carry on its shoulders, ethics is also in danger of being crushed by its own weight.

But the emergence of ethical issues in health care, given recent events in the field, was entirely predictable. Fast-moving developments that have reconfigured not only how we pay for health care, but also how we provide it, have unbalanced the fragile teeter-totter arrangement through which the United States—admittedly in a disorganized fashion—was able to provide at least some health care to most of its residents, most of the time. Equally revolutionary events in health care technology have led many people to question whether health care is always good for you. Whereas we once debated, in private, simple issues such as whether or not to tell a patient he had a terminal illness, we now, in the glare of both electronic and print media, debate the value of the artificial heart. In the words of David Willis, editor of the *Milbank Memorial Fund Quarterly,* our ability to develop medical technology has outstripped our ability to internalize it.

Winston Churchill reportedly once said that Americans could be counted on to do the right thing, once they had exhausted all possible alternatives. An American physician recently observed, paraphrasing Walter Heller, that an ethicist was a person who, having seen that something works in practice, wonders whether it will work in theory. Those two satirical rules actually serve quite well as bookends for the quandaries facing American health care providers. On the one hand, they often must act long before any theory is available to govern that act; on the other hand, they always want to do the right thing, even if no one knows what the right thing is. As the cocktail party participant in a classic *New Yorker* cartoon laments, "I'd like to take the easy way out—if I knew what the easy way out was."

It was in the hope of lighting some of these darkened pathways that this book was undertaken, in full knowledge of the fact that many volumes preceded it and many others will follow. We developed the content, which includes both prepublished and original material, with one goal in mind: to guide policy development and decision making in the health care institution. Ethics is a dim science even under the best of circumstances, and it was not our intention to curse the darkness further with yet another book that raised more questions than it answered. We therefore reviewed the literature and consulted with leading theorists and practitioners of health care ethics with an eye toward helping those institutions and practitioners who are daily on the front lines of ethical decision making.

We knew, going in, that the questions outnumbered the answers by a goodly margin; but we also knew that health care professionals have an astonishing ability to synthesize workable solutions to problems, with only the thinnest of theories to help them. This book, then, only hopes to thicken the basis of decision making, because it presumes that most people working in health care, even in this volatile and sometimes chaotic environment, will still choose to follow the dictates of the heart and the mind as well as those of the purse.

There are many individuals who contributed to this book. Many of their names appear in it and many do not. Among the latter are Mary Layne Ahern, assistant general counsel, American Hospital Association; Albert Jonsen, Ph.D., chief, Division of Medical Ethics, University of California, San Francisco; and Frederick Abrams, M.D., director, Center for Applied Biomedical Ethics, Rose Medical Center, Denver.

This book would not have come about had it not been for the determined professionalism and patience of Audrey Young Kaufman, who is the real editor of this tome, and for Dorothy Saxner, Vice-President, Books, American Hospital Publishing, Inc., who has been my mentor and guide throughout this project and for much of my professional life.

Finally, some thanks are due to those who put me on the road to ethics in health care in the first place. I owe both gratitude and respect to Judith P. Swazey, Ph.D., who, in a brilliant presentation at the American Public Health Association's annual meeting many years ago, introduced me to the subject; to Albert Jonsen, Ph.D., whose intellectual fireworks continue to stimulate me; to Alexander M. Capron and Joanne Lynn, M.D., to whom the American public as a whole owes a debt of gratitude for their yeoman work on the President's Commission; to Glenn Richards, who helped me understand that emotional wrenching is necessary in order to produce good work in ethics; to James F. Childress, whom I have never met, but who has provided us with many of the answers; to Roger W. Evans, Ph.D., and George J. Annas, J.D., who keep me honest; to Jack Wennberg, M.D., and Phil Caper, M.D., who have taught me that reallocation of what we have is a far more moral solution than rationing care to the vulnerable; and to Corrine Bayley, who combines ethical theory and practice every day of her life with both passion and intelligence and thereby serves as an example to us all.

If this book helps even a few of those who must live and work on the firing line, it will have fulfilled its purpose.

Emily Friedman
December 1985

The Hospital within Society:
Theory

For as long as they have existed, hospitals have been perceived as social institutions. Even today, with new incentives associated with the competitive marketplace exerting a stronger influence on health care and hospitals than ever before, the hospital still holds a special place in society. Indeed, the collision of hospitals' traditional social responsibilities with the realities of the marketplace has been one of the strongest forces bringing ethical issues in health care to the fore.

There have been other forces at work as well. The legacy of the civil rights movement of the 1950s and 1960s has come to wield a powerful influence on what patients expect of their hospitals and physicians. The development of technology that prolongs life without restoring health has led to a different relationship between the historically technology-loving American public and health care providers who offer them that technology. An aging society is already exerting stress on social programs that were designed to protect the elderly in an era when relatively few Americans lived to see the age of 70. In terms of what economist Richard Rahn says is a question of "intergenerational equity," the United States must now try to determine who has the best claim on limited health resources: the retired elderly, the nonworking youth, or the employed who are being asked to subsidize health care for both groups.

There is no "right answer" to guide us in these murkiest of waters. However, even if there is no natural law waiting to be discovered that will provide the truth, there are broad ethical frameworks within which we can begin to make decisions, or at least formulate the right questions.

In this section, Howard H. Hiatt, M.D., sets the agenda: what are the limits of the health care practitioner's responsibility, and what constitutes appropriate health care when resources are limited? The wide-ranging and penetrating conclusions of the President's Commission for the Study of Ethical Problems in Medicine and Biomedical and Behavioral Research are offered next. Rogert W. Evans, Ph.D., then argues that the issues of rationing health care services must be expressed in terms of how, *not,* if, *and that technology assessment and optimal use of health care dollars could diminish the pain that American society will have to undergo in the process.*

Rudolf Klein reminds us that culture plays a significant part in how we structure our health care systems and how we ration their services. H. Tristram Engelhardt, M.D., Ph.D., uses organ transplantation as a paradigm for the entire issue of allocation of scarce health care resources and warns us that we should not be deterred from combating unfairness simply because some tragedies will occur regardless of what we do. Finally, Emily Friedman explores whether two tiers of care are acceptable in American health care, and who should decide what that really means.

Protecting the Medical Commons: Who Is Responsible?

Howard H. Hiatt, M.D., Department of Medicine, Brigham and Women's Hospital, Boston

I n 1968, in an article called "The Tragedy of the Commons," Garrett Hardin discussed a class of human problems that in his view had no technical solution.[1] Focusing on the population problem, Hardin likened our present dilemma to that of a group of herdsmen whose cattle shared a common pasture. As long as the number of animals was small in relation to the capacity of the pasture, each herdsman could increase his holdings without detriment to the general welfare. As the number of cattle approached the capacity of the land, however, each additional animal contributed to overgrazing. Any single herdsman attempting to maximize his own gain could reasonably project that the addition of one or a few cattle to his holdings would have minimal effect on the general welfare. All herdsmen reasoning and acting individually in this fashion, however, would destroy the commons. "Ruin," concluded Hardin, "is the destination toward which all men rush, each pursuing his own best interest in a society that believes in the free-

dom of the commons. Freedom in a commons brings ruin to all."

The total resources available for medical care can be viewed as analogous to the grazing area on Hardin's commons, and the practices drawing on those resources to Hardin's grazing animals. Surely, nobody would quarrel with the proposition that there is a limit to the resources any society can devote to medical care, and few would question the suggestion that we are approaching such a limit. Yet there is almost universal recognition that among the additional demands that must be made on our resources are those designed to address the current inadequacy of medical care for large sectors of the population. The dilemma confronting us is how we can place additional stress on the medical commons without bringing ourselves closer to ruin.

In our society, demands from both preventive and curative medicine are made upon the same commons and therefore must be regarded as in competition with each other and with needs

Reprinted, with permission, from *The New England Journal of Medicine* 1975 July 31. 293(5):235–241.
Based on the keynote address at the First Annual Conference on Progress and Prospects in Health Care Distribution Systems, Miami, FL, November 25–27, 1974.
Supported by grants from the Robert Wood Johnson Foundation and the Commonwealth Fund.
When this article was written, Dr. Hiatt was at the Center for Analysis of Health Practices, Harvard School of Public Health, Boston.

for research and teaching. Priority setting is further complicated by the inadequacy of data that are critical to intelligent decision-making. Failure to recognize these realities has in the past often led to unwise policy setting, without due consideration of long-term consequences. We need to consider problems arising from ways in which the medical commons has traditionally been used and the need for alternative approaches.

First of all, let us look at a principle on which medical practice has been based—that one should do everything possible for the individual patient. Let us then examine this principle in the context of our system, in which few constraints are placed upon the introduction of new medical practices. I believe this is a luxury we can no longer afford. As we develop more and more practices that may be beneficial to the individual but not to the interests of society, we risk reaching a point where marginal gains to individuals threaten the welfare of the whole.

Secondly, we must examine another consequence of freedom of access to the medical commons: the utilization of precious resources for practices that benefit neither the individual nor society, and that indeed are frequently harmful to both. Such practices are especially important in a campaign to reduce demands on the medical commons, for their elimination would benefit both individual and society.

Thirdly, there is a widely accepted but narrow interpretation of health as an exclusively medical concern, which, together with a failure to appreciate fully the limitations of curative medicine, contributes to continuing raids on the commons by expensive practices. At best, many of these deal imperfectly with conditions that could be prevented by less costly approaches.

Although no one should be optimistic that we can rapidly change existing practices and thereby redirect resources to other pressing needs, an examination of a few of our present problems may be useful, especially in preventing their replication, and possibly in contributing to their amelioration.

Medical Practices That Pose Conflicts between the Interests of the Individual and Those of Society

An infant born with agammaglobulinemia has markedly reduced resistance to and may die from infection. The test for detecting the condition is simple and relatively inexpensive. Once the condition is diagnosed, one can immediately institute treatment that will prevent or ameliorate serious infections. However, the condition is so rare that in a society with limited resources it would be difficult to argue for a universal screening campaign, even though it might prevent serious illness and occasionally even death among a few infants.

Detection of agammaglobulinemia may be an extreme case, but a sensitive one nonetheless. Even more troubling are questions that arise concerning more prevalent conditions. A most poignant example today may be kidney dialysis and transplantation, access to which has been largely determined by economic and geographic considerations. Other procedures pose similar questions. If coronary-artery bypass graft operations were shown to be effective for all patients with coronary-artery disease, if an effective artificial heart were found, if the artificial pancreas now being investigated were shown to be potentially useful to the estimated four million Americans with diabetes, what fraction of our resources should be given to these measures, and at what cost to others dependent on the commons?

A decision that may shortly be before us provides another example. A recent report[2] suggested that trained pre-hospital rescue units may contribute to increased survival of patients with cardiac arrest. The report described 301 subjects with prehospital ventricular fibrillation for whom the rescue units were used. For the 42 who survived to leave the hospital, the mean survival period was 12.7 months (and five of the survivors required long-term care for brain damage). For discussion purposes, let us grant that such an approach to patients with cardiac arrest did save these lives. Reasoned decision making would then require that society first ascertain the cost per life saved and determine whether a universal program of implementation were worthy of further consideration. Two critical questions would be: What can really be achieved? Are the benefits of wide application such as to warrant displacing something else? In raising such questions, it is essential to recognize the needs for continuing research in medical care, such as that represented by the study on the rescue units, on the one hand, and for decision making regarding the dissemination of new practices, once proved effective, on the other.

A deeply troubling (and perhaps insoluble)

ethical dilemma comes sharply into focus when we attempt to set a monetary value on a human life. However, the dilemma is unnecessarily intensified by a widespread misconception that the principal objective of medical practice is the prevention of death. Bunker[3] points out that only a small fraction of surgery and a much smaller fraction of nonsurgical encounters involve life-and-death decisions, most being directed at the provision of relief from physical or emotional discomfort or disability. In these circumstances we must think in such terms as which measures will provide greater relief, which conditions are more burdensome, and which patients are in greater need of help. Although these quesions are obviously thorny ones, they provide a more common framework for discussion of tradeoffs than attempts to relate the value of a life to the resources of the commons. The latter question, too, must be dealt with, but much less often than the former.

The issues that arise with regionalization of medical resources seem so much easier to resolve that one wonders why they are so prevalent. Early in the 1960's, for example, it was found that of almost 800 hospitals in the United States equipped for closed heart surgery, over 90 per cent did fewer than one case per week, and 30 per cent had done none in the year studied.[4] Although regionalization may sometimes lead to inconvenience and questions of "status" (some take pride in having "everything" locally available), the drawbacks seem trivial when compared, first, to the medical advantage of having such complicated procedures carried out by specialists whose skills are honed on a continuous basis and, second, to the obvious economic benefits.

Medical Practices of No Value or of Undetermined Value

Nancy Mitford[5] may have been indulging in literary license when she predicted that "in another two hundred and fifty years present day doctors may seem to our descendants as barbarous as Fagon and his colleagues seem to us . . . In those days, terrifying in black robes and bonnets, they bled the patient; now, terrifying in white robes and masks, they pump blood into him." Wholesale bloodletting disappeared from our "therapeutic" kit long ago, but within my own professional lifetime, I recall seeing patients "treated" for multiple sclerosis by having blood pumped into them until they were polycythemic.

How do we determine which practices should be discarded and which continued? More than 20 years ago the British statistician Sir Austin Bradford Hill demonstrated the importance to medical investigation of the randomized controlled trial, which had been developed earlier in agriculture by R. A. Fisher. It was used for testing the Salk vaccine, and partly as a result, when the field trials of the vaccine were completed, the vaccine's usefulness has been unequivocally proved.

One could cite a substantial number of procedures that were at one time practiced rather widely in this country, many of them within relatively recent years, but that have now been virtually abandoned. Such a list might include gastric freezing for peptic ulcer, colectomy for epilepsy, bilateral hypogastric-artery ligation for pelvic hemorrhage, renal-capsule stripping for acute renal failure, sympathectomy for asthma, internal-mammary-artery ligation for coronary-artery disease, the "button" operation for ascites, adrenalectomy for essential hypertension, complete dental extraction for a variety of complaints thought to be the result of focal sepsis, lobotomy for many mental disorders, and wiring for aortic aneurysm. It is interesting that most of these practices disappeared not because better procedures came along (which would have been an appropriate reason) but because they were found ultimately to be without value. No careful pilot studies were undertaken to evaluate them at the time they were introduced. As a result, even though some merited introduction on an experimental basis, they remained on the medical commons much too long, at costs that went beyond those of the economic resources inappropriately used.

A number of other medical practices, shown or suggested to be without merit, remain with us. For example, treating critical phases of acute illnesses in intensive-care units has become an established practice in many general hospitals over the past decade. Griner[6] compared adult patients suffering from pulmonary edema of nonsurgical causes who were admitted to the intensive-care unit of a university hospital with those admitted to a general medical floor immediately before the opening of the special unit. His studies revealed no difference in mortality and a slightly but no significantly increased duration of stay for patients in the unit. In Griner's words, "The most noticeable change in the overall experience of adult patients hospitalized with acute pulmonary edema . . . since the opening of an intensive care unit has been a marked increase in the cost of rendering care to these patients." (Note that charges for a day of care on the general medical services of one Boston teaching hospital at present average $250; charges for a day on the intensive-care unit exceed $400!) The Griner study requires confirmation, particularly since his "control" group may have differed from the experimental. But if it were proved valid, what steps might be taken to protect the commons?

Although tonsillectomy surely has a place in medical practice, some pediatricians suggest that over 90 per cent of the one million children who underwent tonsillectomies last year in the United States did so unnecessarily. Consistent with this estimate, one study showed a greater than 10-fold difference in the procedure from one area to another in the same state.[7] If 90 per cent is a reasonable approximation, the $400 million taken from the medical commons for this purpose might have been reduced to less than $40 million, the number of hospital days required for people undergoing this operation might have been reduced proportionately, and the number of deaths, using only a conservative estimate of deaths expected from general anesthesia alone, might have been cut from 70 to seven. The reduction in human suffering, of course, cannot be described in such quantitative terms.

Oral hypoglycemic agents were initially hailed as an alternative to insulin injections for many diabetic patients. Randomized clinical trials, however, gave evidence, first published over five years ago,[8,9] of increased cardiovascular disease, which in the view of most experts outweighs any possible short-term benefits of the drugs. Nonetheless, according to a rough estimate based on the number of prescriptions written and the prescription renewal rate, 1.4 million Americans were taking these compounds last year. This figure has gone up progressively over the years despite increasing adverse evidence concerning the usefulness of the drugs.[10]

It is important to recognize that randomized trials cannot always be done,[11,12] but the problem is compounded in dealing with practices already adopted. Once disseminated, a practice is not quickly abandoned, even after it has been shown ineffective—another strong reason for careful evaluation before widespread adoption of new procedures. Let us consider the drain on resources resulting from a few practices whose true usefulness still remains to be established.

At present, there are few hospitals without coronary-care units. There is no disputing the cost they have added to our medical bills, but there is much debate about their effects on mortality from myocardial infarction.[13,14]

Cytologic examination of uterine cervical secretions is commonly assumed to be responsible for the acknowledged recent decline in deaths from carcinoma of the uterine cervix. However, this cause-and-effect connection has by no means been conclusively demonstrated. Since the death rate began falling some years before there was widespread use of the examination, and, further, since the rate of decline has been much the same in different areas, irrespective of the proportion of women screened,[15,16] serious questions must be raised concerning the role of the procedure.

These data emphasize the need for further evidence and cast considerable doubt on the justifiability of the enormous drain of resources. However, both the coronary-care unit and cervical cytologic examination are so much a part of the medical culture that it now seems impossible to carry out proper evaluation. Indeed, one effect of premature adoption is to place ethical difficulties in the way of truly controlled trials.

A present case in point may be coronary-artery bypass graft operations. It is estimated that 38,000 such procedures were carried out in the United States in 1973, at a cost in excess of $400 million. Almost 400 hospitals are believed to have bypass teams, and one of the strongest proponents for this approach to management of coronary-artery disease was recently quoted as having said that the United States should prepare to do 80,000 coronary arteriograms a day.[17] Rough calculations indicate that such a radiologic assessment alone would cost in excess of $10 billion a year and would average one catheterization for every American every 10 years. If today's ratio of arteriograms to bypass surgery were to prevail, the cost of the resultant surgery would exceed $100 billion a year, a figure almost equivalent to the total resources now on the commons!

The current absence of regulatory mechanisms for dissemination of such procedures offers little hope for restraints, even long enough for proper evaluation. Ironically enough, in the absence of regulatory mechanisms, national health insurance, particularly if limited to catastrophic events, could accelerate premature application of this and similar costly procedures.

At an earlier stage of utilization is the computerized axial tomograph machine for radiologic examination. The capital cost of each machine is nearly $400,000. It permits extremely sophisticated diagnostic studies of the brain without the need for invasive procedures, and may prove an important addition to the diagnostic armamentarium. However, its role remains to be established. Furthermore, it requires more highly specialized personnel, and there already is evidence of its being used for purposes for which much simpler equipment is adequate. Will we be able to establish guidelines for the purchase and use of this machine before it, too, becomes a prominent and unregulated occupant of the medical commons?

Medical Practices for Potentially Preventable Conditions

There are at present substantial claims on our resources that could be reduced appreciably on the basis of existing knowledge. The savings in lives, disability, and money resulting from polio vaccine are often and appropriately cited as evidence of a triumph of modern medical research. However, carelessness in prophylactic programs has recently led to a recrudescence of poliomyelitis. Another striking example was the increased incidence of measles that followed a decrease in distribution of measles vaccine (at least in part the result of decreased federal support). The annual number of reported cases of measles decreased from almost 500,000 in 1962 to 22,000 in 1968,[18] but, with lessening of attention to control programs, rose again to a high of 75,000 in 1971. The incidence has since receded, but the need for constant attention is apparent. It has been estimated that the economic benefit of measles vaccine over a 10-year period exceeded $1.3 billion. The savings in terms of lives saved and cases of mental retardation averted[19] are even more important.

Fluoridation provides another example of how preventive measures can spare our resources. There is persuasive evidence that we could halve dental decay among children by fluoridation, at an annual cost of less than 20 cents per person. Nevertheless, less than 60 per cent of the United States water supply was artificially fluoridated in 1972.[4]

Compensation paid last year in the United States by the Social Security Administration alone for victims of black lung exceeded $500 million. The physician, lacking specific treatment for this condition, is largely limited to treating compli-cations and providing the emotional support required by patient and family. Although it is admittedly difficult to estimate the cost of preventing this condition, it seems likely that it would not begin to approach present costs in economic, let alone human, terms.

Although preventive medical care often has little effect where poor social conditions are allowed to persist,[20] this is not always the case.[21,22] Gordis,[22] for example, has shown that over a three-year period in an urban area with comprehensive medical care, rheumatic fever was about one third lower than in comparable parts of the same city without such care. The implications for reductions in valvular heart disease and nephritis are apparent, and the long-term economic effects would probably be highly beneficial.

There is, perhaps, even more evidence of how changes in social conditions can reduce demands on medical resources. For example, it is well known that, probably in large part because of improved nutrition, deaths from tuberculosis had fallen 10-fold in Britain in the century before the first effective medical measures became available.[23] Also highly relevant, although difficult to quantitate in terms of economic effects on the commons, are conclusions drawn from an examination of birth certificates for New York City for the year 1968. If a New York mother was white, native born, and a college graduate, her infant's chances of dying before his first birthday were 9 per thousand. Corresponding chances for the infants of black, native-born mothers with an elementary-school education were 51 per thousand.[24]

Also difficult to deal with are conditions whose prevention requires changes in individual behavior. This year 70,000 American males will die of lung cancer—more than the total number of victims of the three next most common forms of cancer, well over 90 per cent of all people with lung cancer, and approximately the same proportion killed by it more than 25 years ago. The admittedly impressive advances in cancer surgery, radiotherapy, chemotherapy, and anesthesia and in our understanding of certain aspects of carcinogenesis have had no effect on this or, in fact, on most prevalent forms of cancer. It is estimated that as much as 90 per cent of all cancer in this country is the result of environmental factors. In lung cancer, cigarette smoking has unquestionably been implicated. How to respond to that information, thereby sparing the medical commons, remains a challenge. So far as other forms of cancer are concerned, has an adequate fraction of the massive resources committed to cancer programs been allocated to identifying carcinogens and to reducing exposure?

Progress and Prospects in Health Care Distribution Systems

While we must draw further upon our resources to increase access to medical care for the people who are now underserved, the commons is clearly approaching depletion. This fact makes it the more urgent that new demands be limited to practices that have been conclusively demonstrated to meet well defined needs. New practices must also be shown to be more important than whatever will be displaced as a result of their adoption.

McKeown[25] points out that too often in medicine tasks are approached without any adequate survey of the nature of the most important problems. Now that there is generally successful management of infectious diseases, he emphasizes, the currently most pressing problems in Western societies are congenital disabilities, including mental defects, mental illness, and diseases of aging. Any approach designed to provide access to health care for an underserved population cannot purport to be comprehensive if it does not give serious attention to these problems. McKeown's list was neither offered as all-inclusive nor in fact was it intended to describe needs specific to the United States. In a study of children in a large urban American community, Kessner, Snow, and Singer[26] found a shockingly high prevalence of all the conditions being investigated. More than one fourth of children six months to three years old had anemia, and more than one fourth of children four to 11 years of age failed a comprehensive vision screening examination. Twenty per cent of all children had evidence of middle-ear disease, and 7 per cent of those four to 11 years old had hearing loss in speech frequencies that could interfere with learning. Illustrating yet another kind of need, the studies of Brook et al.[27] have shown that even by minimal criteria, only two thirds of the patients discharged from a highly respected American teaching hospital had adequate follow-up care during the six months after discharge. For most of the other patients, any benefit derived from hospitalization had been lost by the time of the six-month evaluation interview. All these diverse needs point to the necessity of attention to deficiencies frequently found in planning the delivery of health care—deficiencies in collecting and evaluating information, in analyzing results, in determining costs, and in using valid data as a basis for action.

Admittedly, not all needs of an adequate medical-care delivery system can be described in quantitative terms. One example in my view is the security implicit in the existence of an organized medical-care system to which people can quickly and easily turn. There must be a telephone number that can be called at any time of day or night and that offers access to enlightened advice, and, if needed, entry into the system. The voice on the telephone need not be that of a physician; indeed, that would be wasteful. However, it is not too much to expect it to be that of a person who is concerned, compassionate, and informed, who has access to the caller's medical record, and who can offer practical and sensitive responses—that is, suggestions for effective action and reassurance appropriate to the problem. My own experience with a prepaid group practice left a strong impression that this service was as much appreciated as any other.

Like most contemporary medical dilemmas, assessing the quality of medical performance is easier to identify as a problem than to deal with. Economic as well as sociologic, psychologic, and other considerations suggest that medical-care systems be arranged so that the skills of the medical-care provider are matched to the job undertaken. Methods for continuing evaluation of performance would help to achieve this end and to promote flexibility as our capabilities improve.

Of course, medical care, no matter how well delivered, is not the sole solution to most of the health problems that confront us. Kessner's population was an urban one, and many of the deficiencies that he and his colleagues observed could be attributed more to the social, economic, or demographic characteristics of the children than to how or where they received medical care.[26] This is not an argument against the need for greater access to better medical care, for it would surely be possible to improve the medical situation described. Rather, it is a way to emphasize that changes in social factors—housing, nutrition, education, etc.—are necessary in any comprehensive and effective approach to health problems.

The innovations that are needed or that are in prospect must be preceded by pilot tests. Not only is pre-testing an integral part of any research endeavor, but as has been indicated, the difficulties of eliminating medical practices once they are widely disseminated make it imperative that there be rigorous evaluation.

Who Will Protect the Commons?

It was not so long ago that the commons bore relatively few expensive practices, there were no well defined limits, and the conscientious physician took from it what he deemed essential for his patient. Recently, however, we have witnessed major advances in expensive technology, greater complexity of medical problems, greater expertise in medical and health matters on the part of nonmedical professionals, and greater participation by consumers in dealing with major issues. These developments have all taken place in a short time and appear to be accelerating. Meanwhile, no well conceived methodology for governing access to the medical commons has evolved, despite the ever increasing need for setting priorities, particularly as we approach the institution of national health insurance. Certainly, our failure to confront these very difficult problems has not meant that problems have not been dealt with. However, when we had relatively limited capabilities and seemingly unlimited resources, the consequences of a largely laissez-faire policy were not so visible and so painful as they now are. Unless safeguards not in view are conceived and applied, the priorities for use of the commons will continue to be set as they have been—at best by well intentioned policy makers with information of limited quantity and quality, and at worst in anarchic fashion.

How should priorities be set in the United States? Who should set them? How much should be allocated for health in toto? Of that total, how much should be allocated for medical care? How much for research, and in that category, how much for basic science and how much for applied? How much for medical education? How much for educating the public? Of each fraction, how should apportionments be made? And what, in each case, should be the quid pro quo? If a hypertension management program can receive only a limited sum, how should that money be optimally used? If renal dialysis cannot be universally available, who should qualify for treatment? What kinds of people should make these decisions? On what basis should their decisions be made?

Although there are no simple answers to these questions, let me first emphasize how I believe national priorities cannot and should not be set. It is surely not fair to ask the physician or other medical-care provider to set them in the context of his or her own medical practice. A physician or other provider must do all that is permitted on behalf of his patient. In that sense the physician is and should be responsible, with his patient and the patient's family, for setting priorities for that patient's management, within the limits available. The patient and the physician want no less, and society should settle for no less. For example, if society has set no ground rules for the use of kidney dialysis other than medical ones, and if in a physician's judgment his 80-year-old patient's overall condition warrants dialysis, everything must be done to see that he is so treated. On the other hand, the physician can, however reluctantly, accept society's constraints regarding eligibility requirements for kidney dialysis, even if he does not consider them to be in the best interests of his patient.

I believe it is as inappropriate to indict physicians for the depletion of resources on the commons as it is to expect physicians alone to determine priorities. The challenge for the medical profession is how to join with others in effective decision making. In this context, let us return to the three problem areas of the commons described earlier.

In the face of conflicts between the interests of the individual patient and of society, choices must be made concerning how much of (or whether) our resources should, for example, be spent for kidney dialysis and for heart transplants, and if so, who is eligible. Physicians must help gather and present as realistically and comprehensively as possible scientific and medical information about kidney dialysis and heart transplants, and then join with a variety of other professionals, including statisticians, epidemiologists, economists, policy analysts, lawyers and ultimately, politicians and the public in setting priorities. Clearly, decisions will heavily depend on both the quality and the quantity of information provided by the medical profession.

To protect the commons from useless, prematurely introduced, or otherwise inappropriate practices, the physician must join statisticians, epidemiologists and economists to ensure that no practice is widely adopted without prior evaluation. As reported by Cochrane,[28] the British National Health Service encourages examination of new diagnostic and therapeutic practices, often by randomized clinical trial, and then submits them for approval by an officially appointed board. (Thus, for example, at the time of Cochrane's presentation neither the carcinoembryonic antigen test for cancer nor coronary-artery bypass graft operations had yet been approved.) As Cochrane has stressed,[29] clinical validation of a practice is not by itself adequate reason for its dissemination. It must be shown to be more effective than other practices available for the same medical problem. And even if this second requirement is satisfied, its value should be manifestly greater than that of those other practices that its adoption would displace.

It is in the third area, prevention, that long-term opportunities are greatest for protecting the resources of the commons. Here, too, the physician must join with others, including consumers, if programs are to be maximally effective. The example of the costs and our therapeutic limitations in the management of black lung was earlier stressed. Although the physician by himself can do little to prevent the condition, his effectiveness in prevention could be amplified many times if he were joined by the mine operator, the union official, the politician, the lawyer, the chemist, the engineer and others. In addition, a more widespread understanding of the limitations of therapeutic medicine could generate greater attention to the need for campaigns directed at preventing black lung and the myriad other conditions for which we can now do so little.

It cannot be overemphasized that our successes in prevention of disease reflect in large part the fruits of research. If these successes are to be followed by the many others we and future generations so badly need, a substantial and predictable fraction of our resources must be set aside for basic scientific research, and for education of research scientists. In my view it is essential that society create mechanisms that separate the demands on the commons of research and of education from those of medical care, for these should not be forced to compete with each other on a continuing basis.

In conclusion, two points seem to me worthy of special emphasis. The first is that the critical question confronting the medical professions is not whether society will find ways to govern access to and control the use of the medical commons. (A people that was sufficiently aroused to create a Food and Drug Administration to control pharmaceutical preparations will surely find mechanisms for controlling medical and surgical procedures when the effects of inadequate restraints become more widely evident.) The question, rather, is how physicians will participate in the creation of control mechanisms in a manner that reflects both enlightened self-interest and the public interest. Physicians must join with educators and others to find ways to encourage the general public to understand more about not only their bodies but also the limitations and uncertainties of medical care, so that society's decision-making can be as fully informed as possible. Indeed, only if physicians assume a major role can they contribute adequately to the protection of the public interest.

Secondly, it is essential that the process of decision making with respect to the medical commons be maximally flexible. Many technical approaches to medical care that were acceptable a decade ago are inadequate today; the same thing must be said about medical judgments and even ethical and moral decision making. Much of what we physicians and our fellow members of society agree is appropriate for 1975 will probably be inadequate for the conditions of 1980. Although it is unfortunately true that existing data are inadequate in most cases to permit fully enlightened decision making today, decision making must and does go on, nonetheless, sometimes by default. This fact makes it more urgent that the process undergo continuing review and revision, to permit us to deal with the issues that inevitably emerge from any reordering of priorities and from continuing progress.

I am indebted to Drs. Herbert Sherman, John Bunker, Harvey Fineberg, and Donald Berwick for many helpful discussions, and to Ms. Cordelia Swain and Miss Constance West for technical assistance.

References

1. Hardin G: The tragedy of the commons. Science 162:1243–1248, 1968

2. Liberthson RR, Nagel EL, Hirschman JC, et al: Prehospital ventricular defibrillation: prognosis and follow-up course. N Engl J Med 291:317–321, 1974

3. Bunker J: Risks and benefits of surgery, From Benefits and Risks in Medical Care: A symposium held by the Office of Health Economics. Edited by D Taylor. Luton, England, White Crescent Press, Ltd, 1974

4. Maxwell RJ: Health Care: The growing dilemma. New York, McKinsey and Company, Inc., 1974

5. Mitford N: The Sun King. New York, Harper and Row, 1966

6. Griner PF: Treatment of acute pulmonary edema: conventional or intensive care? Ann Intern Med 77:501–506, 1972

7. Wennberg J, Gittelsohn A: Small area variations in health care delivery. Science 182:1102–1108, 1973

8. The University Group Diabetes Program. A study of the effects of hypoglycemic agents on vascular complications in patients with adult-onset diabetes. Diabetes 19:Suppl 2:747–830, 1970

9. Knatterud GL, Meinert CL, Klimt CR, et al: Effects of hypoglycemic agents on vascular complications in patients with adult-onset diabetes. IV. A preliminary report on phenformin results. JAMA 217:777–784, 1971

10. Report of the Committee for the Assessment of Biometric Aspects of Controlled Trials of Hypoglycemic Agents. JAMA 231:583–608, 1975

11. Jaffe N, Frei E III, Traggis D, et al: Adjuvant methotrexate and citrovorum-factor treatment of osteogenic sarcoma. N Engl J Med 291:994–997, 1974

12. Weinstein MC: Allocation of subjects in medical experiments. N Engl J Med 291:1278–1285, 1974

13. Astvad K, Fabricius-Bjerre N, Kjaerulff J, et al: Mortality from acute myocardial infarction before and after establishment of a coronary care unit. Br Med J 1:567–569, 1974

14. Martin SP, Donaldson MC, London CD, et al: Inputs into coronary care during 30 years: a cost effectiveness study. Ann Intern Med 81:289–293, 1974

15. Mitchell JW: Exfoliative cytology in screening for cervical cancer—a critique. Can Med Assoc J 105:833,836, 1971

16. Kinlen LJ, Doll R: Trends in mortality from cancer of the uterus in Canada and in England and Wales. Br J Prev Soc Med 27:146–149, 1973

17. Does the U.S. need 80,000 coronary angiograms a day? Med World News 15(34):14–16, 1974

18. Landrigan PJ, Conrad JL: Current status of measles in the United States. J Infect Dis 124:620–622, 1971

19. Barkin RM, Conrad JL: Current status of measles in the United States. J Infect Dis 128:353–356, 1973

20. McDermott W, Deuschle KW, Barnett CR: Health care experiment at Many Farms. Science 175:23–31, 1972

21. Alpert JJ, Heagarty MC, Robertson L, et al: Effective use of comprehensive pediatric care: utilization of health resources. Am J Dis Child 116:529–533, 1968

22. Gordis L: Effectiveness of comprehensive-care programs in preventing rheumatic fever. N Engl J Med 289:331–335, 1973

23. McKeown T, Lowe CR: An Introduction to Social Medicine. Second edition. Oxford, Blackwell Scientific Publications, 1974

24. Institute of Medicine, Panel on Health Services Research. Infant Death: An analysis by maternal risk and health care (Contrasts in Health Status, Vol 1), Washington, DC, Institute of Medicine, National Academy of Sciences, 1973

25. McKeown T: A conceptual background for research and development in medicine. Int J Health Serv 3:17–28, 1973

26. Institute of Medicine, Panel on Health Services Research. Assessment of Medical Care for Children (Contrasts in Health Status, Vol 3). Washington, DC, Institute of Medicine, National Academy of Sciences, 1974

27. Brook RH, Appel FA, Avery C. et al: Effectiveness of inpatient follow-up care. N Engl J Med 285:1509–1514, 1971

28. Cochrane AL: The feasibility of relating quality control to medical outcomes: a critical appraisal. Presented at the fall meeting of the Institute of Medicine, National Academy of Sciences, Washington, DC, November 6, 1974

29. *Idem:* Effectiveness and Efficiency: Random reflections on health services. London, Nuffield Provincial Hospitals Trust, 1972

Introduction to *Securing Access to Health Care*

President's Commission for the Study of Ethical Problems in Medicine and Biomedical and Behavioral Research

In November, 1978, the United States Congress passed legislation establishing the President's Commission for the Study of Ethical Problems in Medicine and Biomedical and Behavioral Research, which was charged with investigating and reporting on key ethical issues in health care. Among those issues were the definition of death, several areas of biomedical research, access to health care, making decisions as to the course of treatment, deciding to forego life-sustaining treatment, and genetic problems. This chapter is taken from the introduction to volume I, Securing Access to Health Care, a Report on the Ethical Implications of Differences in the Availability of Health Services. *It was published in March 1983.*

The prevention of death and disability, the relief of pain and suffering, the restoration of functioning: these are the aims of health care. Beyond its tangible benefits, health care touches on countless important and in some ways mysterious aspects of personal life that invest it with significant value as a thing in itself. In recognition of these special features, the President's Commission was mandated to study the ethical and legal implications of differences in the availability of health services.[1] In this Report to the President and Congress, the Commission sets forth an ethical standard: access for all to an adequate level of care without the imposition of excessive burdens. It believes that this is the standard against which proposals for legislation and regulation in this field ought to be measured.

In fulfilling its mandate from Congress, the Commission discusses an ethical response to differences in people's access to health care. To do so, it is necessary both to examine the extent of those differences and to try to understand how they arise. This focus on the problems of access ought not to obscure the great strengths of the American health care system. The matchless contributions made by America's biomedical scientists to medical knowledge and techniques, the high skill and compassionate devotion of countless physicians and other health professionals, the extensive financial protection against health care costs available to most people, the great generosity with time and funds of many individuals and organizations—these are the hallmarks of health care in the United States. Therefore, the objective here is not to disparage the system but merely to encourage responsible decisionmakers—in the private sector and at all levels of government—to strive to ensure that every American has a fair opportunity to benefit from it.

Health care is a field in which two important American traditions are manifested: the responsibility of each individual for his or her own welfare and the obligations of the community to its members. These two values are complementary

This chapter is an excerpt from the Introduction to *Securing Access to Health Care,* a Report on the Ethical Implications of Differences in the Availability of Health Services. Washington, D.C.: Government Printing Office, March 1983.

rather than conflicting; the emphasis on one or the other varies with the facts of a particular situation. In the field of health care, personal responsibility is a corollary of personal self-determination, which the Commission discussed in its recent report on informed consent.[2] At the same time, ill health is often a matter of chance that can have devastating consequences; thus, concern has long been expressed that health care be widely available and not unfairly denied to those in need.

Since the nineteenth century, the United States has acted—through the founding of the Public Health Service and of hospitals for seamen, veterans, and native Americans, and through special health programs for mothers and infants, children, the elderly, the disabled, and the poor— to reaffirm the special place of health care in American society. With the greatly increased powers of biomedical science to cure as well as to relieve suffering, these traditional concerns about the special importance of health care have been magnified.

In both their means and their particular objectives, public programs in health care have varied over the years. Some have been aimed at assuring the productivity of the work force, others at protecting particularly vulnerable or deserving groups, still others at manifesting the country's commitment to equality of opportunity. Nonetheless, most programs have rested on a common rationale: to ensure that care be made accessible to a group whose health needs would otherwise not be adequately met.[3]

The consequence of leaving health care solely to market forces—the mechanism by which most things are allocated in American society—is not viewed as acceptable when a significant portion of the population lacks access to health services. Of course, government financing programs, such as Medicare and Medicaid as well as public programs that provide care directly to veterans and the military and through local public hospitals, have greatly improved access to health care. These efforts, coupled with the expanded availability of private health insurance, have resulted in almost 90% of Americans having some form of health insurance coverage. Yet the patchwork of government programs and the uneven availability of private health insurance through the workplace have excluded millions of people. The Surgeon General has stated that "with rising unemployment, the numbers are shifting rapidly. We estimate that from 18 to 25 million Americans—8

to 11 percent of the population—have no health insurance coverage at all."[4] Many of these people lack effective access to health care, and many more who have some form of insurance are unprotected from the severe financial burdens of sickness.

Nor is this a problem only for the moment. The Secretary of Health and Human Services recently observed that despite the excellence of American medical care, "we do have this perennial problem of about 10% of the population falling through the cracks."[5] What is needed now are ethical principles that offer practical guidance so that health policymakers in Federal, state, and local governments can act responsibly in an era of fiscal belt tightening without abandoning society's commitment to fair and adequate health care.

Summary of Conclusions

In this Report, the President's Commission does not propose any new policy initiatives, for its mandate lies in ethics not in health policy development. But it has tried to provide a framework within which debates about health policy might take place, and on the basis of which policymakers can ascertain whether some proposals do a better job than others of securing health care on an equitable basis.

In 1952, the President's Commission on the Health Needs of the Nation concluded that "access to the means for the attainment and preservation of health is a basic human right."[6] Instead of speaking in terms of "rights," however, the current Commission believes its conclusions are better expressed in terms of "ethical obligations."

The Commission concludes that society has an ethical obligation to ensure equitable access to health care for all. This obligation rests on the special importance of health care: its role in relieving suffering, preventing premature death, restoring functioning, increasing opportunity, providing information about an individual's condition, and giving evidence of mutual empathy and compassion. Furthermore, although life-style and the environment can affect health status, differences in the need for health care are for the most part undeserved and not within an individual's control.

In speaking of society, the Commission uses the term in its broadest sense to mean the collective American community. The community is made up of individuals who are in turn members of many other, overlapping groups, both public and private: local, state, regional, and national units; professional and workplace organizations; religious, educational, and charitable institutions; and family, kinship, and ethnic groups. All these entities play a role in discharging societal obligations.

The societal obligation is balanced by individual obligations. Individuals ought to pay a fair share of the cost of their own health care and take reasonable steps to provide for such care when they can do so without excessive burdens. Nevertheless, the origins of health needs are too complex, and their manifestation too acute and severe, to permit care to be regularly denied on the grounds that individuals are solely responsible for their own health.

Equitable access to health care requires that all citizens be able to secure an adequate level of care without excessive burdens. Discussions of a right to health care have frequently been premised on offering patients access to all beneficial care, to all care that others are receiving, or to all that they need—or want. By creating impossible demands on society's resources for health care, such formulations have risked negating the entire notion of a moral obligation to secure care for those who lack it. In their place, the Commission proposes a standard of "an adequate level of care," which should be thought of as a floor below which no one ought to fall, not a ceiling above which no one may rise.

A determination of this level will take into account the value of various types of health care in relation to each other as well as the value of health care in relation to other important goods for which societal resources are needed. Consequently, changes in the availability of resources, in the effectiveness of different forms of health care, or in society's priorities may result in a revision of what is considered "adequate."

Equitable access also means that the burdens borne by individuals in obtaining adequate care (the financial impact of the cost of care, travel to the health care provider, and so forth) ought not to be excessive or to fall disproportionately on particular individuals.

When equity occurs through the operation of private forces, there is no need for government involvement, but the ultimate responsibility for ensuring that society's obligation is met, through a combination of public and private sector arrangements, rests with the Federal government. Private health care providers and insurers, charitable bodies, and local and state governments all have roles to play in the health care system in the United States. Yet the Federal government has the ultimate responsibility for seeing that health care is available to all when the market, private charity, and government efforts at the state and local level are insufficient in achieving equity.

The cost of achieving equitable access to health care ought to be shared fairly. The cost of securing health care for those unable to pay ought to be spread equitably at the national level and not allowed to fall more heavily on the shoulders of particular practitioners, institutions, or residents of different localities. In generating the resources needed to achieve equity of access, those with greater financial resources should shoulder a greater proportion of the costs. Also, priority in the use of public subsidies should be given to achieving equitable access for all before government resources are devoted to securing more care for people who already receive an adequate level.[7]

Efforts to contain rising health care costs are important but should not focus on limiting the attainment of equitable access for the least well served portion of the public. The achievement of equitable access is an obligation of sufficient moral urgency to warrant devoting the necessary resources to it. However, the nature of the task means that it will not be achieved immediately. While striving to meet this ethical obligation, society may also engage in efforts to contain total health costs—efforts that themselves are likely to be difficult and time-consuming. Indeed, the Commission recognizes that efforts to rein in currently escalating health care costs have an ethical aspect because the call for adequate health care for all may not be heeded until such efforts are undertaken. If the nation concludes that too much is being spent on health care, it is appropriate to eliminate expenditures that are wasteful or that do not produce benefits comparable to those that would flow from alternate uses of these funds. But measures designed to contain health care costs that exacerbate existing inequities or impede the achievement of equity are unacceptable from a moral standpoint. Moreover, they are unlikely by themselves to be successful since they will probably lead to a shifting of costs to other entities, rather than to a reduction of total expenditures.

Notes

1. 42 U.S.C. § 300v-1(a)(1)(D)(Supp. 1981).

2. President's Commission for the Study of Ethical Problems in Medicine and Biomedical and Behavioral Research, *Making Health Care Decisions,* U.S. Government Printing Office, Washington (1982).

3. Although public programs have generally rested on this rationale, some have been structured so as to include people who could obtain adequate care on their own without excessive burdens. Medicare, for example, covers virtually all of the elderly, not only those who cannot afford the cost of care.

4. Interview with Dr. C. Everett Koop, U.S. Surgeon General, U.S. *News & World Report* 35, 36 (June 28, 1982). The Director of the Congressional Budget Office recently stated that almost 11 million former workers and their dependents have already lost their coverage under their employers' health insurance plan because of unemployment, and that more will lose coverage as their extended benefits expire. This is in addition, she points out, to roughly 20 million persons who are uninsured for other reasons. Alice M. Rivlin, *Health Insurance and the Unemployed,* Statement before the Subcomm. on Health and the Environment, Comm. on Energy and Commerce, U.S. House of Representatives (Jan. 24, 1983).

5. Larry Frederick, Schweiker on Health Policy, *Medical World News* 61, 69 (July 19, 1982).

6. *President's Commission on the Health Needs of the Nation,* U.S. Government Printing Office, Washington (1953) at 3.

7. Although the Commission does not endorse devoting public resources to individuals who already receive adequate care, exceptions arise for particular groups with special ethical claims, such as soldiers injured in combat, to whom the nation owes a special debt of gratitude.

Health Care Decisions: A Summary of the Conclusions of the President's Commission

Alexander M. Capron, LL.B., Department of Law, University of Southern California, Los Angeles

In this chapter, Alexander M. Capron, executive director of the President's Commission for the Study of Ethical Problems in Medicine and Biomedical and Behavioral Research, now the Norman Topping Professor of Law at the University of Southern California, Los Angeles, summarizes the findings that the President's Commission published in Making Health Care Decisions *(1982)* and Deciding to Forego Life-Sustaining Treatment *(1983).*

Introduction

Making Health Care Decisions[1] and *Deciding to Forego Life-Sustaining Treatment*,[2] two of the 11 reports of the President's Commission for the Study of Ethical Problems in Medicine and Biomedical and Behavioral Research, explore the ways that decisions about health care, in areas such as preventive care, surgery, family planning, and life-sustaining treatment, are shaped by moral, ethical, and legal constraints. Although the complexity of the subject makes it "exceptionally difficult to summarize the Commission's conclusions" and "the synopsis provided here should be read in the context of the reasoning, elaboration, and qualifications"[3] set forth in the reports themselves, this chapter provides a brief summary of these reports.

Three major interests are implicated in health care decision making: (1) the patient's right of self-determination and (2) the patient's well-being, as reflected in (3) the health professional's expert judgment. In addition, when it becomes necessary to prevent suicide, to protect third parties, or the like, the state's interest may also be activated. Yet, despite the importance of these interests, no one answer can be given for most health problems. Because of incomplete knowledge, the attendant uncertainty of treatment outcome, and the diversity of personal values and objectives, each course of treatment is accompanied by its own benefits and risks, the balance of which will shift depending on a patient's health status. As a result, the roles of the physician and the patient in the decision-making process have been matters of debate.

Advances in medical technology and increased medical consumerism have led to changing expectations, requiring a redefinition of the roles of health care professionals. Two models have been used to describe the poles of health care decision making: medical paternalism and patient sovereignty. In each model the moral authority has been assigned to one side, while the other side assumes a compliant role. On the one hand, medical paternalism portrays the professional as the patient's moral surrogate, with the authority and the responsibility to make health

Professor Capron was executive director of the President's Commission for the Study of Ethical Problems in Medicine and Biomedical and Behavioral Research.

care decisions in what the professional regards as the patient's best interests. On the other hand, patient sovereignty assigns to the professional the role of technician, providing the requisite information and performing those steps desired by the patient.

The President's Commission found that neither of these extreme positions adequately addresses the nature and needs of health care today. Instead, the extreme diversity of health problems and possible treatments requires a cooperative relationship between the patient and the health care professional. Such a relationship provides the context for shared decision making based on "mutual respect and participation, not a ritual to be equated with reciting the contents of a form that details the risks of particular treatments."[4]

Informed Consent

Although health care professionals have traditionally been accorded great deference and authority, limits have also been present. The long-recognized obligation of professionals to seek consent from their patients before a physical intervention—in legal terms, a "touching"—has evolved over the past quarter century into the legal doctrine of informed consent. In addition to requiring voluntary consent, the informed consent doctrine mandates that a professional engage in discussion and disclosure in order to "inform" the patient.

The President's Commission was asked by Congress to report on the subject of "informed consent." Rather than focus solely on the legal technicalities of the rule, the Commission decided to examine the subject within the broader context of relations and communication between patients and providers.

> Fundamentally, informed consent is based on respect for the individual, and in particular, for each individual's capacity and right both to define his or her own goals and to make choices designed to achieve these goals. But in defining informed consent (and its exceptions) the law has tempered this right of self-determination with respect for other values, such as promotion of well-being, in the context of an expert-layperson relationship.[5]

Through a large national survey, the Commission found that a desire for information, choice in treatment decision, and respectful communication (values that underlie the concept of informed consent) were present among Americans regardless of age, sex, race, income, education, and subculture. However, when questioned as to what informed consent meant, both the public and health care providers produced a range of responses, leading the Commission to conclude that informed consent is "only dimly perceived—and perhaps even misunderstood—by many people."[6]

Legal Background

Doctrine

Early consent-to-treatment cases were concerned with unauthorized procedures and were prosecuted as "battery." Battery consists of the harmful or offensive touching of another person without that person's consent. In addition to express consent, permission may also be implied by a person's acts or words. Battery cases generally involve situations in which a surgeon has exceeded the agreed-upon limits of an operation, or where a professional actually has acted against the patient's expressed wishes.

In contrast, informed consent deals with disclosure and discussion, and is prosecuted as negligent nondisclosure. The term "informed consent" first appeared in *Salgo v. Leland Stanford Jr., University Board of Trustees*,[7] and *Natanson v. Kline*.[8] This "duty to warn," which imposes an affirmative obligation on the health care provider, is a legal obligation in many states that recognize a legal right of recovery for failure to obtain informed consent.

> [S]uch cases typically involve allegations by an injured patient that a practitioner's improper failure to warn of specific risks led the patient to accept medical procedures that resulted in harm the patient would have avoided if warned. The courts must determine whether such allegations are true and, if so, whether the practitioner should be legally liable to the injured patient.[9]

In deciding what must be disclosed, states have adopted different standards of care. Some states utilize professional custom, which requires the patient to produce expert testimony, and some use patient-based criteria, which do not require expert testimony.

Litigation Process
One of the Commission's reasons for looking beyond the law of informed consent was to overcome the distorting effect that the litigation process has had on achieving the goals of ethical theory in this field. First, when a case gets to court, the patient's complaint is that *something* went wrong. The court is faced with a patient whose treatment resulted in an injury that was distressing enough to generate a lawsuit. This leaves judges with a different perspective from that of physicians, most of whose patients have experienced good outcomes, are pleased with their treatment, and thus seldom make an issue of the formal rules of informed consent. Second, the legal rule in most states that the injury suffered must have resulted from a risk that the professional failed to disclose narrows the court's attention to the specific nondisclosure in the patient's complaint, generally to the exclusion of a broader inquiry regarding the overall course of care and the process of discussion and decision making and whether it properly respected the patient's right of self-determination.

Third, the court is faced with judgments made in hindsight. For example, would the patient have refused treatment if he or she had known of the risk, or did the professional's failure to disclose the risk "cause" the patient to accept the treatment that led to the injury? Although the law usually prescribes an "average, reasonable person" standard, the jurors, in fact, may consider the special circumstances of a particular patient, as the nondisclosed risk did materialize and did result in injury.

Fourth, the court must determine what was disclosed. Although oral testimony based on the patient's and the professional's memories may be unsatisfactory, the introduction of an informed consent form may be equally so. Often, these forms become substitutes for real consent; the risks are merely recited and a signature obtained without any discussion and shared decision making.

Finally, in naming defendants in the suit, the patient is likely to name those with "deep pockets"—the physician and the hospital—who are most financially responsible, regardless of the responsibility of other members of the health care team.

Ethical Foundations

The rules developed by the law are actually a manifestation of an ethical imperative that "pa-tients who have the capacity to make decisions about their care must be permitted to do so voluntarily and must have all relevant information regarding their condition and alternative treatments."[10]

Whereas the scholarly literature and legal commentary may seem to suggest that only articulate, well-educated people are suitable candidates for active participation in informed treatment decisions, the Commission's national survey revealed a universal preference for choice, respectful communication, and information. As an ethically based concept, rather than a mere legal regulation, informed consent should remain flexible, so as to accommodate the various professional-patient relationships.

> Such variations might take any of several directions; in one relationship, the patient might prefer not to be burdened by detailed discussion of risks unlikely to arise or to affect the decision; in another relationship, a patient might request unusually detailed information on unconventional alternative therapies; in a third, a patient with a longstanding and close relationship of trust with a particular physician might ask that physician to proceed as he or she thinks best, choosing the course of therapy and revealing any information that the physician thinks would best serve the interests of the patient. Inherent in allowing such variations is the difficulty of ensuring they are genuinely agreeable to both parties and do not themselves arise out of an imbalance in status or bargaining power.[11]

Although patient choice is essential, it is not absolute. It is important to recognize that the patient's wishes may conflict with the professional's own moral beliefs, violate some standard of acceptable practice, or require resources to which the patient has no right.

Institutional and Professional Responsibilities

Hospitals and other health care institutions have major responsibilities in facilitating good physician-patient decision making. Although the Commission placed the initial responsibility for developing shared decision making on health care professionals, in institutional settings especially the risk arises that care will be provided by various medical teams of professionals acting independently, resulting in a fragmentation of responsibility. This leads to dehumanization of care; the patient has no central figure to look to for information, advice, or reassurance.

Such situations pose a far more serious threat to patient well-being and autonomy than any formal disclosure of remote risks on informed consent forms could possibly remedy. Indeed, the Commission believes that serious efforts by health care institutions to ensure that patients have one identifiable and reliable source of information concerning their care would do far more to remedy the current ills of the health care system than would legal prescriptions with which compliance can be neither assumed nor enforced.[12]

Also, institutions should adopt procedures to enhance patients' decision-making capacity, by treating them as well-informed adults who want to participate in choosing their treatment, not as passive children. Determining whether a person has the capacity to make health care decisions is not an all-or-nothing proposition. A person may be capable of making some but not all decisions. This determination should be made at the time the need for a decision arises. Out of respect for self-determination, it should be assumed that the person has the capacity, unless its lack has been shown. "Decision-making incapacity should be found to exist only when people lack the ability to make decisions that promote their well-being in conformity with their own previously expressed values and preferences."[13] Even then, to the extent possible, the individual should be consulted and kept involved in decisions.

Health care professionals and institutions should serve as resources, both providing information and referring people to other relevant sources, for example, libraries, universities, hospices, and other hospitals.

The expanded potential of medicine has also widened the range of choices about health care. Increasingly, the question is not simply whether to accept a single intervention that is available for a particular condition, but which intervention to choose. Often the alternatives vary markedly in their prospects for success, their intrusiveness, their potential side effects, and their other implications for patients'

ability to conduct their lives as they see fit. A determination of what is "indicated" is thus inextricably intertwined with the needs and values of the particular patient.[14]

Patients must be given access to information that allows them to assess the costs and benefits for themselves, and arrive at informed decisions. Withholding information from patients is acceptable only if (1) they request that information be withheld, or (2) their well-being would be directly threatened by its disclosure. Withholding information only because it is unpleasant is unacceptable; the Commission found that most people want to know the worst.

Finally, health care institutions should establish means for surrogate decision making when patients are unable to make decisions themselves. When decisions must be made by others, the decisions should be those the patient would have made or, if the patient's wishes are not known, the decision must be made in the patient's best interests. This means that the surrogate decision maker will be limited to a range of reasonable decisions that is narrower than what the surrogate might choose for himself or herself, based on personal, idiosyncratic values.

With the idea of shared decision making in mind, families and professionals should collaborate; judicial pronouncements on medical treatment should be sought only when no consensus can be reached or if specifically required by state law. Institutions should also investigate the usefulness of ethics committees, which can be used to review the decision making process that has been employed for patients who lack the capacity to decide. Such a committee can also consult with patients and physicians on difficult health care matters.

The role of the family should also be recognized. Although patient privacy should be respected, judicious involvement of family members can promote patient understanding and decision making. At the same time, professionals must recognize that the situation also has the potential for coercion and must be on guard for its occurrence.

Education, Research, and Implementation

In order to prepare health care providers to assume their new roles in sharing decision making, the Commission recommended that more attention be devoted to formal study of this subject during medical and nursing educational and training programs. Classes should be added to the curriculum, and examinations and evaluations ought to test for these skills, both in the schools and at the national level.

The model of health care decision making proposed by the Commission clearly entails a considerable commitment of time. However, because of the importance of promoting well-being and self-determination, along with the positive therapeutic side effects of increased patient participation, all treatment interventions should include a discussion component, with appropriate reimbursement for the time spent. Patient involvement can easily be incorporated through techniques such as written or oral expressions of understanding. Institutions can encourage further research to determine the effectiveness and efficiency of these and other techniques of improving the quality of decision making.

Decisions About Life-Sustaining Treatment

In its report on *Deciding to Forego Life-Sustaining Treatment,* the Commission applied its conclusions about informed consent and shared decision making to the special problems of death and dying. Advances in medical technology have altered the underlying causes of death.

> Frequent dramatic breakthroughs—insulin, antibiotics, resuscitation, chemotherapy, kidney dialysis, and organ transplantation, to name a few—have made it possible to retard and even to reverse many conditions that were until recently regarded as fatal. Matters once the province of fate have now become a matter of human choice, a development that has profound ethical and legal implications.[15]

As a result, the dying patient is likely to be older and subject to health problems that can be combatted. "In this age of surgical derring-do and widespread use of drugs, almost no disease can be said any longer to have a 'natural history'."[16] Concomitantly, the setting for medical care has shifted from the home to the institution. Unfortunately, this has resulted in the alienation of many terminally ill patients.

Patients who are known to be dying are segregated as much as posisble from all the others, and . . . doctors spend as little time in attendance as they can manage . . . When [doctors] avert their eyes it is not that they have lost interest, or find their attendance burdensome because wasteful of their talents; it is surely not because of occupational callousness. Although they are familiar with the business, seeing more of it at first hand than anyone else in our kind of society, they never become used to it. Death is shocking, dismaying, even terrifying. A dying patient is a kind of freak. It is the most unacceptable of all abnormalities, an offense against nature itself.[17]

Thus, the patient faced with chronic, uncontrolled, or overwhelming pain, which in turn exacerbates the fear the patient already has of the symptoms and conditions of the dying process, is left unsupported and isolated. The hospice movement has been particularly responsive to these problems, demonstrating methods, such as manipulation of drug dosage and schedules that can reduce pain to manageable levels without unacceptable side-effects.

The Commission found that informed decision making by competent patients regarding decisions about life-sustaining treatment should be respected, enhanced, and promoted by health care professionals. While there should be a presumption in favor of sustaining life, the right of competent patients to reject even life-sustaining treatments should be recognized.

However, just as in the case of general decision making, the patient should have no right to demand options that violate the professional's moral beliefs or the bounds of acceptable medical practice. Neither should the patient be able to demand resources to which he or she has no legitimate claim. Yet, while resources may be rationed in the interest of equity, life-sustaining treatments for "dying" patients should not be singled out for these limitations. Finally, information regarding any policies and limitations of this sort adopted by an institution should be readily available to the patient and surrogate decision makers.

Because of the effects of medical technology over when and how a person will die, there is an enormous concern for finding the appropriate balance between making death "too easy" and prolonging death "too long."

Under modern conditions, to achieve some harmony between an individual's death and personal values throughout life will probably entail not only awareness of personal values but also the sensitivity and compassion of others and the tolerance of a society willing to allow a fair range of choice—both for people to find and create meaning in living while dying, and for survivors to incorporate and interpret their loss.[18]

Each patient must be considered on an individual basis, but guidelines can greatly facilitate achieving a good decision-making process.

Philosophical Considerations

Health care providers often believe themselves to be prevented from doing the right thing for patients by certain ethical or legal constraints or, sometimes, both. The Commission showed that many of these are based on a misunderstanding of the applicable principles and rules. Particularly notable in this regard are the philosophical distinctions sometimes drawn between withdrawing and withholding treatment, between killing and allowing to die, and between ordinary and extraordinary interventions.

Withholding versus Withdrawing Treatment

At heart, this distinction has more to do with psychology than with philosophy. Of course, it would be easy to belittle it by reciting hypothetical occurrences—such as the respirator that is accidentally unplugged—where it is hard to know whether the case is one of stopping or not starting. But the real point is simply that, unless a special expectation of continued treatment has been created, it ought to be no more significant—morally or legally—to cease a treatment in a patient than not to start the same treatment in the same patient.

> Adopting the opposite view—that treatment, once started, cannot be stopped, or that stopping requires much greater justification than not starting—is likely to have serious adverse consequences. Treatment might be continued for longer than is optimal for the patient, even to the point where it is causing positive harm with little or no compensating benefit.[19]

Even more troubling is the restrictive effect that the distinction—particularly if embodied explicitly in legal rules—can have on initial treatment decisions. A serious wrong occurs when a treatment that might save life or improve health is withheld from a gravely ill patient because the health care personnel are afraid that they will find it very difficult to stop the treatment if, as is fairly likely, it proves burdensome rather than beneficial for the patient. Hospitals and physicians should be aware that the law rejects the distinction. Indeed, in the *Eichner* decision in New York, Justice Meade noted that "it is important that the law not create a disincentive to the fullest treatment of patients by making it impossible for them . . . to choose to end treatment which has proven unsuccessful."[20]

Killing versus Allowing to Die

Although some writers have tried to rest this distinction on an alleged difference between acts and omissions, most philosophers—as well as lawyers and judges—recognize that what is really at stake here is the notion of *duty*, rather than any artificial line between certain human conduct labelled an "act" and other conduct called an "omission." Therefore, it is more useful to describe the distinction as one between killing and allowing to die, because to do so brings out the moral impact that people intend when they contrast acting and omitting as causes of death: actions leading to death are more closely scrutinized than omissions with the same result because, in general, they are more likely to be serious wrongs. This generalization does not derive from an alleged difference between acts and omissions as such but from such factors as whether the decision reflects the pursuit of the patient's ends and values, whether health care providers and others have fulfilled their duties to the patient, and whether the risk of death—from the action or nonaction—has been appropriately weighed.

> [T]he recognized duty of physicians to treat patients with appropriate technologies and methods means that criminal sanctions may be imposed on a physician whose patient died because of the physician's failure to act in circumstances under which no liability would attach for nonphysicians. The *omission* of a duty to take protective action by someone obligated to do, such as a physician or a parent, is regarded by the law in the same way that an *action* would be that led to the same result.[21]

Although the criminal prosecution of health care professionals for killing patients is rare, the threat of criminal prosecution doubtless serves as a strong deterrent to abuse, as well as an affirmation of the value of life and the special role of physicians and nurses as life-protecting professionals. The courts and legislatures attempt to balance the value society places on protecting life with the value of self-determination; this has led them to distinguish between suicide and allowing refusal of treatment by, or on behalf of, terminally ill patients. Some earlier cases declined to allow withdrawals of treatment (because of doubts about patients' competence), but all the recent cases have allowed competent patients to refuse life-prolonging treatment and have declined to attach any liability to the health care personnel for the deaths that followed.

Ordinary versus Extraordinary Treatment

Physicians and lay people alike often contrast "ordinary" and "extraordinary" (or "heroic") measures, but the terms often create confusion because people mean different things when they use them. For some the contrast is statistical (how common or unusual a treatment is), for others it is technological (how simple or complex a treatment is), for some it is historical (how novel or innovative a treatment is), and for still others, the distinction is economic (how cheap or expensive the treatment is). As the Commission concluded,

> [T]he distinction between ordinary and extraordinary treatments has now become so confused that its continued use in the formulation of public policy is no longer desirable. . . . Clarity and understanding in this area will be enhanced if laws, judicial opinions, regulations, and medical policies speak instead of terms of the proportionate benefit and burdens of treatment as viewed by particular patients. With the reasoning thus clearly articulated, patients will be better able to understand the moral significance of the options and to choose accordingly.[22]

Legal Considerations

As already suggested, the law has not been misled by these sometimes confused distinctions but instead has turned to the real bases that underlie them. As mentioned, the courts have not drawn an artificial line that would make it more difficult to withdraw treatment than to withhold it; like-

wise, they have emphasized physicians' fulfilling their duties to their patients (rather than acts versus omissions) in evaluating the rightness of physicians' allowing a patient to die, and have looked to the benefits and burdens for patients of interventions rather than to the mere label "ordinary" or "extraordinary."[23]

In addition to these substantive rules, the law has also recently clarified the procedures needed to protect patient's authority to decide about the extent and limits of their medical care, even in life-and-death situations. Furthermore, beginning with the New Jersey Supreme Court's decision in the *Quinlan* case, judges have used the constitutional right of privacy as the base for recognizing the authority of a surrogate decision maker (Karen's father) to refuse medical treatment on behalf of an incompetent patient. This authority must, however, be exercised in light of the "interests of the State in . . . preservation and sanctity of human life and defense of the right of the physician to administer medical treatment according to his best judgement."[24]

Advance Directives

The President's Commission examined methods provided by statutes as well as by the judge-made common law to facilitate patient-centered decision making. The major methods are two types of "advance directives" that let people

> anticipate that they may be unable to participate in future decisions about their own health care—an "instructive directive" specifies the types of care a person wants (or does not want) to receive; a "proxy directive" specifies the surrogate a person wants to make such decisions if the person is ever unable to do so; and the two forms may be combined.[25]

These directives may be used for any health care situation, and have been used to express desires concerning life-sustaining treatment. Although an advance directive serves the values of self-determination and well-being, in the actual process of "shared decision making" it, of course, is not the same as *active* moral agency.

> Consequently, although self-determination is involved when a patient establishes a way to project his or her wishes into a time of anticipated incapacity, it is a sense of self-determination lacking in one important attribute: active, contem-

poraneous personal choice. Hence, a decision not to follow an advanced directive may sometimes be justified even when it would not be acceptable to disregard a competent patient's contemporaneous choice. Such a decision would most often rest on a finding that the patient did not adequately envision and consider the particular situation within which the actual medical decision must be made.[26]

Health care providers should, however, respect and implement these decisions whenever possible.

Advance directives may be implemented through "living wills," through "directives to physicians" under state "natural death" acts, and through durable powers of attorney pursuant to state law. These devices vary in specificity, usefulness, and legal force.

Living Wills

Living wills are instruction directives that have been developed by medical and legal commentators as well as religious, educational, and professional groups, through which a person can indicate a preference for no "heroic" or "extraordinary" treatments.

> There have been many versions proposed, varying widely in their specificity. Some explicitly detailed directives have been drafted by physicians—outlining a litany of treatments to be foregone or disabilities they would not wish to suffer in their final days. The model living wills proposed by educational groups have more general language.[27]

Although living wills are increasingly popular with the public, they are of questionable legal force and effect. Because of the legal rule that a person's incompetency terminates any agency he or she may have created, health care professionals have not felt themselves bound to carry out the terms of a living will; at the same time it is also unclear whether those who do follow the dictates of the living will will be immune from criminal or civil liability. Additionally, living wills are vulnerable to abuse; there are no penalties for misuse, forgery, concealment, or destruction. At the very least, however, drawing up a living will encourages a patient to discuss the subject of care at the end of life with family members and physicians, and the document itself provides evidence of a formerly competent patient's wishes; further, the document will even have legal effect in those states that have recognized the authority of surrogates to decline life-prolonging care when there is "clear evidence" of the patient's views.

Directives to the Physician

To overcome the uncertain legal status of living wills, since 1976 "natural death acts" have been enacted by about 40 states and the District of Columbia to establish the legal requirements for binding "directives to physicians" regarding the termination of care when death is imminent. The President's Commission was critical of the effect, if not the intent, of these acts because of their limiting definitions. Further, it found that some health care professionals view the statutes as the exclusive mechanism for life-sustaining decision making, meaning that people who are unaware of the statutes, do not understand them, or have failed for any other reason to sign a directive, may be subject to unwanted treatment, whereas in the absence of the statute physicians in at least some cases would have been comfortable allowing a surrogate to refuse treatment.

Durable Powers of Attorney

The Commission suggested that physicians and health care facilities encourage patients to make use of "durable power of attorney" statutes, which can be found in 42 states.

> A "power of attorney" is a document by which one person (the "principal") confers upon another person (the "agent") the legally recognized authority to perform certain acts on the principal's behalf. . . . Such actions by agents are as legally binding on principals as if the latter had performed the acts themselves.[28]

Since the common law power of attorney becomes ineffective when the principal becomes incapacitated, the statutes have allowed for a "durable" power of attorney, which continues an agent's authority after the principal becomes incapacitated. These statutes are flexible enough to allow the principal to draft directives that reflect the complex nature of health care decision making, especially by proxies. However, special safeguards will need to be developed to adapt durable powers specifically to the health care context and to protect from the possibility of abuse.[29]

Institutional Responsibilities

The Commission urged health care facilities to improve the options available to dying patients, specifically that responsive and respectful care be provided for those who have chosen to reject life-sustaining treatment and for those who have no options. In elaborating on institutions' responsibilities to adopt "appropriate procedures to enhance patients' competence, to provide for designation of surrogates, to guarantee that patients are adequately informed, to overcome the influence of dominant institutional biases, to provide review of decision making, and to refer cases to the courts appropriately,"[30] the President's Commission paid special attention to three categories of patients whose care presents special problems.

Patients with Permanent Loss of Consciousness

Once permanent loss of consciousness has been reliably diagnosed, the patient's family should be allowed to determine the care provided. Other than ensuring the provision of basic nursing services, the law does not (and should not) prescribe any specific treatments. Denial of access to certain treatments may be justified, if providing a scarce resource to the one patient would deny access to another who would benefit significantly more, or if carefully implemented policy indicated that serious inequities would be created.

Seriously Ill Newborns

The parents of a child are the best decision makers for the child, unless they disqualify themselves, have a manifest conflict of interest, or choose a course of action that goes against the child's best interests. While an infant's comfort must be assured, futile treatments need not be provided. In evaluating whether a treatment would be beneficial, the infant's current and future status, the availability of special services, and the state of medical science must be considered. In order to make an informed decision, all necessary tests and consultations should be conducted, and their results discussed with the decision makers.

The Commission recommended that institutions have review policies and clear and explicit criteria for decisions about life-sustaining treatment for seriously ill newborns. Whereas an infant's best interests must be pursued when the outcome is clear, the parents should be allowed to decide when the outcome is ambiguous. If the physician or the institution concludes that the parents should be disqualified, the matter should be referred to public agencies for a judgment and the appointment of another surrogate decision maker for the baby.

Cardiopulmonary Resuscitation

Institutions should have clear policies regarding "do not resuscitate" (DNR) orders; most will require that cardiopulmonary resuscitation (CPR) be performed in the absence of any orders against it. Physicians should assess the potential benefit of CPR for patients, when indicated, and all patients who are at risk for cardiac arrest should, if competent, be informed of the risks and benefits of CPR in their case and be given an opportunity to decide whether CPR will be performed; if the patient is incompetent, the surrogate should be allowed to decide whether CPR will be applied.

If a physician's assessment disagrees with a patient's wishes, the physician, after further discussion, should either comply with the patient's wishes or transfer the patient to a physician who will comply. When a physician disagrees with a surrogate's wishes, the physician after further discussion should refer the matter to the institution's ethics committee, and if necessary to the court. Institutional policy should also make clear how DNR orders are to be incorporated into a patient's record and by whom, and how and when such orders are to be reviewed and revised.

The policy should also establish that DNR orders have no implications for any other treatments; that is, it may be appropriate to continue vigorous, intensive care to achieve a cure or alleviate an illness or injury even though resuscitation would not be attempted should cardiopulmonary arrest occur despite such efforts. Finally, the institution's DNR policies should be readily available to patients and their surrogates.

Notes

1. President's Commission for the Study of Ethical Problems in Medicine and Biomedical and Behavioral Research. *Making Health Care Decisions.* Washington, D.C.: U.S. Government Printing Office, 1982 (hereinafter cited as *Health Care Decisions*).

2. President's Commission for the Study of Ethical Problems in Medicine and Biomedical Research. *Deciding to Forego Life-Sustaining Treatment.* Washington, D.C.: U.S. Government Printing Office, 1983 (hereinafter cited as *Deciding to Forego*).

3. *Deciding to Forego*, p.3.

4. *Health Care Decisions*, p. 2.

5. *Health Care Decisions*, p. 17.

6. *Health Care Decisions*, p. 17.

7. 154 Cal. App. 2d 560, 317 P.2d 170 (1957).

8. 186 Kan. 393, 350 P.2d 1093, *Opinion on denial of motion for rehearing*, 187 Kan. 186, 354 P.2d 670 (1960).

9. *Health Care Decisions*, p. 24.

10. *Health Care Decisions*, p. 2.

11. *Health Care Decisions*, p. 39.

12. *Health Care Decisions*, p. 33.

13. *Health Care Decisions*, p. 3.

14. *Health Care Decisions*, p. 34.

15. *Deciding to Forego*, p. 1.

16. Lasagna, L. The prognosis of death. In: Brim, O. G. Jr., and others, editors. *The Dying Patient.* New York: Russell Sage Foundation, 1970, pp. 67, 76.

17. Thomas, L. Dying as failure. *Annals Amer Acad Pol & Soc Science.* 1980 477:2.

18. *Deciding to Forego*, p. 22.

19. *Deciding to Forego*, p. 75.

20. *In re* Eichner, 102 Misc. 2d 184, 423 N.Y.S. 2d 580, 594 (1979), aff'd, 73 A.D. 2d 431, 426 N.Y.S. 2d 517 (1980), Modified sub Nom. *In re* Storar, 52 N.Y. 2d 363, 438 N.Y.S. 2d 266, 420 N.E. 2d 64 Cert. denied, 454 U.S. 858 (1981).

21. See above, p. 34.

22. See above, pp. 88–89.

23. See, for example, *In re* Conroy, 98 N.J. 321, 486 A.2d 1209 (1985); Barber v. Superior Court, 147 Cal. App. 3d 1006, 195 Cal. Rptr. 484 (1983); Satz v. Perlmutter, 379 So.2d 359 (Fla. 1980).

24. *In re* Qinlan, 70 N.J. 10, 355 A.2d 647, 663, cert. denied, 429 U.S. 922 (1976).

25. See above, p. 136.

26. See above, p. 137.

27. See above, p. 139.

28. See above, p. 146.

29. After the Commission issued its report, *Deciding to Forego Life-Sustaining Treatment,* the California legislature amended its law to create a Durable Power of Attorney for Health Care, Calif. Civil Code SS2410-2443, 1984.

30. See above, p. 4.

Health Care Technology and the Inevitability of Resource Allocation and Rationing Decisions

Roger W. Evans, Ph.D., Health and Population Study Center, Battelle Human Affairs Research Centers, Seattle

Part 1

Discussions regarding the high cost of medical care in increasing numbers now include commentaries on the possibility that the resources available for medical care must be allocated across medical care programs. While in the past, resources available for the medical needs of the nation have at least been perceived as unlimited, the appearance of numerous large and small medical technologies and their indiscriminate use among some physicians has thrust resource allocation decisions into the forefront.[1] It is questionable whether it will be possible, in the future, to redistribute to medical programs resources available for other purposes. For example, resources earmarked for defense could be reallocated to meet health care needs. Meanwhile, it is now obvious that the health care of the nation is being jeopardized in at least two ways, both of which have implications for resource allocation. First, resources available to health care programs for the needy and disadvantaged have been threatened by budget cuts or have already been reduced substantially. Second, funds available for health-related research are being subjected to budgetary reductions.

These cuts also may affect both public and private insurance programs. These actions have heralded a renewed concern over which groups of beneficiaries are likely to be adversely affected.[2] For example, it is possible that resource limitations and ad hoc rationing systems could threaten the benefits currently derived through Medicare for patients with end-stage renal disease (ESRD) and various categories of Medicaid beneficiaries.[3] Accompanying these developments have been decisions by private insurers to revise coverage policies. Recently, some major insurers have begun to consider the possibility of limiting coverage to only those situations in which a physician providing treatment has performed a given procedure, such as coronary artery bypass surgery, a specified number of times. Policy initiatives such as this certainly raise questions about how persons with catastrophic illnesses will be treated in the future. Will medical care be regionalized or will the current, relatively fragmented delivery system remain in place?[4-6]

In past months there has also been a substantial reduction in funds made available for health-related research. Iglehart,[7] in a review of

Reprinted, with permission, from the author and the *Journal of the American Medical Association* 1983 Part 1. Apr. 15. 249(15):2047–2053; Part 2. Apr. 22/29. 249(16):2208–2219.

the status of the National Institutes of Health (NIH), concluded that "the NIH seems destined to face bleaker real budgets in fiscal 1983 and beyond." Thus, biomedical research is being given a lower priority, and, consequently, it is reasonable to expect that in the long run, the health of the population will be adversely affected. For example, it is becoming increasingly difficult to earmark sufficient resources for clinical trials, one of the major methods by which the efficacy and safety of new technological innovations are assessed.[8-12]

A picture is now beginning to emerge in which, in the future, resource constraints are likely to make allocation decisions inevitable.[13] Consequently, the tasks of both the clinician and policymaker are likely to become more difficult. For example, in the absence of formal resource allocation rules and the failure to test new health technology adequately and to assess its broader social implications completely, clinicians to an increasing degree find themselves being forced to confront problems that traditionally have been reserved for biomedical ethicists.[14-19] Unfortunately, clinicians are often ill prepared to deal with complex bioethical issues. Few clinicians have previously been asked to participate proactively in the allocation, let alone the rationing, of health care resources. Many would argue that, in principle, this activity represents a conflict of interest and is contrary to the Hippocratic oath.

Policymakers, perhaps surprisingly, seem to be equally inept at resolving ethical dilemmas. As described by myself and co-workers,[20] this was particularly true of the End-Stage Renal Disease Program, in which it was decided that in a country where resources appeared almost limitless, the ethical and moral dilemma of selecting patients for treatment, based on a perceived need to limit treatment, was resolved rather easily by making additional resources available to treat people with ESRD. In describing the process by which Medicare benefits were extended to ESRD patients, my co-workers and I concluded the following:

> The federal government appears to have been more concerned with ridding itself of the moral dilemma of indirectly deciding who could live and who would die in a country of almost unlimited resources. The easiest way to eradicate this problem was to treat everyone equally by making everyone eligible for the same benefits.

Today, it is now apparent that this decision has only staved off the inevitable—deciding which patients should be treated under public and private insurance programs. The prospect that such decisions may become inevitable raises a number of important medical, social, ethical, legal, and economic questions. To the surprise and chagrin of many, such decisions are not completely foreign to the medical profession.[21,22] Problems of medical triage and the treatment of patients in intensive care units (including neonatal intensive care) and other "high-cost" users of medical care raise similar questions.[23-33]

Life Expectancy, Chronicity, Disability, Medical Technology, and Medical Care Costs

The reason that bioethical issues have emerged among the more predominant issues in medicine today becomes clear when one considers the increased prevalence of chronic disease, the changing age distribution of the population, notable increases in life expectancy, the increased prevalence of disability, the introduction and widespread availability of new medical technology, and the high cost of medical care. The interrelationships among these are obvious. For example, the longer people live, the greater the likelihood that they will exhibit chronic disease, have subsequent disability, make use of new and expensive medical technology, and, ultimately, fall into the category of high-cost users of medical care.[34-38]

Life Expectancy

The percentage of persons older than 65 years has steadily risen in all industrialized countries during the past century.[39] While the proportion of elderly persons in the United States has doubled since 1900, their numbers have increased sevenfold. Today, the life expectancy of males, regardless of race, is approximately 70 years and for females is 77 years.[40] The average life expectancy for both groups is about 71 years. Overall, males are expected to outlive their earlier (1900) counterparts by 22 years, and females, their counterparts by 29 years (Table 1). While the longevity of nonwhites lags behind whites, the gains achieved by nonwhites have been even more dramatic as minority life expectancy in this country has doubled.

The composition of the population is also changing. In 1950, 12.3 million persons in the

Table 1. Life Expectancy at Birth According to Race and Sex, United States, Selected Years
from 1900 through 1978*

	Total, yr			White, yr			All Other, yr†		
	Both Sexes	M	F	Both Sexes	M	F	Both Sexes	M	F
1900‡	47.3	46.3	48.3	47.6	46.6	48.7	33.0	32.5	33.5
1950	68.2	65.6	71.1	69.1	66.5	72.2	60.8	59.1	62.9
1960	69.7	66.6	73.1	70.6	67.4	74.1	63.6	61.1	66.3
1970§	70.8	67.1	74.7	71.7	68.0	75.6	65.3	61.3	69.4
1975§	72.5	68.7	76.5	73.2	69.4	77.2	67.9	63.6	72.3
1976§	72.8	69.0	76.7	73.5	69.7	77.3	68.3	64.1	72.6
1977§	73.2	69.3	77.1	73.8	70.0	77.7	68.8	64.6	73.1
1978§	73.3	69.5	77.2	74.0	70.2	77.8	69.2	65.0	73.6

*Data from Department of Health and Human Services.[40]
†For 1900 through 1902, data for the "all other" category were for blacks only.
‡Death registration area only. The death registration area increased from ten states and the District of Columbia in 1900 to the coterminous United States in 1933.
§Excludes deaths of nonresidents in the United States.

United States, or 8.1% of the total population, were older than 65 years. By 1960, this group had grown to 16.6 million persons, or 9.2%. The number reached 23.5 million in 1977, an increase of 91.1% from 1950, and this figure represented 10.9% of the total population. It is now projected that the number of persons older than 65 years will be 31.8 million by the year 2000—12.2% of the total population and a 157% increase in 50 years.[40] As the population ages, chronic disease and disability are becoming increasingly visible problems. Chronic rather than acute diseases are now the most prevalent causes of death in industrial societies.[22,41]

Chronic Disease and Disability

Since the early 1900s, there has been a substantial decline in those infectious diseases that have proved to be so intractable in past years.[42] Heart attack, stroke, cancer, and leukemia are but a few of those retrogressive chronic diseases, often of slow insidious onset, that have replaced infections, viruses, and tubercular fatalities in the United States.

Given current available data sources, it is difficult to estimate the true prevalence of chronic disease. Few population-based epidemiologic studies have been undertaken to estimate explicitly the prevalence of all chronic diseases.[43] The Framingham Heart Study represents but one exemplary population-based epidemiologic study of cardiovascular disease. Results of this study have shown the now apparent decline in the prevalence of cardiovascular disease.[39,44,45]

Other statistics on chronic disease that have been published by the National Center for Health Statistics are based on self-reported illness and disability in the Health Interview Study. These reports indicate that in the early years of life, only about six of 1,000 persons endure chronic conditions. During young adulthood (age 25 or so), the rate increases to 35, and by the fourth decade that figure has almost tripled to 100 persons of every 1,000. By age 65, this number has again doubled and then doubled yet another time after age 75, until almost 90% of all persons older than 90 years live with a chronic illness.[46] Again ignoring the age factor, it has at times been estimated that approximately 50% of the civilian population, excluding residents in institutions, have one chronic condition or more.[47] As for the number of chronic conditions per person, one study has shown this to be 2.2.[47]

It is currently estimated that 80% of health care resources in the United States, including facilities, services, and biomedical research, are now devoted to chronic disease.[34] During 1978, an estimated 10.3 million persons, or 45%, of the civilian population aged 65 years and older not residing in institutions were reported in health interviews to have some degree of activity limitation caused by chronic disease or impairment (Table 2).[48] Of these 10.3 million persons, fully 85.2% indicated that they were limited in or unable to carry on major activities, affecting their ability to work or manage a household.[48] The remainder were limited but not in major activity.

Ignoring the age factor, 30 million Americans (14% of the total population) were reported to have dysfunction caused by chronic diseases, and, of these, 23 million, or 74.6%, were limited in or unable to carry on major life activities, affecting their ability to work, manage a household, or attend school.[48]

Table 2. Distribution of Persons with Limitation of Activity Because of Chronic Conditions, According to Age and Degree of Limitation, United States, 1978*

Age of Both Sexes, yr	No. of Persons, in Thousands			%			
	Total Population	With Activity Limitation (in Major Activity)	With no Activity Limitation	Total Population	With Activity Limitation	Limitation in Major Activity	With no Activity Limitation
All ages	213,828	30,306 (22,598)	183,523	100.0	14.2	10.6	85.8
<17	59,012	2,309 (1,178)	56,703	100.0	3.9	2.0	96.1
17–44	88,627	7,501 (4,621)	81,126	100.0	8.5	5.2	91.5
45–64	43,403	10,244 (8,063)	39,159	100.0	23.6	18.6	76.4
≥65	22,788	10,252 (8,736)	12,535	100.0	45.0	38.3	55.0

*Data from Givens.[48]

Medical Technology

Over the years, medical technology has been most successful in dealing with infectious diseases. Thomas,[49,50] in his analysis of technology, notes that much of the technology germane to the treatment of infectious diseases "comes from a genuine understanding of disease mechanisms, and when it becomes available, it is relatively inexpensive, relatively simple, and relatively easy to deliver." This technology is exemplified by modern methods for immunization against diphtheria, pertussis, and the childhood virus diseases and the contemporary use of antibiotics and chemotherapy for bacterial infections.[51] Other examples cited by Thomas[50] include the treatment of endocrinologic disorders with appropriate hormones, the prevention of hemolytic disease of the newborn, and the treatment and prevention of various nutritional disorders.

Major technological advances, however, have been made specifically for treating incurable chronic diseases, many of which have varying implications for the level of functional ability patients are able to regain. Since many of these interventions do not cure disease, they are frequently referred to as "halfway technologies,"[50,51] and the extent to which a patient is able to cope and regain maximum function becomes all important. As described by Crane,[22] technological changes have affected the very character of illness, permitting the physician to have greater control over the process of dying and the timing of death. She also notes that in less obvious ways, improvements in medical technology have produced increasing levels of disability in western society.[52] Moreover, technology has permitted the survival of more or less severely disabled persons such as diabetics and infants with myelomeningocele who would otherwise have died.

It is now estimated that each year, hundreds—perhaps thousands—of new technologies enter the medical care system. These include drugs, procedures, devices and instrumentation, all constituting preventative, diagnostic, and therapeutic tools.[53] Many of these technologies have undoubtedly contributed to the substantial improvement in the health status of the American people. Also, relief of pain, amelioration of symptoms, and rehabilitation now have become possible for many patients with diseases that cannot be successfully prevented or treated.[53] The benefits of medical technology, in some instances, have been found to be more apparent than real.[54] For example, various inefficacious procedures have been practiced and then abandoned in this country. These include gastric freezing for peptic ulcer, colectomy for epilepsy, hypogastric artery ligation for pelvic hemorrhage, sympathectomy for asthma, internal mammary artery ligation for coronary artery disease, adrenalectomy for essential hypertension, and wiring for aortic aneurysm.[51,54-57]

While efficacy and safety (that is, medical technology's medical benefits and risks) have traditionally been the primary focus of health technology assessment,[51,53,58-62] attention has begun to focus on other aspects of health care technology.[63,64] For example, on June 12, 1980, Patricia Roberts Harris, then secretary of the Department of Health and Human Services, announced that new health technologies must be evaluated not only on the basis of their medical efficacy and safety but also on the basis of their "social consequences" before "financing their wide distribution."[65] As noted by Knox,[65] the approach being suggested by Harris was even more comprehensive than that used by, for example, the Environmental Protection Agency in dealing with pesticides, the Food and Drug Administration in its treatment of pharmaceuticals, and the Occupational Safety and Health Administration's approach to carciongens in the work place.[66-69] New health technology was to be evaluated concerning its cost-effectiveness, cost-benefit ratios, ethical implications, and "long-term effects on society." The all-encompassing intent of technology assessment has been characterized by Banta and Behney[59] as follows:

> Technology assessment is seen as a comprehensive form of policy research that examines short- and long-term social consequences (e.g., societal, economic, ethical, legal) of the application of technology. Technology assessment is an analysis of primarily social rather than technical issues, and is especially concerned with unintended, indirect, or delayed social impacts.

It is now becoming more evident that the assessment of any emerging or existing technology must, at least, include consideration of the following parameters: (1) the potential need for the procedure, device, instrument, or drug, (2) the relevant constraints on the availability of the technology (e.g., absence of donor organs for transplantation, location of treatment facilities, shortage of trained personnel), (3) the cost-effectiveness-cost-benefits of the technology assessed in terms of both economic and social costs, including lives saved, (4) the legal issues pertaining to the adoption and availability of the technology, including risks associated with its use (e.g., where will the technology be made available?; who is eligible to receive the technology?; what risks does the recipient incur in the use of the technology?), and (5) the ethical issues concerning the selection of recipients of the technology, the allocation of resources to health care programs, and individual patient rights to health care regardless of cost and availability. Failure to consider these issues will make it extraordinarily difficult to anticipate the long-term implications of any emerging or existing technology.[70-73]

Cost of Medical Care

In 1980, expenditures for medical care consumed 9.4% of the gross national product (GNP).[74] In this same year, health care spending increased by 15.2%, representing a moderate acceleration over the 12.5% increase during 1979. This figure is substantially higher than the 13.4% growth rate between 1978 and 1979 and is certainly much higher than the average of 12.2% annually over the period of 1965 to 1979.[74] Gross national product increases have averaged 9.2%

per year for the same period. This substantially greater growth rate in the health care sector compared with the rest of the economy resulted in the health care share of the GNP rising from 6.1% in 1965 to the 9.4% level seen today. Between 1950 and 1978 alone, in the United States, total annual expenditures for health care and other forms of health-related activities increased 1,500%.[75] In 1950, medical care expenditures constituted 4.5% of the US gross GNP.

In analyzing these increased health expenditures, it is obvious that third-party payers have, in many respects, contributed to the rise in health care costs, primarily because they have traditionally placed few constraints on expenditures. In 1979, personal health care funds supplied by third parties amounted to $147.0 billion of the $217.9 billion in personal health expenditures, or 68%.[74] Federal, state, and local governments financed the largest portion of that amount—about 40% of the total. Private health insurance payments covered an additional 27% of personal health care. In 1980, private insurers, including Blue Cross and Blue Shield plans, commercial insurance companies, and independent plans, paid benefits amounting to $58.1 billion, or 27% of personal health care expenditures. In 1980, approximately 76% of the US population was covered by private hospital insurance.[74]

Often the cost of disability is ignored as a health-related factor. This is somewhat misleading, since every chronic disease requires a certain level of expenditure for medical care, but, at the same time, the person may be disabled and, consequently, draws on disability programs for various cash benefits. The total cost of illness should reflect not only actual medical treatment costs but the cost of services and other benefits the person receives because of his illness.[76-83]

Table 3 gives a complete breakdown of government expenditures for illness-tested welfare programs for fiscal year 1975.[84,85] As shown here, in 1975, cash payments to disabled persons under these public programs amounted to more than $23 billion. The growth of the disability program is also interesting. As noted by Stone,[84] disability benefits administered through the Social Security program, although smaller than retirement benefits in total dollar amount, are increasing at a much higher rate, and the number of disability beneficiaries is also growing faster than the number of retirement beneficiaries (Table 4). A close examination of the Supplemental Security Income program presents a similar picture—fed-

Table 3. Government Expenditures for Illness-Tested Welfare Programs for Fiscal Year 1975*

Program	Amount, In Billion Dollars		
	Federal	State-Local	Total
Disability insurance			
(Social Security Administration)	7.6	. . .	7.6
Civil service disability	1.4	. . .	1.4
Railroad disability	0.2	. . .	0.2
Black lung benefits	0.6	. . .	0.6
Uniform services			
Veterans Administration and military disability	4.7	. . .	4.7
Other (income-tested)	0.5	. . .	0.5
Temporary disability insurance	. . .	0.9	0.9
Workers compensation	1.3	3.2	4.5
Public assistance			
Supplemental Security Income-disabled	2.3	. . .	2.3
Aid to families with dependent children			
(disabled male head of household)	0.6	. . .	0.6
Total			23.3†

*Data from Stone[84] and Skolnik and Dales.[85]

†Total does not include payments made through various private insurance arrangements or payments made for medical services.

Table 4. Growth of Disability and Retirement Programs under Old Age, Survivors, Disability, and Health Insurance, 1965 through 1979*

Program	No. of Beneficiaries, in Millions		% of Increase	Amount of Benefits, in Billion Dollars		% of Increase
	1965	1979		1965	1979	
Retirement	13.9	22.4	61	12.5	59.3	374
Disability	1.7	4.8	182	1.6	12.5	681

*Data from the Department of Commerce, Bureau of the Census.[106]

eral payments to disabled persons grew by 13.6% between 1977 and 1980, as compared with an increase of only 8.0% in payments to the aged (Table 5).

The rapidly rising costs of health care have served to spur interest in health care technology assessment.[51,55,86-90] Recently, much blame has been placed on health care technology as the "culprit" behind high health care costs.[10,11,91-101] Although the total contribution of new technology to rising costs is controversial, estimates of the effect of technology on increased per diem

Table 5. Growth of Expenditures under Supplemental Security Income, 1979 and 1980*

	Federal Payments, in Billion Dollars		% of Increase
	1979	1980	
Aged	2.5	2.7	8.0
Disabled	4.4	5.0	13.6

*Data from the Department of Commerce, Bureau of the Census.[105]

hospital costs range from 33% to 75%, with 50% being an average figure.[51,54,99,101-103] Detailed case studies have been undertaken that illustrate the variable effect of technology on the treatment of chronic disease.[54] Scitovsky and McCall,[104] for example, looked at the changing cost of treating 11 different conditions at the Palo Alto Medical Clinic in California during a period of several years.[104] They found the real cost of treating five conditions fell, while the cost of treating six actually increased. Closer examination of these six conditions showed that there had been a notable increase in the use of diagnostic tests and therapeutic procedures per diagnosis. Laboratory tests per case of perforated appendicitis rose from 5.3 in 1951, to 14.5 in 1964, to 31.0 in 1971. Inhalation-therapy procedures for myocardial infarction rose from 12.8 per case in 1964 to 37.5 in 1971.[51,54,104]

Fineberg and Hiatt[89] have noted that, for several reasons, rising medical costs can be attributed to technology. First, although the trend is toward shorter hospital stays, this is accompanied by an increased consumption of resources during hospitalization. Second, more advanced equipment design may improve efficiency, but, with increased use of the equipment and other "induced costs," potential savings are never realized. Third, many new technologies do more than simply perform old services more efficiently—they provide new and expensive services. The intensive care unit, for example, is but a single innovation that in 1974 was found to account for 10% of all hospital costs.[87]

It is often argued that big, expensive technologies contribute disproportionately to the high cost of medical care, although the costs and benefits of a new technology largely depend on how and to which patients it is applied.[89,105,107] Moloney and Rogers,[92] however, have argued that the big and highly visible technologies such as the computed tomographic scanner "actually account for far less of the annual growth in medical expenditures than do the collective expense of thousands of small tests and procedures that are more frequently used by physicians and that individually cost little."

The use of a technology is directly related to reimbursement for its use.[10,51,107–109] Moloney and Rogers[92] suggest that one approach, although problematic, to slowing the use of a technology is to develop protocols "that instruct physicians to use technologies only when less expensive methods cannot provide adequate information on patient care; limit reimbursement to use according to these standards." At present, policies with regard to the reimbursement of new technologies, if they exist, are often inconsistent. Under the Medicare program, the major reason for excluding a technology for reimbursement is when it has not been demonstrated to be safe and effective.[110,111] As described by Bunker and associates,[10] "the government's reimbursement policy has been left largely to the commercial and non-profit carriers to whom the government, by contract, has delegated the responsibility for processing claims." To accomplish this objective, some carriers, such as California and Massachusetts Blue Shield, have organized their own technology assessment committees and procedures. California Blue Shield has only recently placed limitations on procedures that are considered experimental. Previously, the carrier was committed to reimbursing for services that were "reasonable and necessary."[10] At present, there seems to be no satisfactory uniformly applied approach to limiting the growth of technology through alternative reimbursement policies.

Table 6. Growth in the Medical Technology Industry*

	1958	1977
Sales, billion dollars	1.0	8.1
No. of companies	1,366	1,442
No. of establishments	2,802	3,203

*Data from Wenchel.[113]

Controlling the growth and distribution of technology is complicated by the fact that the medical technology industry is large and multinational.[51,68,112] To slow its growth through regulation surely would have a multitude of political ramifications. Since World War II, the medical technology industry has experienced dramatic growth in sales, firms, and establishments (Table 6).[113] Wenchel[113] attributes much of the growth to the increased demand for health services supported by private, voluntary health insurance and government programs such as Medicare and Medicaid, Hill-Burton, and Regional Medical Programs. The roentgenography and electromedical industries have seen the greatest increase in sales, showing an increase of $1.8 billion between 1958 and 1977.[113] Consequently, it is difficult to imagine that the medical technology industry is willing to sit idle as new regulations are introduced to slow the growth of technology. Perhaps this is most true in those situations in which existing rather than emerging technologies are being scrutinized.

Summary

The foregoing discussion points to several problems and developments that indicate the inevitability of resource allocations to health care programs. The US population is aging; chronic disease is becoming more prevalent, disability a common occurrence. To meet the needs of an aging, chronically ill, and disabled population, a complex array of expensive and sophisticated medical technologies has emerged. The cost of these technologies will make it necessary to develop elaborate plans not only to enable them to be used but to ensure that people receiving them derive the maximum expected benefits. Thus, it is apparent that resource allocation decisions are likely not only to become a necessity but to become routine.[114,115]

In short, in the future, the demand for health care will doubtlessly outstrip available resources.[116,117] The problem then becomes one of determining how best to allocate the available resources to optimize the health of the population. To accomplish this objective, it will be necessary to study carefully new and existing technology to determine the magnitude of potential benefits.[10,11,51,58] At the same time, it will be necessary to increase the efficiency of the existing health care delivery system in an attempt to ensure that maximum benefits are being derived.[118] During this process, it is probable that some types of medical care can no longer be provided, or, if provided, they will be done so on a limited basis, since the derived benefits are too costly for all to benefit. The question then becomes one of determining the best method of implementing allocation decisions.[119,120] In doing this, it subsequently will become necessary to ration care within health care programs that have been spared from complete extinction. Although advanced technology will provide many persons with a new lease on life, not all are expected to benefit equally, if at all. As these allocation and rationing exercises are undertaken, a new appreciation of medical ethics will come about, accompanied by a more careful assessment of the nature of death and dying within this society.[121,122] These issues as they apply to this analysis are more completely delineated in part 2.

Part 2

Allocation and Rationing of Health Care Resources

Of all the resource-shortage crises this nation is expected to confront in the future, the problem of resource distribution is likely to be most acute and problematic in medicine.[23,29,123] Persons will be recognized as in need of, and then denied, benefits that the medical care provision system is capable of providing. Instead of an unidentified mass of persons being denied access to a needed resource, persons whose names have become known to the public will be declared ineligible for a treatment or service they are known to require.[124] Perhaps this scenario is inhumane, but it is undoubtedly a true representation of reality. As already noted, technology now permits to be saved the lives of persons who less than a decade ago would have surely died. Moreover, technology has made it exceedingly difficult to specify at precisely what point life ceases. This has prompted Crane[22] to conclude that both medicine and law are moving toward a "social interpretation" of life.

It should come as no surprise that the resources available to meet the demand for health care are limited.[125–130] Weinstein and Stason,[127] for example, have pointed out that decisions are already being made—physicians allocate their time, hospitals ration beds, fiscal intermediaries devise reimbursement policies—all of which suggest that priorities are being set. This is not to deny the recency of problems associated with resource constraints. Even a few decades ago, before the proliferation of medical technology and the pervasiveness of insurance, constraints on health care resources were largely unheard of. In the past, the distribution of health care resources has been accomplished by implicitly limiting their availability or, when available, restricting people's access to them.[131] Thus, the concepts of availability and accessibility are critical to the problem of resource distribution.[132,133] *Rationing* is the term often used to describe the process of differentially distributing resources. *Rationing* has become a value-laden term—one that implies that persons are likely to be treated unequally.[134] *Allocation* is another term often used to describe the unequal distribution of resources. While *Webster's New World Dictionary* defines *rationing* as "a fixed portion; share; allowance," *allocation* is to "set apart for a specific purpose, to distribute according to a plan."

As suggested by the definitions of rationing and allocation, there is merit in distinguishing between the allocation and the rationing of health care resources. Other have used the terms *macroallocation* and *microallocation* to make a similar distinction.[134,135] Regardless of the terms used, it should be recognized that allocation and rationing differ with regard to temporality and level. First, allocation decisions are likely to precede rationing decisions. Second, allocation is a concept that does not apply well at the level of the individual patient but rather is more appropriately applied at the aggregate or health care program level.

In a period when resources available for health care have become increasingly constrained, attention is directed toward making the provision of health care more efficient. For example, although much attention has recently focused on the enormous cost of the End-Stage Renal Disease Program, the question being addressed is not whether patients should have their Medicare benefits cut off but rather how treatment can be provided at less cost. (The total cost of the kidney program in fiscal year 1982 is expected to be $1.8 billion. Stated in other terms, patients with end-stage renal disease [ESRD], representing <0.25% of all Medicare part B beneficiaries, now account for >9% of total Medicare part B expenditures.[136]) Thus, the debate over which type of therapy (primarily home or in-center dialysis) is least costly is again being hotly debated.[137-147] At the same time, there is renewed interest in methods by which donor organ availability can be increased.[148-151] Recent hearings once again have indicated that home dialysis is probably less costly than in-center dialysis but that kidney transplantation is a greater bargain since the cost is not only lower in the long run, but the quality of life of renal transplant recipients is generally thought to be better than that of patients receiving dialysis.[152-155] Since there seems to be room for improving the provision of ESRD services, there is only minimal consideration being given to reduction or discontinuation of benefits that patients with renal disease currently receive. Thus, resources will continue to be allocated to the End-Stage Renal Disease Program, but, in the future, greater attention will focus on the *intraprogram* allocation of resources. It will be expected that the agency responsible for administering the program, the Health Care Financing Administration (HCFA), will write regulations that will maximize the use of those resources made available to the program; that is, the HCFA will be expected to promote the least costly treatment modalities by providing incentives for their adoption.[138]

Should the resources available for health care become increasingly constrained, the Department of Health and Human Services will be put in a position wherein *interprogram* allocation decisions will become necessary. These allocation decisions would concern how to distribute resources across health and, perhaps, social and other publicly financed programs. For example, a question might be raised as to whether the resources currently used to treat kidney disease might better be allocated to prevention activities or to a maternal and child health care program in which the derived benefits are likely to surpass those currently received by patients with ESRD.[55] In the future, competition for the available resources is likely to be great. The high cost of some new technologies might well make their widespread use prohibitive. Should this prove to be the case, it will then be necessary to consider the

rationing of resources within health care programs.

Resources are rationed at the individual level, while allocation occurs at the aggregate level. Once it is apparent that all who are in need cannot be treated, the question then becomes one of which potential recipients are going to derive the greatest benefits. Again, this is precisely what occurred during the early years of dialysis, when there was substantial patient selection by physicians or committees. At that time, it was decided that although all patients with ESRD had a terminal condition, some had better prospects for treatment than others.[20,156] The preferred candidates were selected on the basis of a variety of criteria, e.g., age, medical suitability, mental acuity, family involvement, criminal record, economic status (income, net worth), employment record, availability of transportation, willingness to cooperate in the treatment regimen, likelihood of vocational rehabilitation, psychiatric status, marital status, educational background, occupation, and future potential.[20,156-158] These criteria served as the basis on which scarce resources were rationed. Similar criteria currently are used to select potential heart transplant recipients and, thus, also serve as a rationing mechanism.[159-162] The decision to extend Medicare benefits to patients with ESRD resolved the rationing problem for the federal government. However, as noted by myself and associates,[20] the federal government "appears to have been more concerned with ridding itself of the moral dilemma of indirectly deciding who could live and who would die in a country of almost unlimited resources" than with simply trying to deal with the more general problem of costly medical care.

Now that the federal government is at least willing to entertain the possibility of differentially allocating resources to health care programs, it inevitably will also have to entertain the need to ration health care resources once interprogram allocation has occurred and the efficient use of available resources is maximized. Should resources be constrained further and no greater efficiency attained, it would become necessary to ration the available resources to certain persons based on some uniform set of guidelines.

The foregoing raises two important questions that have yet to be addressed—(1) On what basis will resource allocation decisions be made? (2) How are criteria for rationing likely to be developed?

Establishing Criteria for Explicit Resource Allocation

In the medical literature, one increasingly finds medical procedures, practices, and technology subjected to what is commonly referred to as "cost-effectiveness and cost-benefit analysis."[51,126–130,163–167] Although the two are related, they are different approaches to the assessment of health practices and technology. Nevertheless, both cost-effectiveness analysis (CEA) and cost-benefit analysis (CBA) are presented as tools that can be used by the policymaker to make resource allocation decisions.

A CBA or a benefit-cost analysis requires that both costs and benefits be assigned monetary values.[168] Various methods have been proposed to measure the resource value of health care benefits. These include, for example, expected productivity loss based on discounted future earnings at the age of death or disability.[82,169,170] The benefit-cost framework thus converts decreased deaths and disability into increases in productivity and treats them as the indirect benefits of a health intervention. Thus, indirect benefits are then combined with any direct savings in health resource consumption (the direct benefits) to yield a net value.

A CEA, unlike a CBA, does not require that both costs and benefits be assessed in monetary terms. Instead, the aim of a CEA is to measure benefits in nonmonetary terms using mortality, morbidity, or quality-adjusted life years. To this extent, a CEA preserves a sense of intangible health care benefits, whereas a CBA typically notes these but fails to assess them.[168] A CEA is particularly useful for comparing alternative approaches with the treatment of a given medical condition. For example, in-center hemodialysis, home hemodialysis, continuous ambulatory peritoneal dialysis, and kidney transplantation all represent alternative approaches to the treatment of ESRD. A CEA allows one to compare these treatments to determine which provides the greatest benefits at the least cost.[170] Similarly, heart transplantation might be compared with its alternative—traditional medical and surgical management—as approaches to the treatment of end-stage cardiac disease (ESCD).[76] Finally, percutaneous transluminal coronary angioplasty might be compared with coronary artery bypass surgery as alternative approaches to the treatment of atherosclerosis.[171,172] In all these instances, the goal of a CEA is the same—to determine which treatment approach to a given condition yields the greatest benefits at the least cost.

Both CEA and CBA can be applied on a larger scale than described herein. This application is critical to both intraprogram and interprogram allocation decisions. A CEA can be used to compare the benefits derived from various health care programs to determine which program (not specific treatment approach) yields the greatest benefit at the least cost, provided the benefits of each program being compared are expressed in the same terms (M. C. Weinstein, PhD, written communication, April 14, 1982). For example, kidney dialysis can be compared with heart transplantation to see which has the greatest benefits, with benefits expressed in terms of mortality, morbidity, or quality-adjusted life years. Weinstein describes this process as follows:

> The comparison of cost-effectiveness ratios serves as a basis for allocating resources if the objective is to maximize health benefits. Thus, if kidney dialysis has a cost-effectiveness ratio (relative to the next best alternative for ESRD) of $60,000 per quality-adjusted life year, and cardiac transplant has a cost-effectiveness ratio (relative to the next best alternative) for ESCD) of $50,000 per quality-adjusted life year, then resources should be allocated to the latter ahead of the former.

In this case, the proposed interprogram analysis strictly applies to health care programs. Another pertinent example might be to compare the cost of a potential maternal and child health program with the End-Stage Renal Disease Program or a potential ESCD program.

If the goal of the interprogram analysis is to compare the expenditure of health care resources with other socially desirable uses of resources, such as a public assistance program, a cost-benefit analysis is appropriate. Within the CBA framework, all expenditures and benefits are converted to monetary terms, which permits direct comparisons to be made among various diverse programs. The results of such an analysis may indicate that resources should be reallocated from social and other publicly financed programs to support health programs and vice versa. The problem with the CBA framework, however, is the requirement that human lives and quality of life be valued in dollars.[117,127]

Ultimately, the major objective of an inter-program analysis that involves only health programs or health and other publicly financed programs is to ensure that those programs that produce the greatest benefit will be those that receive the greatest support from the federal government. In this regard, it is apparent that, given limited resources and a need to allocate them in the most effective manner possible, a CEA or a CBA allows programs to be ranked according to their effectiveness or benefits derived or both. Weinstein and Stason[127] have summarized how this is done in the case of CEA as follows:

> Alternative programs or services are then ranked from the lowest value of the cost-effectiveness ratio to the highest, and selected from the top until available resources are exhausted. The point on the priority list at which the available resources are exhausted, or at which society is no longer willing to pay the price for the benefits achieved, becomes society's cut-off level of permissable cost per unit effectiveness. Application of this procedure ensures that the maximum health benefit is realized, subject to whatever resource constraint is in effect.

Thus, it is now possible to see that the allocation of health care resources and resources available to other programs as well can be subjected to a formalized set of procedures. By requiring that all assumptions are clearly stated, it is possible to perform the necessary quantitative analyses required to make the appropriate allocation decisions. In those areas where the data are least secure, it is possible to undertake sensitivity analyses to explore further the impact of decisions under differing assumptions.

Table 7 summarizes which type of analysis can be applied to various allocation decisions. If possible to achieve, a CEA should be the method of choice. In only one instance is it likely that a CEA would be inappropriate. This is in the case wherein an interprogram analysis is required to compare health program expenditures and benefits with non-health-related program expenditures and benefits. In this case, it would be necessary to express in monetary terms the benefits derived from the program. If an intraprogram allocation decision is required, a CEA should always be the method of choice, while, in principle both a CBA and CEA could be applied to making an interprogram *health* allocation decision.

Establishing Criteria for Explicit Rationing

The resource rationing problem is different from the resource allocation problem. Although, in many respects, allocation decisions set the parameters and constraints within which rationing occurs, it is somewhat more difficult to submit the rationing process to a formalized set of procedures. The literature on clinical decision making, although not solely intended to be a framework for rationing, does provide an excellent framework with which to view rationing.

Once resources have been allocated to programs, and should these not be sufficient to meet the demand of all in need, clinicians are left with the problem of deciding which patients to treat.[173-176] The problems that were faced in the early days of kidney dialysis already have been described, pointing to obvious problems with any system that basically discriminates among people in the distribution of health care resources.[177,178] According to many, all people have a "right to health care" and, in a country as wealthy as the United States, no one should go untreated.[179-185] Yet, people often fail to recognize that with every right there also is an obligation.[186,187] People have a responsibility, an obligation as it were, to care for themselves in a manner that will maximally ensure good health (e.g., eat a good diet and exercise daily). Unfortunately, a vast majority of the population fails to fulfill its end of the "social contract" and chooses to engage in practices and behavior that are known to be detrimental to their

Table 7. Applying Cost-Effectiveness and Cost-Benefit Analysis to Program Allocation Decisions

Type of Decision Required	Cost-Effectiveness Analysis (CEA)	Cost-Benefit Analysis (CBA)	Method of Choice
Intraprogram allocation decision	Yes	Yes	CEA
Interprogram health allocation decision	Yes	Yes	CEA
Interprogram health *v* other publicly financed program allocation decision	No	Yes	CBA

health (e.g., excessive smoking, drinking, eating, and failure to exercise). Therefore, it could be argued that if everyone has a right to health care, then appropriate contracts should be drawn up to ensure that everyone keeps their end of the bargain.[186] This, of course, would require regulatory reform and strict enforcement, something that would be difficult and costly to undertake. Ultimately, however, the limits of the broad humanistic concept of a right to health care must be recognized. Within the context of rationing, those persons who have done the most to preserve their health could conceivably be the first to benefit from the available resources.[187,188]

The problem grows in complexity when it is recognized that the final decision concerning the rationing of resources will be the shared responsibility of the clinician or medical team, the patient, and any other representative of the patient (e.g., family or nearest of kin).[189] It is unlikely that explicit exclusion criteria will be developed that are equally palatable to all involved.[190,191] Thus, any criteria for rationing would be interpreted and practiced by individual clinicians.[192-194] This is consistent with the concept of the "clinical mentality" advanced by Freidson,[195] which suggests that clinicians see each patient as a special case and treat each accordingly. Medical practice is typically occupied with the problems of individuals rather than of aggregates or statistical units. To impose a set of rationing criteria that must be strictly adhered to implies that patients need not be considered as unique individuals but rather as aggregates. This would, in fact, represent a radical restructuring of the process of rendering clinical judgment.[196]

In the final analysis, it is possible to establish some general *guidelines* on, perhaps, a condition-by-condition basis, to be applied to decide whether a patient should be treated.[197] The problem, however, is that all cases will have to be reviewed individually, with explicit attention given to the manner in which each patient deviates from the guidelines. These decisions are likely to be made when any of the following conditions are met: (1) the treatment is determined to be futile, (2) the patient declines treatment, (3) the quality of the patient's life is unacceptable, or (4) the cost of providing care is too great.[197,198] In evaluating each case, what people decide to do will be subject to considerable variability. What is presented as a formal policy may be informally practiced in a variety of ways. Policy and practice can differ remarkably.

As described here, rationing is the process by which criteria are applied to selectively discriminate among patients who are eligible for resources that have been previously allocated to various programs. Rationing criteria, although conceivably developed at the aggregate level, are likely to be interpreted and implemented at the individual level. Thus, there are two major problems associated with rationing. These are (1) the development of acceptable criteria for withholding treatment on a condition-by-condition basis and (2) identifying that person or those persons who should make the decision not to treat.

Childress,[134] in his discussion of rationing, has distinguished between what he refers to as "rules of exclusion" and "rules of final selection." The first set of rules establishes the pool from which the final selections are made. The final selections are then based on the rules of final selection. Childress[134] provides the following advice: "The best approach to determining the pool for final selection is to forget that the resource is limited and to exclude only those patients whose medical and psychological condition would certainly prevent successful treatment." The rules for final selection, however, are more controversial. Major alternatives include social worth criteria or some form of chance (e.g., randomization, lottery, or "first come, first treated"). Rescher,[123] pursuing this same line of thought, has suggested that there are two biomedical and three social factors relevant to final selection. Relative likelihood of successful treatment and life expectancy are the relevant biomedical factors, while the social factors include family role, potential future contributions, and past services. All of these criteria are difficult to quantify and evaluate.

At this point, it is again important to reiterate that the most critical decisions that must be confronted today are those involving the allocation of resources across health care programs.[117] Once these decisions have been made, it will then become important to consider whether rationing will be necessary and what form it will take. It is precisely at this point that the nature and requirements of clinical decision making will become increasingly subjected to public and professional scrutiny.[198-200] Furthermore, it is at this point that patients and their next of kin will become increasingly involved in the decision-making process, and quantity and quality of life trade-offs will become important.[174,201-203] The decision-making process is well described in the literature.[21,22,128,198,204-211]

Resource Allocation in Perspective

Most discussions of resource allocation and rationing are narrowly focused and lack perspective. Attention is often directed to how health care resources are spent and not how a reallocation of resources from other government programs, such as defense and other publicly financed programs, might produce considerable gains in the health status of the population. Take, for example, the controversy that currently surrounds the End-Stage Renal Disease Program. This program is obviously costly, and the benefits derived by many patients have been reported to be few.[20,212] Policymakers now question whether this program will be allowed to continue in its current form.[20,143]

Unfortunately, excessive attention has probably focused on the kidney program. The problems associated with providing medical care to patients with ESRD is only symptomatic of a more widespread problem—health care costs continue to escalate as a larger number of people increasingly benefit from new and expensive health care technology. However, it must be recognized that other health and social programs are equally costly. For example, in 1981, an estimated 100,000 to 125,000 Americans underwent coronary artery bypass surgery, first performed in 1968, and the numbers continue to rise.[213] Yet those who have the surgery amount to only 0.4% of the nation's population. At $2.0 billion per year (a conservative estimate according to Randal), coronary artery bypass surgery accounts for about 1.0% of the total annual US health bill.[214,215] The growth in the number of coronary artery bypass procedures performed each year has been substantial. In 1973, it was estimated that 38,000 such procedures were carried out in the United States at a cost in excess of $400 million.[55] Collectively, coronary artery bypass surgery is the most costly operation performed in this country and has boosted private health insurance premiums for the population as a whole.[213]

Interestingly, for most patients, the efficacy of coronary artery bypass surgery is questionable.[56,214-221] There is evidence that the procedure is effective in prolonging the life of patients who suffer from a major blockage of the main trunk of the left coronary artery, but evidence of the efficacy of the procedure on patients with "three-vessel disease" or in whom all three arteries are blocked is less clear. These patients presumably make up 30% to 40% of the total. Moreover, the rate of return to work among patients who have coronary artery bypass surgery is not impressive.[216,222-227]

The costs associated with neonatal intensive care are also high and are comparable with the costs of ESRD and coronary artery bypass surgery. A recent case study on the costs and effectiveness of neonatal intensive care estimates that the average expenditures per patient in 1978 were about $8,000, with costs for some patients well over $40,000.[228] Since there are no national data on the volume of neonatal intensive care being provided in the United States, only rough estimates can be produced, based on studies with small sample sizes and varying definitions of levels of care. Burdetti and associates provide the following estimates of neonatal intensive care supply and use:

1. Neonatal intensive care unit admissions—6% of all live births go to intensive care, accounting for 200,000 admissions each year.

2. Estimated average length of stay—eight to 18 days per patient.

3. Number of hospitals with neonatal intensive care units—600.

4. Number of intensive care beds—7,500.

5. Total cost of neonatal intensive care—$1.5 billion each year.

Thus, based on the foregoing, questions being asked about the treatment of patients with ESRD could also be asked of coronary artery bypass surgery and neonatal intensive care. Since Medicare finances only a small percentage of these procedures and services (perhaps 20.0% nationwide in the case of coronary artery bypass surgery, with Medicaid paying for another 5.0%), the amount of publicity they have attracted remains small. In the case of coronary artery bypass procedures, the majority of patients rely on third-party payers, but, even so, their out-of-pocket expenses may equal 20% of the total bill.[213]

To provide even greater perspective for this discussion, the current level of defense spending as well as expenditures associated with the federal corrections system should be examined. It is well recognized that the resources devoted to national defense dwarf those available to health and social programs.[229] It is less well recognized, however, that it now costs as much per year to support a convicted felon in the federal correctional system as it does to keep a person alive on home hemodialysis. It seems a paradox that producing and maintaining the means to destroy life and warehousing in correctional facilities people who have outright taken the lives of others continues to absorb enormous resources that might justifiably be used otherwise. Why is it that when health care programs are criticized as being too costly, no attempt is made to put this in perspective by looking at other, less desirable uses of resources?

Table 8 gives budget authority and Table 9 budget outlays as provided in the fiscal year 1983 budget of the US government.[230] National defense expenditures are more than twice those available for government-financed health care programs. The size of the budget for the administration of justice is minuscule when compared with either the budgets for national defense or health; yet, when one examines that portion of the justice budget devoted to corrections, it is not inconsequential, considering how the resources are used. In 1978, the average daily population in federal correctional facilities peaked at 29,347. Today, the average daily population has dropped to approximately 27,000. The cost per person per year (fiscal year 1981) for supporting persons convicted of violating federal laws as well as persons charged with crimes and detained for trial or sentencing is approximately $13,000 ($352 million per year for 27,000 persons). Yet, as the prison population is declining, inflation is driving up the costs of operations to a point where outlays for operating correctional facilities are expected to be about $367 million in 1982 and $386 million in 1983.

Iglehart[7] has recently summarized the proposed budget (fiscal year 1983) for major federal departments and agencies. Figures for defense and military functions and those for health and human services are given in Table 10. In reviewing the total budget, Iglehart concluded that, insofar as research and development funds are concerned, "research in physics, engineering, and other fields with potential military and industrial applications fared considerably better than did medical research."

For fiscal year 1984, the Reagan administration has requested a National Institutes of Health (NIH) budget of $4.1 billion, representing an increase of $73 million, or 1.8% over last year's proposal. Once the projected 4.9% inflation rate for 1983 is considered, however, the NIH will end up losing this modest gain in terms of real dollars.

Not surprisingly, the Department of Defense (DOD) is expected to fare well in 1984. Since his election, President Reagan has increased annual outlays for the DOD by 33%, with plans to increase the DOD budget by another 14% in 1984. As of this date, the administration has requested $274 billion for the DOD, with some congressmen indicating that this figure will be reduced by at least $15 billion. Overall, despite pending cuts in the DOD budget, it is still expected to increase by 30.0%, reaching a total of $29 billion, or 65% of the total US budget for research and development.

In the final analysis, it is apparent that resources directed to health care programs and health-related activities are not excessive when compared with other publicly financed programs of somewhat dubious value.[12] At the same time, it is evident that some health care programs have been unjustly critized when it is recognized that

Table 8. Budget Authority by Function

Function (Budget Code)	Actual, in Billion Dollars, 1981	Estimates, in Billion Dollars					
		1982	1983	1984	1985	1986	1987
National defense (050)	182.4	218.9	263.0	291.0	338.0	374.9	408.4
Health (550)	68.9	79.2	77.8	81.4	93.6	115.7	128.3
Administration of justice (750)	4.3	4.3	4.5	4.6	4.5	4.6	4.6

Table 9. Budget Outlays by Function

Function (Budget Code)	Actual, in Billion Dollars, 1981	Estimates, in Billion Dollars					
		1982	1983	1984	1985	1986	1987
National defense (050)	159.8	187.5	221.1	253.0	292.1	331.7	364.2
Health (550)	66.0	73.4	78.1	84.9	93.5	102.4	111.9
Administration of justice (750)	4.7	4.5	4.6	4.6	4.5	4.5	4.6

Table 10. Conduct of Research and Development in Defense and Health*

Department or Agency	Obligations, in Billion Dollars			Outlays, in Billion Dollars		
	1981	1982	1983	1981	1982	1983
Defense and military functions	16.5	20.6	24.5	15.7	18.8	22.7
Health and human services	4.0	4.0	4.1	4.0	3.9	4.0

*Data from Inglehart.[7]

other medical procedures are equally as costly as those currently receiving careful scrutiny, such as the End-Stage Renal Disease Program. Thus, the following conclusion is unequivocal—resource allocation decisions must be viewed in perspective.

Facing the Inevitable—Death and Dying

As described previously, numerous ethical issues surround the allocation and rationing of health care resources. When not all will benefit, the dilemma becomes one of choosing who will. The ethical problems inherent in CBA and CEA are by no means resolved.[19,231] It is apparent, however, that should these procedures be applied to resource allocation decisions, this society will become acutely aware of mortality.[232-237]

Historically, within this society, there is a preoccupation with health, almost to the point where death is observed as the ultimate of all evil. Major social surveys of the population have continuously shown that health is highly valued.[238] Interestingly, however, it has become increasingly difficult to define the parameters of health. Even a person's need and ability to interact with others has been designated as "social health."[239-241] Perhaps this is because of the fact that the most commonly accepted definition of health is that provided in the Constitution of the World Health Organization,[242] which states that "health is a state of complete physical, mental and social well-being and not merely the absence of disease or infirmity." Consequently, at least three types of health are found in the literature—physical health, mental health, and social health. It is now difficult to determine what is and what is not health.

Preoccupation with health is obviously an unacknowledged preoccupation with death and, perhaps, the process of dying. While many people fear death, the overriding concern is with dying, i.e., the process by which death comes about. For the most part, this society seems to be fully committed to the preservation of life at all costs, despite the quality of life the afflicted is likely to lead. It has only been in recent years that clinicians and the public have been willing to straightforwardly acknowledge and verbalize their concern with what might be called the "quantity v quality of life trade-off."[21,22,128,156,164,173,201-203,210,243] Accompanying this, of course, have been open discussions of the value of human life.[78,81,83,244-251] The uncertainty of what follows death has led many to eschew death in favor of living, regardless of the quality of their existence. Recent studies, however, show that persons, when faced with the prospect of a long-term chronic illness, are at least willing to consider the prospects of a shorter but higher quality of life.[128,201,202]

This in itself suggests that people have come to grips with the notion of death. Nevertheless, widely held religious beliefs and convictions would suggest that a large proportion of the population is unwilling to entertain the possibility of voluntary euthanasia or passive suicide as solutions to prolonged suffering.[235] Some religious groups would, in fact, consider life with catastrophic long-term illness an act of God and the illness a test of their religious conviction. In fact, they may believe that illness enhances their ability to demonstrate their religious faith to others in a testimonial fashion.

Over the years, technology has evolved to a point where the determination of death is increasingly problematic.[252-261] In fact, the new understanding of death is largely a consequence of technological advances in life-support systems. The President's Commission has now grappled with the problem of translating the current physiological understanding of death into acceptable statutory language. The Commission was also interested "in the dispute between 'whole brain' and 'higher brain' formulations of death and appraising currently used brain-based tests for death, which have become increasingly varied and sophisticated."[257] A set of guidelines has been established for the determination of death, but these are not accepted by all.[254,255,257]

Thus, the ability of technology to stave off premature death through a variety of means makes it increasingly likely that this society will be unable to fully come to grips with death in a manner that facilitates the withholding of treatment when the expected outcomes are negligible or counterindicative to the well-being of the patient and his or her next of kin. Surprisingly, however, there is considerable interest in hospice care in the United States, which, in effect, suggests that a decision to discontinue vigorous treatment is acceptable.[262–264] As described by Saunders,[262] "The hospice movement sets out to ensure that every person who can no longer benefit from the increasing complexity of the general hospital will have the support he and his family need. The whole family is the unit of care and should also be seen as part of the caring team." By most standards, the hospice concept is not a new innovation; it dates back to as early as 1983, when St. Luke's Hospital was established in London.

Perhaps unfortunately, it is rarely the case that the similarity between hospice care and the voluntary withholding of treatment is recognized.[198] The parallel is close, yet it is currently argued that patients, under all circumstances, should receive every extraordinary means of care available to prolong life. Only when society is fully able to come to grips with death and dying is it likely that "policies and procedures for decisions not to treat" not only will be formulated but will also be followed. This period is likely to be hastened as financial constraints force the issue. Putting this in prespective, Manning[236] has stated:

> Somewhere along the way, consciously or unconsciously, explicitly or implicitly, society will have to make some basic decisions about the allocation of economic resources as between human beings of advanced years and those who are younger . . . We have not begun to consider the violent social dislocation that would be brought about if a large fraction of the population were to be kept alive for significantly longer periods of time.

As noted previously, the problems that must be addressed are essentially ethical or, perhaps, ethical-legal.[189] New medical technology has not only dramatically changed the practice of medicine, but it has also raised a variety of issues with which clinicians are rather uncomfortable. The problem, however, is that these issues are relatively new and must be worked through carefully. Many of the issues surrounding the allocation and rationing of resources are almost metaphysical in nature. There is no clear-cut solution to the problems they instill for society. Ethics are relative to time, place, and perhaps most importantly, culture. The anthropologist Ruth Benedict,[265] in describing the "cultural relativist" perspective on culture, made a profound observation. She stated:

> No man ever looks at the world with pristine eyes. He sees it edited by a definite set of customs and institutions and ways of thinking. Even in his philosophical probings he cannot go behind these stereotypes; his very concepts of the true and the false will still have reference to his particular traditional customs.

The cultural relativist perspective nicely summarizes the problems inherent in making resource allocation and rationing decisions. Even though based on explicit and hopefully rational criteria, any plan that is eventually adopted is certainly debatable from the perspectives of others. To adopt a set of criteria is to make a decision about limiting treatment. On the other hand, to treat all patients with a given disorder or within a given disease category, regardless of derived benefits, necessarily implies the withholding of treatment from patients with other disorders. The question is truly one of priorities. Data can be used to set priorities, but human judgment must be exercised to determine which priorities will hold.

The future is likely to be interesting. The conscious development of explicit allocation criteria, as a first step in the direction of wisely using limited resources, will be controversial. Questions must be raised as to how resources will be allocated not only to health programs but social programs as well. There are certainly many patients with diseases and esoteric medical conditions who could benefit from additional resource allocations. In 1972, it was decided that patients with ESRD would be eligible for Medicare benefits, yet there were and are many other patients with diseases and conditions who could have sustained the prolonged attention of government agencies.

Allocation issues will obviously be submitted to a complex sociopolitical decision-making process. Decisions can be made on the basis of allocation tools such as CEA or CBA, or a grim political battle could be waged between different lobbying groups, each representing the special interests of patients with specific diseases or conditions. In either case, the first decision will be as to which patient groups will receive support (i.e., the resource allocation decision); then, as resources continue to dwindle, allocations will be made within programs and decisions will be made as to how clinicians *might* ration the limited resources made available to them. Increasingly, it is apparent that this scenario approximates the situation of the kidney disease program today. As already noted, people at all levels of government are concerned about the amount spent on the kidney program and are looking for ways to stretch what seems to be increasingly finite resources. In this regard, it could be stated that the "battle" has just begun and that the "war" is yet to be fought.

While the dilemmas created by resource allocation and rationing decisions are undeniable, it would seem that they have and will continue to provide an impetus for a reconsideration of the meaning of death and the essence of life. Reasonably acceptable criteria have been established for the determination of death, yet the very essence of life continues to be elusive. People do seem to be on the verge of seriously valuing their lives, not only in terms of longevity but in terms of quality.[117,201,202]

Although Condorset envisioned that a "period must one day arrive when death will be nothing more than the effect either of extraordinary accidents, or the slow gradual decay of vital powers; and that the duration of the interval between the birth of man and his decay will have no assignable limit," Choron[232] has aptly pointed out that "the postponement of death is not a solution to the problem of the fear of death. . . . There still will remain the fear of dying prematurely."

In his treatise on death, Ernst Becker[234] shows that the fear of death is universal and that this fear "haunts the human animal like nothing else; it is a mainspring of human activity—activity designed largely to avoid the fatality of death, to overcome it by denying in some way that it is the final destiny of man." He argues that far too much effort is put into establishing immortality, in his words, into establishing a "formula for triumphing over life's limitations." People have failed to take life and its limitations seriously. He concludes his discourse, as follows, with a challenge for those who have used science to define the very essence of life:[234]

> The problem with all the scientific manipulators is that somehow they don't take life seriously enough; in this sense, all science is "bourgeois," an affair of bureaucrats. I think that taking life seriously means something such as this: that whatever man does on this planet has to be done in the lived truth of the terror of creation, of the grotesque, of the rumble of panic underneath everything. Otherwise it is false. Whatever is achieved must be achieved from within the subjective energies of creatures, without deadening, with the full exercise of passion, of vision, of pain, of fear, and of sorrow. How do we know that our part of the meaning of the universe might not be a rhythm in sorrow?

Had Becker devoted his attention to an analysis of the full implications of life-prolonging, advanced biomedical technology, it is difficult to speculate what he would have concluded. It is likely, however, that he would have concluded that western society has become too infatuated with the fear of death and has failed to realize the true essence and value of life, despite its length.

Comment

I have attempted to put modern technology into perspective by noting that technological innovation is in response to the demand created by the increased life expectancy and changing age distribution of the population and the increased prevalence of chronic disease and its concomitant diability. Increasingly, it is recognized that sophisticated medical technology, however, is not without its price. In recent years, it has been argued that technology has been a major contributor to rising health care costs in this country. Whether technology will continue to be viewed as the culprit behind rising health care costs is yet to be seen.

Efforts are now being made to control technology by a more thorough, comprehensive, and ongoing assessment of new, emerging, and existing technological innovations.[51,266–274] In this regard, Relman[90,275] has correctly argued that one effective method of moderating the cost of medical care, while improving its quality, is to initiate "a major new national program of support for the evaluation of medical procedures of all kinds." From his perspective, it is the cost of ignorance associated with medical technology that is too great, not medical progress. In Relman's words, "The cost culprit is not technology per se, but only technology that is ineffective, superfluous, or unsafe."[257,276] In short, the goal of technological assessment should not be to curb the development of technologies but rather to provide the means for an unbiased evaluation of new technology before it becomes too widely diffused in practice. To meet this goal, Bunker and associates[10,11] have proposed the establishment of a private, nonprofit corporation for the collection, analysis, and dissemination of data on medical procedures and for the support of new clinical trials. The Institute for Health Care Evaluation, as they refer to it, would be intended to fill partially the void created by the abolition of the ill-fated National Center for Health Care Technology.[277] This Institute would have neither policy-making nor regulatory functions. At the present time, the HCFA has taken on an increasingly visible role in the assessment and regulation of new health care technology.[278] This role is evidenced by two generic types of policy decisions that the HCFA must make, namely, (1) coverage decisions—whether an item or service is one for which the program can pay—and (2) reimbursement decisions—how much is appropriate to pay for a covered item or service.

Despite Bunker's proposal for an Institute for Health Care Evaluation and the remarkable and noteworthy efforts of the Office of Technology Assessment, the foregoing discussion concludes that technological assessment, although likely to increase the efficiency of the health care provision system, will not be sufficient to wholly resolve impending budget constraints proposed by the Reagan administration. There are, indeed, limitations on the resources that can be allocated to health care programs, although some reallocation decisions would serve to stave off the inevitable. In preparation for the inevitable, plans must be made and techniques developed for the effective allocation and rationing of health care resources. Various suggestions have been offered as to how cost-effectiveness and cost-benefit analytic techniques can be applied to the making of intraprogram and interprogram *allocation* decisions. Clinical decision analysis, although imperfect, is offered as a possible approach to dealing with the resource *rationing* dilemma.

The increasingly apparent need to allocate and ration health care resources has led to a careful scrutiny of medical care costs. Health economists continue to point out that health care costs are almost out of control and that a major solution to this problem is to make the current service provision system more efficient through various competitive strategies, despite the fact that recent reports indicate that competition can have a negative impact on the quality of care patients receive.[279] Taking a differing viewpoint, other commentators have correctly pointed out that the health care industry, employing approximately 4.3 million workers, is the second largest industry in the United States and that reductions in health care through competition or other strategies would serve to displace a large number of persons in this industry.[280] The effect would be dramatic as displaced health care workers "would either displace others from their jobs or go on the welfare rolls. Either way one looks at it, a shrinkage of the health-care industry would create a ripple effect throughout our economy."[280] This has led Kolff to suggest that efforts to control health care costs through careful technology assessment "totally neglects the notion that we should move towards a service oriented economy instead of towards an industrial production directed economy" (W. J. Kolff, MD, PhD, written communication, Feb 22, 1983). He asks, "What are we to do with our unemployed? Unless we expand our 'services,' there is no solution."

The causes and cure of medical cost inflation are only partially understood and, thus, remain debatable. Jellinek and others,[280–283] however, believe that there are factors other than the "delivery of health care or the marketing of illness" that have led to increased spending in the health care sector. Jellinek[281] believes that the continued rise in health care expenditures is a result of increased alienation and depersonalization associated with post-World War II society. The response of society is to compensate by aggressive attention to the individual when he or she becomes ill. Jellinek[281] summarizes his position as follows:

Societal willingness to support extraordinarily expensive new medical technology and advanced training, which implicitly communicates a willingness to place a high value on individual human life in contrast to the low value implied by industrial depersonalization, may represent one important form of adjustment of the social contract. The increase in society's expenditures for medical care may constitute a stabilizing force necessary to counter the destabilizing impulses generated by continued economic development.

In the final analysis, however, perhaps Jellinek's[281] assessment of the problem does not go far enough. For example, it seems almost a paradox that defense spending goes unchecked while, at the same time, massive cuts have been made in public health care assistance programs as well as health care research efforts. While public fund-raising may produce the required resources to enable a young child to receive a liver transplant or a middle-aged person to obtain a heart transplant, to date, there remains relatively little public debate over the merits of increased defense expenditures, which obviously pale current health care expenditures.

Unfortunately, the lay public, nevertheless, seems to be either unaware of or has chosen to ignore the key ethical issues implied by resource allocation and rationing decisions. Perhaps not uncharacteristically, people remain willing to come to the aid of identifiable victims of resource scarcity, such as persons in need of organ transplants. At the same time, the lay public finds a special attraction in persons such as artificial heart recipient Barney Clark, who has been honored for "risking his life in order to save it." Thus, in the end, perhaps, the real concern with personal health in today's society is not so much the depersonalization and alienation that many persons feel but rather the fact that destructive forces of an unprecedented magnitude have served to completely threaten human existence.[284-286] Consequently, for many people, the true value of life becomes most apparent either when a person's life is at stake because they are denied medical care that is available but in short supply or when the type of medical care required is unavailable. Although often highly publicized by the mass media, each of the patients who fall into these categories serves to underscore the basic dilemma—health care resources are limited.

The inevitability of resource allocation and rationing decisions has been well characterized by Fuchs.[125] In his discussion of the problems of health and medical care, he notes that an economic approach to these is firmly rooted in three fundamental observations of the world. These are as follows: (1) resources are scarce in relation to human wants, (2) resources have alternative uses, and (3) people have different wants, with considerable variation in the relative importance they attach to them. Yet, the basic economic problem identified by Fuchs[125] is "how to allocate scarce resources so as to best satisfy human wants."

While Fuchs places a great deal of emphasis on the economics of resource allocation and provides only cursory attention to the social, ethical, and legal implications of allocation and rationing decisions, the fact is that without economic constraints, most allocation and rationing decisions would be unnecessary except in situations in which the needed resource, natural or otherwise, is severely limited. In instances of the latter, economic resources would not be sufficient to alleviate scarcity. The basic premise of this discussion, therefore, is that constraints on economic resources will necessitate resource-allocation and rationing decisions, which, in turn, will make the confrontation of various social, ethical, and legal issues inescapable. In the future, the major issues confronting not only medicine but this society as a whole will be the social, ethical, and legal implications of resource allocation and rationing, whether framed in terms of distributive justice,[287-292] discrimination against the poor and disadvantaged,[293] or the withholding of treatment from those with catastrophic illness.[197] All of these share a common underlying theme—the need to confront human finality and purposeful existence.[294]

As described herein, the problems associated with the allocation and rationing of scarce medical resources, economic (e.g., health care dollars) or natural (e.g., organs and tissue for transplantation), are, indeed, related to dying as an experience and death as an event. This discriminatory use of resources (and that is basically what allocation and rationing imply) has a lot to do with the fact that persons are eventually denied something they require—in this case, medical care. Schelling[124] underscores the essential ingredient of rationing decisions when he distinguishes between an "individual death/life" and a "statistical death/life." The two are, in reality, different and he provides the following example to illustrate his point:

Let a 6-year old girl with brown hair need thousands of dollars for an operation that will prolong her life until Christmas, and the post office will be swamped with nickels and dimes to save her. But let it be reported that without a sales tax the hospital facilities of Massachusetts will deteriorate and cause a barely perceptible increase in preventable deaths—not many will drop a tear or reach for their checkbooks.

This distinction is an important one because it highlights the fact that the death of a person is a unique, often private event. Yet, at the local level, the victim and his or her family have an intense interest. In fact, as Schelling[124] notes, if society takes an interest in a local death, it is often because of a general concern that "reasonable efforts are made to conserve life than in whether those efforts succeed."

At this point in time, it is predictable that resource allocation decisions are unlikely to be carefully scrutinized by the public until resource rationing decisions become an inescapable fact of life. When the public is exposed to rationing decisions that it feels are contrary to the interest of the persons involved, despite catastrophic illness, it is likely to call into question the worthiness of allocation decisions. When it becomes apparent that these decisions are based on a mix of medical and social criteria, the latter which the public is much more likely to understand and despise as the basis for differentially valuing human life, the public will become increasingly irritated and resentful.

While selection criteria of any sort are likely to be viewed as unjust, it is a truism that not all people are likely to maximally or optimally benefit from available medical technology. For example, I and associates[20] have shown how dramatically the extension of Medicare benefits to patients with ESRD affected the composition of the patient population. In particular, indicia of patient rehabilitation, such as employment status, show a decline in the overall status of the patient population.

In the future, decisions must be made concerning which patients will maximally and optimally benefit from expensive health care technology, yet a watchful person must focus on such decisions to ensure that "social worth" will not be the criterion of final determination. The problem, however, is that, in many respects, social and medical criteria are inextricably intertwined. People of low socioeconomic status are likely to be in poorer health with multiple disease conditions, which, in part, reflects poor nutritional habits, detrimental lifestyle, and the historical lack of resources to obtain proper health care. Consequently, if medical criteria were to be the basis on which rationing decisions are made, they might exclude the poor and disadvantaged because health and socioeconomic status are highly interdependent. For example, it is not unusual to find that of those persons with ESRD, those of lower socioeconomic status are likely to have multiple comorbid health conditions such as diabetes, hepatitis, and hypertension. Not only are these patients less desirable candidates for dialysis and transplantation, but they are among the more expensive patients to treat.

Without careful planning and evaluation, the cleavage between the haves and have-nots, as evidenced by formal selection criteria, is likely to become substantial. Those with the financial means may be able to purchase the services they require, while those who are disadvantaged and destitute will be denied care. Claims of a right to health care might well serve as a common goal to bind the disenfranchised.[186,295-302] Specific laws have been promulgated to protect the rights of certain classes of persons; examples include Section 504 of the Rehabilitation Act of 1973, the Age Discrimination Act, and Title VII of the Civil Rights Act. Each of these laws has important implications for resource rationing decisions.

It is highly probable that disclosure of the names, by the media, of persons who have been denied the benefits of medicine will set into motion complex sociopolitical manuevering to reprieve those who have reportedly been treated unjustly by those with authority to make and enforce resource-rationing decisions. Arguments that surround these decisions are likely to be similar to those made in connection with abortion and the withholding of medical treatment.[198-200,303-305] The Quinlin, Saikewicz, and Dinnerstein cases will frequently be cited as precedent setting. Analogies are likely to be made between current events and the events that took place in Nazi Germany. To this end, it will be argued that to set forth criteria that deny people treatment, in effect, represents a devaluation of life. As Carroll[306] has noted:

Life has become increasingly cheap in our time. Today, Auschwitz and Dachau are museums; Coventry, Dresden, and Hiroshima, vague memories; the deaths several years ago of hundreds of thousands of Indonesians, a footnote to history; race riots in American cities, a subject of study; and war casualties in Viet Nam, an object of routine reports.

Moreover, the practice of rationing will bring forth cries that the precedent is now set for the "floodgates to be opened" to the "mass slaughter" of persons whom rationing criteria declare to be of "marginal" value.

The point of the matter, however, is that rationing decisions are already being made.[127] The fact that they are not publicized has prevented them from becoming a social issue, despite the fact that they have attracted the attention of bioethicists.[21,22,307,308] Nevertheless, the future is likely to be filled with accounts of persons who have been refused treatment. Within a society that has failed to come to grips with the meaning of death and the essence of life, rationing decisions will seem unusually cruel. Yet, when these decisions are acknowledged as inescapable, this society, this culture, will be more prepared to deal with the one event that is truly inevitable—death.

Preparation of this article has been made possible by grant 95-P-97887/0-01 and contract 500-81-0051, provided by the Health Care Financing Administration.

The author received assistance from Christopher R. Blagg, MD, George L. Maddox, PhD, Carl Josephson, and the entire health care technology assessment team at the Battelle Human Affairs Research Centers. Millie Gregory typed the manuscript and Peg Nadler provided editing assistance.

References

1. Russell L: How much does medical technology cost? *Bull NY Acad Med* 1978;54:124–132.

2. Caper P: Competition and health care: A new Trojan horse. *N Engl J Med* 1982;306:928–929.

3. Iglehart JK: Medicare's uncertain future. *N Engl J Med* 1982;306:1308–1312.

4. McGregor M, Polletier G: Planning of specialized health facilities: Size vs. cost and effectiveness in heart surgery. *N Engl J Med* 1978;299:179–181.

5. Luft HS, Bunker JP, Enthoven AC: Should operations be regionalized?: The empirical relation between surgical volume and mortality. *N Engl J Med* 1979;301:1364–1369.

6. Finkler SA: Cost-effectiveness of regionalization: The heart surgery example. *Inquiry* 1979;16:264–270.

7. Iglehart JK: Health policy report: Prospects for the National Institutes of Health. *N Engl J Med* 1982;306:879–884.

8. Chalmers TC: The clinical trial. *Milbank Mem Fund Q* 1981;59:324–339.

9. Chalmers TC: Who will fund clinical trials? *Sciences* 1982;22:6–8.

10. Bunker JP, Fowles J, Schaffarzick R: Evaluation of medical-technology strategies: I. Effects of coverage and reimbursement. *N Engl J Med* 1982;306:620–624.

11. Bunker JP, Fowles J, Schaffarzick R: Evaluation of medical-technology strategies: II. Proposal for an institute for health-care evaluation. *N Engl J Med* 1982;306:687–692.

12. Frederickson DS: Biomedical research in the 1980s. *N Engl J Med* 1981;304:509–517.

13. Office of Health Economics: Scarce resources in health care. *Milbank Mem Fund Q* 1979;57:265–287.

14. Ramsey P: *The Patient as a Person: Explorations in Medical Ethics.* New Haven, Conn, Yale University Press, 1970.

15. Wertz RW (ed): *Readings on Ethical and Social Issues in Biomedicine.* Englewood Cliffs, NJ, Prentice-Hall Inc, 1973.

16. Beauchamp TL, Childress J: *Principles of Biomedical Ethics.* New York, Oxford University Press, 1979.

17. Stein J: *Making Medical Choices: Who Is Responsible?* Boston, Houghton Mifflin Co, 1978.

18. Callahan D: Shattuck lecture: Contemporary biomedical ethics. *N Engl J Med* 1980;302:1228–1233.

19. Tancredi LR: Social and ethical implications in technology assessment, in McNeil BJ, Cravalho EG (eds): *Critical Issues in Medical Technology.* Boston, Auburn House, 1982, pp 93–112.

20. Evans RW, Blagg CR, Bryan FA Jr: Implications for health care policy: A social and demographic profile of hemodialysis patients in the United States. *JAMA* 1981;245:487–491.

21. Crane D: Decisions to treat critically ill patients. *Milbank Mem Fund Q* 1975;53:1–33.

22. Crane, D: *The Sanctity of Social Life Physician's Treatment of Critically Ill Patients,* New York, Russell Sage Foundation, 1975.

23. Becker EL: Finite resources and medical triage. *Am J Med* 1979;66:549–550.

24. Civetta JM: The inverse relationship between cost and survival. *J Surg Res* 1973;14:265–269.

25. Cullen DJ, Ferrara LC, Briggs BA, et al: Survival, hospitalization charges and follow-up results in critically ill patients. *N Engl J Med* 1976;294:982–987.

26. Turnbull AD, Carlton G, Baron R, et al: The inverse relationship between cost and survival in the critically ill cancer patient. *Crit Care Med* 1979;7:20–23.

27. Thibault GE, Mulley AG, Barnett GO, et al: Medical intensive care: Indications, interventions, and outcomes. *N Engl J Med* 1980;302:938–942.

28. Detsky AS, Stricker SC, Mulley AG, et al: Prognosis, survival, and the expenditure of hospital resources for patients in an intensive care unit. *N Engl J Med* 1981;305:667–672.

29. Martin SW, Donaldson MC, London CD, et al: Inputs into coronary care during 30 years: A cost-effectiveness study. *Ann Intern Med* 1974;81:289–293.

30. Zook, CJ, Moore FD: High-cost users of medical care. *N Engl J Med* 1980;302:996–1002.

31. Schroeder SA, Showstack JA, Schwartz J: Survival of adult high-cost patients: Report of a follow-up study from nine acute-care hospitals. *JAMA* 1981;245:1446–1449.

32. Silverman WA: Mismatched attitudes about neonatal death. *Hastings Cent Rep* 1981;11:12–16.

33. Bridge P, Bridge M: The brief life and death of Christopher Bridge. *Hastings Cent Rep* 1981;11:17–19.

34. Cluff LF: Chronic disease, function and quality of care. *J Chronic Dis* 1981;34:299–304.

35. Reiser SJ: *Medicine and the Reign of Technology*. New York, Cambridge University Press, 1978.

36. Russell LB: *Technology in Hospitals: Medical Advances and Their Diffusion*. Washington, DC, The Brookings Institution, 1979.

37. Brown JHV: *The Health Care Dilemma: Problems of Technology in Health Care Delivery*. New York, Human Sciences Press, 1978.

38. Ellison DL: *The Bio-medical Fix*. Westport, Conn, Greenwood Press Inc, 1978.

39. McGinnis JM: Recent health gains for adults. *N Engl J Med* 1982;306:671–673.

40. Department of Health and Human Services: *Health: United States, 1981,* DHHS publication (PHS) 82-1232. Hyattsville, Md, National Center for Health Statistics, 1981.

41. Lerner M: When, why, and where people die, in Brim OG Jr, Freeman HE, Levine S, et al (eds): *The Dying Patient*. New York, Russell Sage Foundation, 1970, pp 5–29.

42. Dubos R: *Man Adapting*. New Haven, Conn, Yale University Press, 1965.

43. Commission on Chronic Illness: *Care of the Long-term Patient*. Cambridge, Mass, Harvard University Press, 1956, vol 2.

44. Havlik RJ, Feinleib M (eds): *Proceedings of the Conference on the Decline in Coronary Heart Disease Mortality, Bethesda, Md, October 24–25, 1978*. Bethesda, Md, National Institutes of Health, 1979.

45. Dawber TR: *The Framingham Study*. Cambridge, Mass, Harvard University, 1980.

46. Hendricks J, Hendricks CD: *Aging in Mass Society: Myths and Realities*. Cambridge, Mass, Winthrop Publishers Inc, 1977.

47. Strauss A: *Chronic Illness and the Quality of Life*. St Louis, CV Mosby Co, 1975.

48. Givens JD: *Current Estimates From the Health Interview Survey, United States, 1978,* Vital and Health Statistics Series 10, No. 130, Dept of Health, Education, and Welfare publication (PHS) 80-1551. Hyattsville, Md, National Center for Health Statistics, 1979.

49. Thomas L: *The Lives of a Cell: Notes of a Biology Watcher*. New York, The Viking Press Inc, 1974.

50. Thomas L: Notes of a biology-watcher: The technology of medicine. *N Engl J Med* 1977;285:1366–1368.

51. Banta HD, Behney CJ, Willems JS: *Toward Rational Technology in Medicine*. New York, Springer Publishing Co Inc, 1981.

52. Ford AB: Casualties of our time. *Science* 1970;167:256–263.

53. Office of Technology Assessment: *Assessing the Efficacy and Safety of Medical Technologies,* stock 052-003-00593-0. Government Printing Office, 1978.

54. Larson EB: Consequences of medical technology: Controversies and dilemmas. *University of Washington Medicine* 1981;8:2–5.

55. Hiatt HH: Protecting the medical commons: Who is responsible? *N Engl J Med* 1975;293:235–241.

56. Preston T: *Coronary Artery Surgery: A Critical Review*. New York, Raven Press, 1977.

57. Fineberg H: Gastric freezing: A study of diffusion of a medical innovation, in *Medical Technology and the Health Care System,* Committee on Technology and Health Care. Washington, DC, National Academy of Sciences, 1979, pp 173–200.

58. Bunker JP, Hinkley D, McDermott W: Surgical innovation and its evaluation. *Science* 1978;200:937–941.

59. Banta HD, Behney CJ: Policy formulation and technology assessment. *Milbank Mem Fund Q* 1981;59:445–479.

60. Banta D, Sanes J: Assessing the social impacts of medical technology. *J Community Health* 1978;3:245–258.

61. Schwartz WB, Joskow PL: Medical efficacy versus economic efficiency: A conflict in values. *N Engl J Med* 1978;299:1462–1464.

62. Arnstein S, Christakis A: *Perspectives on Technology Assessment*. Jerusalem, Science and Technology Publishers, 1975.

63. Wagner J (ed): *Medical Technology,* Dept of Health, Education, and Welfare publication (PHS) 79-3254. Hyattsville, Md, National Center for Health Services Research, 1979.

64. Wagner JL (ed): *Medical Technology: Research Priorities.* Washington, DC, Urban Institute, 1979.

65. Knox RA: Heart transplants: To pay or not to pay. *Science* 1980;209:570–575.

66. Brooks H, Bowers R: The assessment of technology. *Sci Am* 1970;22:13–21.

67. Coates JF: Technology assessment, in Teich AH (ed): *Technology and Man's Future,* ed 3. New York, St Martin's Press Inc, 1981, pp 229–250.

68. Gordon G, Fisher G: *The Diffusion of Medical Technology.* Cambridge, Mass, Ballinger Publishing Co, 1975.

69. Morrison RS: Visions, in Teich AH (ed): *Technology and Man's Future,* ed 3. New York, St Martin's Press Inc, 1981, pp 7–22.

70. Stocking B, Morrison SL: *The Image and the Reality: A Case Study of the Impacts of Medical Technology.* London, Nuffield Provincial Hospitals Trust, 1978.

71. Committee on Technology and Health Care: *Medical Technology and the Health Care System,* Washington, DC, National Academy of Sciences, 1979.

72. Goldman J (ed): *Health Care Technology Evaluation,* vol 6, in *Lecture Notes in Medical Informatics.* New York, Springer-Verlag, 1979.

73. Frazier H, Hiatt H: Evaluation of medical practices. *Science* 1978;200:875–878.

74. Gibson R, Waldo DR: National health expenditures, 1980. *Health Care Financing Rev,* September 1981, pp 1–54.

75. Herrell JH: Health care expenditures: The approaching crisis. *Mayo Clin Proc* 1980;55:705–710.

76. Evans RW: Economic and social costs of heart transplantation. *Heart Transplantation* 1982;1:243–251.

77. Rice DP: *Estimating the Cost of Illness,* Public Health Service publication 947-6. Government Printing Office, 1966.

78. Rice DP: The economic value of human life. *Am J Public Health* 1967;57:1954–1966.

79. Rice DP: Estimating the cost of illness. *Am J Public Health* 1967;57:424–440.

80. Rice DP, Hodgson TA: *Social and Economic Implications of Cancer in the United States,* Vital and Health Statistics Series 3, No. 20, Dept of Health, Education, and Welfare publication (PHS) 81-1404. Hyattsville, Md, National Center for Health Statistics, 1981.

81. Rice DP, Hodgson TA: The value of life revisited. *Am J Public Health* 1982;72:536–538.

82. Cooper BS, Rice DP: The economic cost of illness revisited. *Soc Secur Bull* 1976;39:21–36.

83. Landefeld JS, Seskin EP: The economic value of life: Linking theory to practice. *Am J Public Health* 1982;72:555–566.

84. Stone DA: Diagnosis and the dole: The function of illness in American distributive politics. *J Health Polit Policy Law* 1979;4:507–521.

85. Skolnik A, Dales S: Social welfare expenditures, fiscal year 1976. *Soc Secur Bull* 1977;40:3–19.

86. Scitovsky A: Changes in the costs of treatment of selected illnesses, 1951–1965. *Am Econ Rev* 1967;53:1182–1190.

87. Russell L: The diffusion of new hospital technologies in the United States. *Int J Health Serv* 1976;6:557–580.

88. Egdahl R, Gertman P (eds): *Technology and the Quality of Health Care.* Germantown, Md, Aspen Systems Corp, 1978.

89. Fineberg HV, Hiatt HH: Evaluation of medical practices: The case of technology assessment. *N Engl J Med* 1979;301:1086–1091.

90. Relman AS: Assessment of medical practices: A simple proposal. *N Engl J Med* 1980;303:153–154.

91. Altman SH, Blendon RJ: *Medical Technology: The Culprit Behind Health Care Costs?* Dept of Health, Education, and Welfare publication (PHS) 79-3216. Government Printing Office, 1979.

92. Moloney TW, Rogers DE: Medical technology: A different view of the contentious debate over costs. *N Engl J Med* 1979;301:1413–1419.

93. Gaus CR, Cooper BS: Controlling Health Technology, in Altman SH, Blendon R (eds): *Medical Technology: The Culprit Behind Health Care Costs?* Dept of Health, Education, and Welfare publication (PHS) 79-3216. Government Printing Office, 1979, pp 242–252.

94. Marks R: Biomedical research and its technological products in the quality and cost problems of health practices, in Altman SH, Blendon R (eds): *Medical Technology: The Culprit Behind Health Care Costs?* Dept of Health, Education and Welfare publication (PHS) 79-3216. Government Printing Office, 1979, pp 235–241.

95. Heyssel RM: Controlling health technology: A public policy dilemma, in Altman SH, Blendon R (eds): *Medical Technology: The Culprit Behind Health Care Costs?* Dept of Health, Education, and Welfare publication (PHS) 79-3216. Government Printing Office, 1979, pp 262–272.

96. Bennett IL Jr: Technology as a shaping force. *Daedalus* 1977;106:125–133.

97. Blendon RJ, Moloney TW: Perspectives on the growing debate over the cost of medical technologies, in Altman SH, Blendon R (eds): *Medical Technology: The Culprit Behind Health Care Costs?* Dept of Health, Education, and Welfare publication (PHS) 79-3216. Government Printing Office, 1979, pp 10–23.

98. Showstack JA, Schroeder SA, Matsumoto MF: Changes in the use of medical technologies, 1972–1977: A study of ten inpatient diagnoses. *N Engl J Med* 1982;306:706–712.

99. Feldstein M, Taylor A: *The Rapid Rise of Hospital Costs*. Government Printing Office, 1977.

100. National Commission on the Cost of Medical Care: *Report of the Task Force on Technology*. Chicago, American Medical Association, 1978, vol 1.

101. Davis K: The role of technology, demand and labor markets in determination of hospital costs, in Perlman M (ed): *The Economics of Health and Medical Care*. New York, John Wiley & Sons Inc, 1974, pp 283–301.

102. Waldman S: Effect of changing technology on hospital costs. *Soc Secur Bull* 1972;35:28–30.

103. Worthington NL: Expenditures for hospital care and physician's services: Factors affecting annual charges. *Soc Secur Bull* 1975;39:3–15.

104. Scitovsky AA, McCall N: *Changes in the Costs of Treatment of Selected Illness, 1951–1964–1971*, Dept of Health, Education, and Welfare publication (HRA) 77-3161. Government Printing Office, 1976.

105. Department of Commerce, Bureau of the Census: *Statistical Abstract of the U.S., 1981*. Government Printing Office, 1981.

106. Fineberg HV: Clinical chemistries: The high cost of low-cost diagnostic tests, in Altman S, Blendon R (eds): *Medical Technology: The Culprit Behind Health Care Costs?* Dept of Health, Education, and Welfare publication (PHS) 79-3216. Government Printing Office, 1979.

107. Stoughton WV: Medical costs and technology regulation: The pivotal role of hospitals, in: McNeil BJ, Cravalho EG (eds): *Critical Issues in Medical Technology*. Boston, Auburn House, 1982, pp 37–50.

108. Derzon RA: Influences of reimbursement policies on technology, in McNeil BJ, Cravalho EG (eds): *Critical Issues in Medical Technology*. Boston, Auburn House, 1982, pp 139–150.

109. Schroeder SA, Showstack JA: Financial incentives to perform medical procedures and laboratory tests: Illustrative models of office practice. *Med Care* 1978;16:289–298.

110. Greenberg B, Derzon RA: Determining health insurance coverage of technology: Problems and options. *Med Care* 1981;19:967–978.

111. Towery OB, Perry S: The scientific basis for coverage decisions by third-party payers. *JAMA* 1981;245:59–61.

112. Elliott D, Elliott R: *The Control of Technology*. London, Wykeham Publications Ltd, 1976.

113. Wenchel HE: *A Summary of the Study of the Medical Technology Industry*, contract 233-79-3011. Hyattsville, Md, National Center for Health Services Research, 1981.

114. Cooper MH: *Rationing Health Care*. London, Croom Helm Ltd, 1977.

115. Katz J, Capron AM: *Catastrophic Diseases: Who Decides What?* New York, Russell Sage Foundation, 1975.

116. Golding AMB, Tosey D: The cost of high-technology medicine. *Lancet* 1980;2:195–197.

117. Mushkin SJ, Dunlop DW (eds): *Health: What Is it Worth?: Measures of Health Benefits*. New York, Pergamon Press Ltd, 1979.

118. Cochrane AL: *Effectiveness and Efficiency: Random Reflections on the National Health Service*. London, Nuffield Provincial Hospitals Trust, Burgess & Son Ltd, 1971.

119. Acton J: Measuring the monetary value of life-saving programs, in *Emergency Medical Services: Research Methodology*, Dept of Health, Education, and Welfare publication (PHS) 78-3195. Rockville, Md, National Center for Health Services Research, 1978.

120. Jones-Lee MW: *The Value of Life: An Economic Analysis*. Chicago, University of Chicago Press, 1976.

121. Fox RC: Ethical and existential developments in contemporaneous American medicine: Their implications for culture and society. *Milbank Mem Fund Q* 1974;52:445–483.

122. Fox RC: *Essays in Medical Sociology: Journeys Into the Fields*. New York, John Wiley & Sons Inc, 1979.

123. Rescher N: The allocation of exotic medical lifesaving therapy. *Ethics* 1969;79:173–186.

124. Schelling TC: The life you save may be your own, in Chase SB Jr (ed): *Problems in Public Expenditure Analysis*. Washington, DC, The Brookings Institution, 1968, pp 127–176.

125. Fuchs VR: *Who Shall Live? Health, Economics, and Social Choice*. New York, Basic Books Inc, 1974.

126. Weinstein MC, Stason WB: *Hypertension: A Policy Perspective*, Cambridge, Mass, Harvard University Press, 1976.

127. Weinstein MC, Stason WB: Foundations of cost-effectiveness analysis for health and medical practices. *N Engl J Med* 1977;296:716–721.

128. Weinstein MC, Fineberg HV, Elstein AS, et al: *Clinical Decision Analysis*. Philadelphia, WB Saunders Co, 1980.

129. Stason WB, Weinstein MC: Allocation of resources to manage hypertension. *N Engl J Med* 1977;296:732–739.

130. Weinstein MC: Estrogen use in postmenopausal women—costs, risks and benefits. *N Engl J Med* 1980;303:308–316.

131. Mechanic D: The growth of medical technology and bureaucracy: Implications for medical care. *Milbank Mem Fund Q* 1977;55:61–78.

132. Mechanic D: *Medical Sociology*, ed 2. New York, Free Press, 1978.

133. Aday LA, Anderson R: *Development of Indices of Access to Medical Care*. Ann Arbor, Mich, Health Administration Press, 1975.

134. Childress JF: Rationing of medical treatment, in Reich WT (ed): *Encyclopedia of Biomedical Ethics*. New York, Oxford University Press, 1979, pp 1414–1419.

135. Blumstein JF: *Constitutional and Legal Constraints on the Rationing of Medical Resources*. Prepared for the President's Commission for the Study of Ethical Problems in Medicine and Biomedical and Behavioral Research, Nashville, Tenn, October 1981.

136. David CK: Hearings of the U.S. House of Representatives Committee on Governmental Operations, Subcommittee on Intergovernmental Relations and Human Resources. *Contemp Dial* 1982;3(April):23–30.

137. Kusserow RP: Hearings of the US House of Representatives' Committee on Governmental Operations, Subcommittee on Intergovernmental Relations and Human Resources. *Contemp Dial* 1982;59:12–18.

138. Iglehart JK: Health policy report: Funding the End-Stage Renal Disease Program. *N Engl J Med* 1982;306:492–496.

139. Relman AS: The new medical-industrial complex. *N Engl J Med* 1980;303:963–970.

140. Rettig RA: The politics of health cost containment: End-Stage renal disease. *Bull NY Acad Med* 1980;56:115–138.

141. Rettig RA: *Implementing the End-Stage Renal Disease Program of Medicare*, Rand publication 2505-HCFA/HEW. Santa Monica, Calif, Rand Corporation, 1980.

142. Kolata GB: NMC thrives selling dialysis. *Science* 1980;208:380–382.

143. Kolata GB: Dialysis after nearly a decade. *Science* 1980;208:473–476.

144. Lowrie EG, Hampers CL: The success of Medicare's End-Stage Renal Disease Program: The case for profits and the private marketplace. *N Engl J Med* 1981;305:434–438.

145. Lowrie EG, Hampers CL: Proprietary dialysis and the End-Stage Renal Disease Program. *Dial Transplant* 1982;11:191–204.

146. Hampers CL, Hager EB: The delivery of dialysis services on a nationwide basis—can we afford the nonprofit system? *Dial Transplant* 1979;8:417–423, 442.

147. Blagg CR: Cui bono?: A response to Drs. Hampers and Hager. *Dial Transplant* 1979;8:501–502, 513.

148. Bart KJ, Macon EJ, Humphries AL: A response to the shortage of cadaveric kidneys for transplantation. *Transplant Proc* 1979;11:455–457.

149. Bart KJ, Macon EJ, Humphries AL Jr, et al: Increasing the supply of cadaveric kidneys for transplantation. *Transplantation* 1981;31:383–387.

150. Bart KJ, Macon EJ, Whittier FC, et al: Cadaveric kidneys for transplantation. *Transplantation* 1981;31:379–382.

151. Steinbrook RL: Kidneys for transplantation. *J Health Polit Policy Law* 1981;6:504–573.

152. Simmons RG, Schilling KJ: Social and psychological rehabilitation of the diabetic transplant patient. *Kidney Int Suppl* 1974;6:S152–S158.

153. Simmons RG, Klein SD, Simmons RL: *The Gift of Life: The Social and Psychological Impact of Organ Transplantation*. New York, John Wiley & Sons Inc, 1977.

154. Poznanski EO, Miller E, Salguero C, et al: Quality of life for long-term survivors of end-state renal disease. *JAMA* 1978;239:2343–2347.

155. Guttmann RD: Rental transplantation: II. *N Engl J Med* 1979;301:1038–1048.

156. Fox RC, Swazey JP: *The Courage to Fail*. Chicago, University of Chicago Press, 1974.

157. Abram HS: Dilemmas of medical progress. *Psychiatr Med* 1972;3:51–58.

158. Katz AH, Proctor DM: *Social-Psychological Characteristics of Patients Receiving Hemo-dialysis Treatment for Chronic Renal Failure: Report of a Questionnaire Study of Dialysis Centers During 1967*. The Kidney Disease Program, Division of Chronic Disease Programs, Regional Medical Programs Service, Health Services and Mental Health Administration, Public Health Service, Dept of Health, Education, and Welfare, 1969.

159. Newman HN: Health Care Financing Administration, Medicare Program: Solicitation of hospitals and medical centers to participate in a study of heart transplants. *Federal Register* 1981;46:7072–7075.

160. Pennock JL, Oyer PE, Reitz BA, et al: Cardiac transplantation in perspective for the future: Survival, complications, rehabilitation, and cost. *J Thorac Cardiovasc Surg* 1982;83:168–177.

161. Copeland JG, Salomon NW, Mammana RB, et al: Cardiac transplantation, a two-year experience. *Health Transplant* 1981;1:67–71.

162. Oyer PE, Stinson EB, Reitz BA, et al: Cardiac transplantation: 1980. *Transplant Proc* 1981;13:199–206.

163. Office of Technology Assessment: *The Implications of Cost-Effectiveness: Analysis of Medical Technology*. Government Printing Office, 1980.

164. Bunker JP, Mosteller CF, Barnes BA: *Costs, Risks and Benefits of Surgery*. New York, Oxford University Press, 1977.

165. Fuchs VR: What is CBA/CEA and why are they doing this to us? *N Engl J Med* 1980;303:937–938.

166. Lashof JC, Behney C, Banta D, et al: The role of cost-benefit and cost-effectiveness analyses in controlling health care costs, in McNeil BJ, Cravalho EG (eds): *Critical Issues in Medical Technology*. Boston, Auburn House, 1982, pp 185–189.

167. Warner KE, Luce BR: *Cost-Benefit and Cost-Effectiveness Analysis in Health Care: Principles, Practice, and Potential*. Ann Arbor, Mich, Health Administration Press, 1982.

168. Fineberg HV, Pearlman LA: *The Implications of Cost-Effectiveness Analysis of Medical Technology: Case Study #11: Benefit-and-Cost Analysis of Medical Interventions: The Case of Cimetidine and Peptic Ulcer Disease*, stock OTA-BP-H-9(11). Office of Technology Assessment, 1981.

169. Klarman HE: Application of cost-benefit analysis to the health services and the special case of technologic innovation. *Int J Health Serv* 1974;4:325–352.

170. Evans RW, Garrison LP, Manninen D: The National Kidney Dialysis and Kidney Transplantation Study; Study description, statement of objectives, and project significance. *Contemp Dial* 1982;3(June):55–58.

171. Gruntzig AR, Senning A, Siegenthaler WE: Nonoperative dilation of coronary-artery stenosis: Percutaneous transluminal coronary angioplasty. *N Engl J Med* 1979;301:61–68.

172. Levy RI, Jesse MS, Mock MB: Position on percutaneous transluminal coronary angioplasty (PTCA). *Circulation* 1979;59:613.

173. Buck RW: Prolonging life in the aged. *N Engl J Med* 1981;305:963.

174. Mazzarella V: An open letter to my mother's nephrologist. *N Engl J Med* 1981;305:175.

175. Parsons V, Lock P: Triage and the patient with renal failure. *J Med Ethics* 1980;6:173–176.

176. Basson MD: Choosing among candidates for scarce medical resources. *J Med Philos* 1979;4:313–333.

177. Childress J: Who shall live when not all can live? *Soundings* 1970;43:339–362.

178. Caplan AL: Kidneys, ethics, and politics: Policy lessons of the ESRD experience. *J Health Polit Policy Law* 1981;6:488–503.

179. Arrow KJ: Uncertainty and the welfare economics of medical care. *Am Econ Rev* 1963;53:941–973.

180. Mechanic D: The right to treatment: Judicial action and social change, in Mechanic D (ed): *Politics, Medicine, and Social Science*. New York, Wiley Interscience, 1974, pp 227–248.

181. Krause EA: *Power and Illness: The Political Sociology of Health and Medical Care*. New York, Elsevier North-Holland Inc, 1977.

182. Strickland SP: *U.S. Health Care: What's Wrong and What's Right*. New York, Universe Books, 1972.

183. Klarman HE: *The Economics of Health*. New York, Columbia University Press, 1965.

184. Fried C: Equality and rights in medical care. *Hastings Cent Rep* 1976;6:29–34.

185. Sidel V: The right to health care: An international perspective, in Bandman EL, Bandman B (eds): *Bioethics and Human Rights*. Boston, Little Brown & Co, 1978, pp 341–349.

186. Bell NK: The scarcity of medical resources: Are there rights to health care? *J Med Philos* 1979;4:158–169.

187. Knowles JH: Responsibility for health. *Science* 1977;198:1103.

188. Allegrante JP, Green LW: When health policy becomes victim blaming. *N Engl J Med* 1981;305:528–529.

189. McCarthy DG, Moraczewski AS (eds): *Moral Responsibility in Prolonging Life Decisions*. St. Louis, Pope John XIII Medical-Moral Research and Education Center, 1981.

190. Winslow GR: *Triage and Justice*. Berkeley, Calif, University of California Press, 1982.

191. Brent L: Deciding who gets what. *Lancet* 1983;1:57.

192. Bell NK (ed): *Who Decides? Conflicts of Rights in Health Care*. Clifton, NJ, Humana Press, 1982.

193. Childress JF: *Who Should Decide? Paternalism in Health Care*. New York, Oxford University Press, 1982.

194. Harron F, Burnside J, Beauchamp T: *Health and Human Values: Making Your Own Decisions*. New Haven, Conn, Yale University Press, 1982.

195. Freidson E: *Profession of Medicine: A Study of the Sociology of Applied Knowledge*. New York, Harper & Row Publishers, Inc, 1970.

196. Feinstein AR: *Clinical Judgment*. Baltimore, Williams & Wilkins Co, 1967.

197. Lo B, Jonsen AR: Clinical decisions to limit treatment. *Ann Intern Med* 1980;93:764–768.

198. Wong CB, Swazey JP: *Dilemmas of Dying: Policies and Procedures for Decisions Not to Treat*. Boston, GK Hall Medical Publishers, 1981.

199. Relman AS: The Saikewicz decision: Judges as physicians. *N Engl J Med* 1978;298:508–509.

200. Barron CH: Medical paternalism and the rule of law. *Am J Law Med* 1979;4:337–365.

201. McNeil BJ, Weichselbaum R, Pauker SG: Speech and survival: Tradeoff between quality and quantity of life in laryngeal cancer. *N Engl J Med* 1981;305:982–987.

202. McNeil BJ, Pauker SG: Incorporation of patient values in medical decision making, in McNeil BJ, Cravalho EG (eds): *Critical Issues in Medical Technology*. Boston, Auburn House, 1982, pp 113–126.

203. McNeil BJ, Pauker SG, Sox HC Jr, et al: On the elicitation of preferences for alternative therapies. *N Engl J Med* 1982;306:1259–1262.

204. Raiffa H: *Decision Analysis: Introductory Lectures on Choices Under Uncertainty.* Reading, Mass, Addison-Wesley Publishing Co Inc, 1968.

205. Keeney RL, Raiffa H: *Decision Making with Multiple Objectives: Preferences and Value Tradeoffs.* New York, John Wiley & Sons Inc, 1976.

206. Brett AS: Hidden ethical issues in clinical decision analysis. *N Engl J Med* 1981;305:1150–1152.

207. Pauker SG, Kassirer JP: The threshold approach to clinical decision making. *N Engl J Med* 1980;302:1109–1117.

208. Schwartz WB: Decision analysis: A look at the chief complaints. *N Engl J Med* 1979;300:556–559.

209. Ransoff DF, Feinstein AR: Is decision analysis useful in clinical medicine? *Yale J Biol Med* 1976;49:165–168.

210. Reich WT: Life: Quality of life, in Reicht WT (ed): *Encyclopedia of Biomedical Ethics.* New York, Oxford University Press, 1979, pp 829–840.

211. Eisenberg JM: Sociologic influences on decision-making by clinicians. *Ann Intern Med* 1979;90:957–964.

212. Gutman RA, Stead WW, Robinson RR: Physical activity and employment status of patients on maintenance dialysis. *N Engl J Med* 1981;304:309–313.

213. Randal J: Coronary artery bypass surgery. *Hastings Cent Rep* 1982;12:13–18.

214. Drunkman WB, Perloff JK, Kaston JA, et al: Medical perspectives in coronary artery surgery: A caveat. *Ann Intern Med* 1974;81:817–837.

215. Stoney WS, Alford WC, Burrus GR, et al: The cost of coronary bypass procedures. *JAMA* 1978;240:2278–2280.

216. Love JW: Employment status after coronary bypass operations and some cost considerations. *J Thorac Cardiovasc Surg* 1980;80:68–72.

217. Mundth ED, Austen WG: Surgical measures for coronary heart disease, part 1. *N Engl J Med* 1975;293:13–19.

218. Coronary artery bypass surgery, editorial. *Lancet* 1976;1:841–842.

219. Kolata GB: Coronary bypass surgery: Debate over its benefits. *Science* 1976;194:1263–1265.

220. Brauwald E: Coronary-artery surgery at the crossroads. *N Engl J Med* 1977;297:661–663.

221. Sanz G, Castaner A, Betriu A, et al: Determinants of prognosis in survivors of myocardial infarction. *N Engl J Med* 1982;306:1065–1070.

222. Hammermeister KE, DeRouen TA, English MT, et al: Effect of surgical versus medical therapy on return to work in patients with coronary artery disease. *Am J Cardiol* 1979;44:105–111.

223. Rimm AA, Barboriak JJ, Anderson AJ, et al: Changes in occupation after aortocoronary vein-bypass operation. *JAMA* 1976;236:361–364.

224. Wallwork J, Potter B, Caves PK: Return to work after coronary artery surgery for angina. *Br Med J* 1978;2:1680–1681.

225. Frick MH, Harjola PT, Valle M: Work status after coronary bypass surgery. *Acta Med Scand* 1979;206:61–64.

226. Barnes GK, Ray MJ, Oberman A, et al: Changes in working status of patients following coronary bypass surgery. *JAMA* 1977;238:1259–1262.

227. Blumlein SL, Anderson AJ, Barboriak JJ, et al: Changes in occupation after coronary arteriography. *Scand J Rehabil Med* 1977;9:79–83.

228. Burdetti P, McManus P, Barrand N, et al: *Neonatal Intensive Care.* Government Printing Office, 1982.

229. Hiatt HH: Sounding board: The physician and national security. *N Engl J Med* 1982;307:1142–1145.

230. Office of the President: *The Budget of the United States Government: Fiscal Year, 1983,* House document 97-124. Government Printing Office, 1982.

231. Tancredi LR, Barsky AJ: Technology and health care decision making—conceptualizing the process for societal informed consent. *Med Care* 1974;12:845–858.

232. Choron J: *Death and Modern Man.* New York, Collier Bros, 1964.

233. Feifel H (ed): *Death in Contemporary America: New Meanings of Death.* New York, McGraw-Hill Book Co, 1977.

234. Becker E: *The Denial of Death.* New York, Free Press, 1973.

235. Maguire DC: *Death by Choice.* New York, Schocken Books Inc, 1973.

236. Manning B: Legal and policy issues in the allocation of death, in Brim OG Jr, Freeman HE, Levine S, et al (eds): *The Dying Patient.* New York, Russell Sage Foundation, 1970, pp 253–274.

237. Veatch RM: *Death, Dying, and the Biological Revolution.* New Haven, Conn, Yale University Press, 1976.

238. Campbell A, Converse PE, Rodgers WL: *The Quality of American Life.* New York, Russell Sage Foundation, 1976.

239. Donald CA, Ware JE Jr, Brook RH, et al: *Conceptualization and Measurement of Health for Adults in the Health Insurance Survey: Social Health,* publication R-1987/4-HEW. Santa Monica, Calif, Rand Corporation, 1978, vol 4.

240. Renne KS: Measurement of social health in a general population survey. *Social Sci Res* 1974;3:25–44.

241. Russell RD: Social health: An attempt to clarify this dimension of well-being. *Int J Health Educ* 1973;74:74–82.

242. Constitution of the World Health Organization, in *The First Ten Years of the World Health Organization*. Geneva, Palais des Nations, World Health Organization, 1958.

243. Sackett DL, Torrance GW: The utility of different health states as perceived by the general public. *J Chronic Dis* 1978;31:697–704.

244. Dorfman NS: The social value of saving a life, in Mushkin SJ, Dunlop D (eds): *Health: What Is it Worth? Measures of Health Benefits*. New York, Pergamon Press, 1979, pp 61–68.

245. Lipscomb J: The willingness-to-pay criterion and public program evaluation in health, in Mushkin SJ, Dunlop D (eds): *Health: What Is it Worth? Measures of Health Benefits*. New York, Pergamon Press, 1979, pp 91–139.

246. Clarke EH: Social valuation of life- and health-saving activities by the demand-revealing process, in Mushkin SJ, Dunlop D (eds): *Health: What Is it Worth? Measures of Health Benefits*. New York, Pergamon Press, 1979, pp 69–90.

247. Fischer GW: Willingness to pay for probabilistic improvements in functional health status: A psychological perspective, in Mushkin SJ, Dunlop D (eds): *Health: What Is it Worth? Measures of Health Benefits*. New York, Pergamon Press, 1979, pp 167–202.

248. Ware JE Jr, Young J: Issues in the conceptualization and measurement of value placed on health, in Mushkin SJ, Dunlop D (eds): *Health: What Is it Worth? Measures of Health Benefits*. New York, Pergamon Press, 1979, pp 141–166.

249. Mooney G: *The Valuation of Human Life*. London, Macmillan Publishers Ltd, 1977.

250. Culyer AJ: *The Political Economy of Social Policy*. Oxford, England, Martin Robertson & Co Ltd, 1980.

251. Culyer AJ: Assessing cost-effectiveness, in Banta HD (ed): *Resources for Health: Technology Assessment for Policy Making*. New York, Praeger Publishers, 1982.

252. Beecher HJ: A definition of irreversible coma: Report of the Ad Hoc Committee of the Harvard Medical School to Examine the Definition of Brain Death. *JAMA* 1968;205:337–340.

253. Mohandas A, Chou SN: Brain death: A clinical and pathological study. *J Neurosurg* 1971;35:211–218.

254. President's Commission for the Study of Ethical Problems in Medicine and Biomedical and Behavioral Research: *Defining Death: Medical, Legal, and Ethical Issues in the Determination of Death*. Government Printing Office, 1981.

255. President's Commission for the Study of Ethical Problems in Medicine and Biomedical and Behavioral Research: Guidelines for the determination of death. *JAMA* 1981;246:2184–2186.

256. Bernat JL, Culver CM, Gert B: On the definition and criterion of death. *Ann Intern Med* 1981;94:389–394.

257. Bernat JL, Culver CM, Gert B: Defining death in theory and practice. *Hastings Cent Rep* 1982;12:5–9.

258. Stahlman MT, Cotton RB: Defining death: Which way? A reply. *Hastings Cent Rep* 1982;12:44.

259. Capron AM, Lyn J: Defining death: Which way? *Hastings Cent Rep* 1982;12:43–44.

260. Parisi JE, Kim RC, Collins GH, et al: Brain death with prolonged somatic survival. *N Engl J Med* 1982;306:14–16.

261. Nagle CE: Brain death with prolonged somatic survival. *N Engl J Med* 1982;306:1361.

262. Saunders C: Hospice care. *Am J Med* 1978;65:726–728.

263. Saunders C (ed): *The Management of Terminal Disease*. London, Edward Arnold (Publishers) Ltd, 1978.

264. Smith DH, Granbois JA: the American way of hospice. *Hastings Cent Rep* 1982;12:8–10.

265. Benedict R: *Patterns of Culture*. Boston, Houghton Mifflin Co, 1934.

266. McNeil BJ, Cravalho EG (eds): *Critical Issues in Medical Technology*. Boston, Auburn House, 1982.

267. Report of a Working Party of the Council for Science and Society: *Expensive Medical Techniques*, London, Council for Science and Society, 1982.

268. Expensive medical techniques, editorial. *Lancet* 1983;1:279–280.

269. Omenn GS, Ball JR: The role of health technology evaluation: A policy perspective, in Goldman J (ed): *Health Care Technology Evaluation Proceedings, Columbia, Missouri, 1978*. New York, Springer-Verlag, 1978, pp 5–32.

270. Sun M: Fishing for a forum on health policy. *Science* 1983;219:37–38.

271. Perry S: Technology assessment proposed. *Health Affairs* 1982;1:123–128.

272. Perry S: Special report: The brief life of the National Center for Health Care Technology. *N Engl J Med* 1982;307:1095–1100.

273. Banta HD (ed): *Resources for Health: Technology Assessment for Policy Making*. New York, Praeger Publishers, 1982.

274. Evans RW, Anderson A, Perry B: The National Heart Transplantation Study: An overview. *Heart Transplant* 1982;2:85–87.

275. Relman AS: The new medical-industrial complex. *N Engl J Med* 1980;303:963–970.

276. Blumenthal D, Feldman P, Zeckhauser R: Misuse of technology: A symptom, not the disease, in McNeil BJ, Cravalho EG (eds): *Critical Issues in Medical Technology.* Boston, Auburn House, 1982, pp 163–174.

277. Relman AS: An institute for health-care evaluation. *N Engl J Med* 1982;306:669–670.

278. Schaeffer LD: Role of the HCFA in the regulation of new medical technologies, in McNeil BJ, Cravalho EG (eds): *Critical Issues in Medical Technology.* Boston, Auburn House, 1982, pp 151–161.

279. Office of Technology Assessment: *Medical Technology Proposals to Increase Competition in Health Care.* Government Printing Office, 1982.

280. Le Maitre GD: Medical cost inflation. *N Engl J Med* 1982;307:1649.

281. Jellinek PS: Yet another look at medical cost inflation. *N Engl J Med* 1982;307:496–497.

282. Jellinek PS: Medical cost inflation. *N Engl J Med* 1982;307:1649–1650.

283. Lee B: Medical cost inflation. *N Engl J Med* 1982;307:1649.

284. Weinberger CW: Shattuck lecture—remarks by the Secretary of Defense to the Massachusetts Medical Society, May 1982. *N Engl J Med* 1982;307:765–768.

285. Relman AS: Physicians, nuclear war, and politics. *N Engl J Med* 1982;307:744–745.

286. Caldicott HM, Walker PF: Preventing nuclear war: The secretary of defense replies to his critics. *N Engl J Med* 1983;308:338–339.

287. Rawls JA: *Theory of Justice.* Cambridge, Mass, Harvard University Press, 1971.

288. Soltan KE: Empirical studies of distributive justice. *Ethics* 1982;92:673–691.

289. Branson R: Theories of justice and health care, in Reich WT (ed): *Encyclopedia of Bioethics.* New York, Free Press, 1978, pp 630–637.

290. Daniels N: Health care needs and distributive justice. *Philos Public Affairs* 1981;10:146–179.

291. Feinberg J: Justice, in Reich WT (ed): *Encyclopedia of Bioethics.* New York, Free Press, 1978, pp 802–810.

292. Daniels N (ed): *Reading Rawls: Critical Studies on Rawl's 'A Theory of Justice.'* New York, Basic Books Inc Publishers, 1975.

293. Piven FF, Cloward RA: *Regulating the Poor: The Functions of Public Welfare.* New York, Vintage Books, 1971.

294. Jonsen AR: Purposefulness in human life. *West J Med* 1976;125:5–7.

295. Englehardt HT Jr: Rights to health care: A critical approach. *J Med Philos* 1979;4:113–117.

296. Beauchamp TL, Faden RR: The right to health and the right to health care. *J Med Philos* 1979;4:118–131.

297. Childress JF: A right to health care? *J Med Philos* 1979;4:132–147.

298. Siegler M: A right to health care: Ambiguity, professional responsibility and patient liberty. *J Med Philos* 1979;4:148–157.

299. Veatch RM: Just social institutions and the right to health care. *J Med Philos* 1979;4:170–173.

300. Daniels N: Rights to health care and distributive justice: Programmatic worries. *J Med Philos* 1979;4:174–191.

301. Ruddick W: Doctor's rights and work. *J Med Philos* 1979;4:192–203.

302. McCullough LB: Rights, health care, and public policy. *J Med Philos* 1979;4:204–215.

303. Curran WJ: The Saikewicz decision. *N Engl J Med* 1978;298:499–500.

304. Relman AS: The Saikewicz decision: A medical viewpoint. *Am J Law Med* 1979;4:233–237.

305. Glantz LH, Swazey JP: Decisions not to treat: The Saikewicz case and its aftermath. *Forum Med* 1979;2:22–32.

306. Carroll C: The ethics of heart transplantation. *J Natl Med Assoc* 1970;62:14–20.

307. Jonsen AR, Siegler M, Winslade WJ: *Clinical Ethics: A Practical Approach to Ethical Decisions in Clinical Medicine.* New York, Macmillan Publishing Co Inc, 1982.

308. Culver CM, Gert B: *Philosophy in Medicine: Conceptual and Ethical Issues in Medicine and Psychiatry.* New York, Oxford University Press, 1982.

Rationing Health Care

Rudolf Klein, University of Bath, Bath, England

In Great Britain, almost all health care is provided through a universal-entitlement, government funded and operated system, the National Health Services (NHS). In 1984, a book on the NHS, The Painful Prescription: Rationing Hospital Care, *by Henry J. Aaron and William B. Schwartz, offered pointed evidence, based on extensive discussions with British physicians and others, that the NHS required physicians to ration hospital and other health care services to the point of allowing patients to die of treatable diseases. The book further suggested that some form of rationing of health care would be inevitable in the United States in the future. The following response by British policy analyst Rudolf Klein to these allegations explores the forces that drive a health care system—need versus demand, the prevailing medical culture, and societal values—and says as much about resource allocation in American health care as it does about the NHS.*

The National Health Service offers a paradox. Seen from within, it is a system which frustrates the aspirations of providers—doctors, nurses, and others—to provide the best possible service and a system where public parsimony compels health care professionals to compromise their own standards. Yet, seen from without, in the context of the health care systems of other advanced Western societies, the NSH is without challenge the best buy model in at least one crucial respect: it provides a comprehensive system of health care at the lowest cost as measured by the proportion of the national income devoted to it.

Not surprisingly, therefore, the NHS is the subject of a major American study by Professors Henry J. Aaron (an economist) and William B. Schwartz (a physician).[1] Given American concern about their health care cost explosion, and given that the obvious policy recipe would be to move towards fixed budgets in place of the present open ended, fee for service system of financing health care in the United States, Britain offers the obvious laboratory for exploring the implications of such a change. Specifically, Aaron and Schwartz address themselves to the question of just how Britain's NHS rations scarce hospital resources. In doing so, they hold up a mirror to the NHS that is of as much interest to British as to American readers—although in some important respects it turns out to be a distorting mirror.

The methodology chosen by Aaron and Schwartz is to compare the performance of the British and American health care systems, using the latter's level of treatment and activity as the benchmark. Thus the starting assumption, only slightly modified in the course of the detailed discussion of the specific procedures and diagnostic processes chosen for investigation, is that the United States provides the optimal level. The conclusion reached is that, while on the whole Britain compares well with the United States in

Reprinted, with permission, from the author and the *British Medical Journal* 1984 July 21. 289(6438):143–144.

dealing with life threatening conditions—particularly when these are, like cancer, "dread diseases" with a high degree of social visibility—the NHS does relatively badly when it comes to procedures designed to improve the quality of life or to investing in equipment designed to improve diagnostic reliability.

In the first category the study notes that bone marrow transplantation is carried out with the same frequency in Britain as in the United States, that all patients with haemophilia obtain high quality treatment, and that megavoltage radiotherapy appears to be readily available to virtually all patients who need it, but that the overall rate of treatment of chronic renal failure—that is, transplantation and dialysis—is less than half that in the United States. In the second category—procedures designed to improve the quality of life—the rate of coronary artery surgery in Britain is only 10% that of the United States, while the rate for hip replacement surgery is between three quarters to four fifths that of the United States. In the third category—investment in diagnostic reliability—Britain has only one sixth of the computed tomography capacity of the United States, and the average British citizen is about half as likely to have x ray examinations as the average American and when he is examined about half as much film is likely to be used. In total, the authors estimate, Britain's expenditure on NHS hospitals would have to go up by almost one fifth if the level of activity and treatment were to approach that of the United States (though it is important to emphasise that over half of this increase is accounted for by a single factor: the much lower level of provision of intensive care beds in this country).

These findings are both predictable and ambiguous. They are predictable in the sense that a service such as the NHS, organised around the philosophy of responding to professionally defined need rather than to consumer demand, is bound to attach higher priority to dealing with life threatening conditions than to those which diminish the quality of life. The study's conclusions might have been stronger still if, for example, it had examined elective surgery. But the findings are ambiguous in so far as they beg the crucial question of how to assess the appropriateness of any given level of activity. The point emerges clearly from the authors' discussion of the use of chemotherapy for cancer in the two countries. Britain spends about 70% less than the United States, per head, on chemotherapeutic agents. The reason for this, the study shows, is that, while British oncologists treat curable cancers just as readily as their American counterparts, they see no reason to treat incurable metastatic cancer by inflicting on patients a "treatment which brings them nothing but unpleasant side effects and is of no benefit," in the words of one British oncologist quoted in the book.

Indeed, perhaps the most useful contribution made by Aaron and Schwartz is to show that differences in the medical cultures of Britain and America are at least as important as differences in the availability of resources. The two are, to an extent, linked. A humane, clinical conservatism in Britain both sustains and is, in turn, reinforced by constraints in resources. A heroic, aggressive style of medicine in the United States helps to explain—and, in turn, to compound—the high rate of spending. Each culture rests on wider differences in the two societies. Britain is an original sin society in which illness and debility are seen as part of the natural order of things and patients tend to be deferential. America is a perfectability of man society in which illness and debility are seen as challenges to action and patients tend to be demanding consumers. Each culture, furthermore, tends to carry its own dangers for the clinicians concerned. In Britain it is—as Aaron and Schwartz argue persuasively in the case of renal dialysis—that doctors will seek to rationalise resource constraints (and make tragic choices more tolerable for themselves) by classifying patients as unsuitable for treatment. In the United States it is that, as Aaron and Schwartz recognise but do not emphasise sufficiently, doctors will seek to rationalise their own desire to maximise their incomes by maximising treatment, and that activity will become an end in itself irrespective of the ultimate outcome for the patient.

The most convincing conclusion drawn by the study for its American audience is, therefore, that the British model is not for export to the United States. But it is important to be clear just why this conclusion is convincing. Its persuasiveness derives from the fact that the dynamics of American society, and its medical system, are incompatible with the organising principle of the NHS, which is—to return to an earlier point—that health care should be rationed according to medically defined needs, not distributed in response to consumer demands. It does not derive from the book's demonstration that the levels of activity are in some respects much lower in Britain than in the United States. This, in itself, tells us little about the overall effectiveness of the two health care systems and risks prompting misleading conclusions (particularly in the United States) about the achievements and weaknesses of the NHS.

Firstly, health care activity should not be confused with health care outcomes. Aaron and Schwartz can hardly be blamed for being unable to measure the effects of the different levels of activity in the two countries on health care outcomes, in terms of either quantity or quality of life. This is a notorious conceptual minefield, where it is difficult to disentagle the effects of medical intervention from the environmental socioeconomic factors. They might usefully, however, have emphasised this problem more in order to avoid possible misinterpretations of their evidence. Certainly, taking such crude, and hard to interpret, indicators as life expectancy and perinatal mortality, Britain does better than the United States.[2]

Secondly, it is a mistake to concentrate exclusively on a number of procuedures—though justifiable as an attempt to explore the problems of rationing scarce resources—for this risks giving a distorted picture of the health care system as a whole. Rationing not only concerns decisions about what resources to devote to individual patients; it also entails decisions about how to ration resources between different groups of patients. The NHS forces explicit choices about the relative priority to be given to the acutely ill, the mentally ill, the old, and the young. Unfortunately, Aaron and Schwartz ignore this dimension, with the result that they present what is at best an incomplete balance sheet.

Finally, rationing is inevitable under any health care system.[3] Aaron and Schwartz rightly warn their American readers that the United States faces the "painful prescription" of rationing if it wishes to put a ceiling on total health care expenditure. But they fail to point out that the United States already rations health care somewhat brutally, although in passing they note that "several million Americans lack adequate insurance or personal means and therefore face obstacles to obtaining hospital care." The issue, in other words, is not whether to ration but how to ration; how best to devise a system which allocates what will always be inadequate resources—in the sense of falling short of permitting the medical providers to do everything technically feasible for all their patients— in the fairest and socially most acceptable way. And on this criterion the NHS, whatever its other failings, must surely be rated a success story.

But it would be wrong to end on a note of complacent self congratulation. This study does raise a major issue for the NHS. As Aaron and Schwartz point out, the dilemmas of rationing are likely to become ever sharper as new techniques and procedures become available. In turn, this may call into question the consensus on which Britain's system of rationing rests. At present this is a system for transmuting collective political decisions about how much money to spend on the NHS into individual clinical decisions about how much care to give to specific patients, thereby transforming tragic choices about who should live and die into technical assessments of the effectiveness of particular courses of action.[4] In return for accepting this responsibility the medical profession enjoys virtually total autonomy in making clinical decisions, certainly greater autonomy than American clinicians. But if the financial constraints within which British clinicians work start biting still more they may come to ask whether the price of freedom—in terms of accepting responsibility for making tragic choices— is not becoming excessive.

References

1. Aaron H. J., and Schwartz, W. B., *The Painful Prescription: Rationing Hospital Care*. Washington, D.C.: The Brookings Institutions, 1984.

2. Maxwell, R. J. *Health and Wealth*. Lexington, MA: Lexington Books, 1981.

3. Fuchs, V. R. *Who Shall Live?* New York: Basic Books, 1974.

4. Calabresi G., Bobbitt, P. *Tragic Choices*. New York: Norton and Co., 1974.

Shattuck Lecture—Allocating Scarce Medical Resources and the Availability of Organ Transplantation: Some Moral Presuppositions

H. Tristram Engelhardt, Jr., Ph.D., M.D., Center for Ethics, Medicine, and Public Issues, Baylor College of Medicine, Houston

The Problem

Some controversies have a staying power because they spring from unavoidable moral and conceptual puzzles. The debates concerning transplantation are a good example. To begin with, they are not a single controversy. Rather, they are examples of the scientific debates with heavy political and ethical overlays that characterize a large area of public-policy discussions.[1] The determination of whether or not heart or liver transplantation is an experimental or nonexperimental procedure for which it is reasonable and necessary to provide reimbursement is not simply a determination on the basis of facts regarding survival rates or the frequency with which the procedure is employed. Nor is it a purely moral issue.[2]

It is an issue similar to that raised regarding the amount of pollutants that ought to be considered safe in the work place. The question cannot be answered simply in terms of scientific data, unless one presumes that there will be a sudden inflection in the curve expressing the relation-ship of decreasing parts per billion of the pollutant and the incidence of disease or death, after which very low concentrations do not contribute at all to an excess incidence of disability or death. If one assumes that there is always some increase in death and disability due to the pollutant, one is not looking for an absolutely safe level but rather a level at which the costs in lives and health do not outbalance the costs in jobs and societal vexation that most more stringent criteria would involve. Such is not a purely factual judgment but requires a balancing of values. Determinations of whether a pol¹ .tant is safe at a particular level, of whether a procedure is reasonable and necessary, of whether a drug is safe, of whether heart and liver transplantations should be regarded as nonexperimental procedures are not simply factual determinations. In the background of those determinations is a set of moral judgments regarding equity, decency, and fairness, cost-benefit trade-offs, individual rights, and the limits of state authority.

Since such debates are structured by the intertwining of scientific, ethical, and political is-

Reprinted, with permission, from *The New England Journal of Medicine* 1984 July 5. 311(1):66–71.
Presented at the annual meeting of the Massachusetts Medical Society, May 12, 1984.

sues, participants appeal to different sets of data and rules of inference, which leads to a number of opportunities for confusion. The questions that cluster around the issue of providing for the transplantation of organs have this distracting heterogeneity. There are a number of questions with heavy factual components, such as, "Is the provision of liver transplants an efficient use of health-care resources?" and "Will the cost of care in the absence of a transplant approximate the costs involved in the transplant?" To answer such questions, one will need to continue to acquire data concerning the long-term survival rates of those receiving transplants.[3-8] There are, as well, questions with major moral and political components, which give public-policy direction to the factual issues. "Does liver or heart transplantation offer a proper way of using our resources, given other available areas of investment?" "Is there moral authority to use state force to redistribute financial resources so as to provide transplantations for all who would benefit from the procedure?" "How ought one fairly to resolve controversies in this area when there is important moral disagreement?"

These serious questions have been engaged in a context marked by passion, pathos, and publicity. George Deukmejian, governor of California, ordered the state to pay for liver transplantation for Koren Crosland, and over $265,000 was raised through contributions from friends and strangers to support the liver transplantation of Amy Hardin of Cahokia, Illinois.[9] Charles and Marilyn Fiske's testimony to the Subcommittee on Investigations and Oversight of the House Committee on Science and Technology provided an example of how fortuitous publicity can lead to treatment[10]—in this case, to their daughter Jamie's receiving payment through Blue Cross of Massachusetts by agreement on October 1, 1982,[11] along with contingency authorization for coverage for liver-transplantation expenses through the Commonwealth of Massachusetts on October 29, 1982.[12] The proclamation by President Reagan of a National Organ Donation Awareness Week, which ran from April 22 through 28, further underscored the public nature of the issues raised.[13] In short, several serious and difficult moral and political dilemmas have been confronted under the spotlight of media coverage and political pressures.[14-17] What is needed is an examination of the moral and conceptual assumptions that shape the debate, so that one can have a sense of where reasonable answers can be sought.

Why Debates about Allocating Resources Go On and On

The debates concerning the allocation of resources to the provision of expensive, life-saving treatment such as transplantation have recurred repeatedly over the past two decades and show no promise of abating.[18-21] To understand why that is the case, one must recall the nature of the social and moral context within which such debates are carried on. Peaceable, secular, pluralist societies are by definition ones that renounce the use of force to impose a particular ideology or view of the good life, though they include numerous communities with particular, often divergent, views of the ways in which men and women should live and use their resources. Such peaceable, secular societies require at a minimum a commitment to the resolution of disputes in ways that are not fundamentally based on force.[22] There will thus be greater clarity regarding how peaceably to discuss the allocation of resources for transplantation than there will be regarding the importance of the allocation of resources itself.[23] The latter requires a more concrete view of what is important to pursue through the use of our resources than can be decisively established in general secular terms. As a consequence, it is clearer that the public has a right to determine particular expenditures of common resources than that any particular use of resources, as for the provision of transplantation, should be embraced.

This is a recurring situation in large-scale, secular, pluralist states. The state as such provides a relatively neutral bureaucracy that transcends the particular ideological and religious commitments of the communities it embraces, so that its state-funded health-care service (or its postal service) should not be a Catholic, Jewish, or even Judeo-Christian service. This ideal of a neutral bureaucracy is obviously never reached. However, the aspiration to this goal defines peaceable, secular, pluralist societies and distinguishes them from the political vision that we inherited from Aristotle and which has guided us and misguided us over the past two millennia. Aristotle took as his ethical and political ideal the city-state with no more than 100,000 citizens, who could then know each other, know well whom they should elect, and create a public consensus.[24,25] It is ironic that Aristotle fashioned this image as he participated in the fashioning of the first large-scale Greek state.

We do not approach the problems of the proper allocations of scarce resources within the context of a city-state, with a relatively clear consensus of the ways in which scarce resources ought to be used. Since the Reformation and the Renaissance, the hope for a common consensus has dwindled, and with good cause. In addition, the Enlightenment failed to provide a fully satisfactory secular surrogate. It failed to offer clearly convincing moral arguments that would have established a particular view of the good life and of the ways in which resources ought to be invested. One is left only with a general commitment to peaceable negotiation as the cardinal moral canon of large-scale peaceable, secular, pluralist states.[26]

As a result, understandings about the proper use of scarce resources tend to occur on two levels in such societies. They occur within particular religious bodies, political and ideological communities, and interest groups, including insurance groups. They take place as well within the more procedurally oriented vehicles and structures that hold particular communities within a state. The more one addresses issues such as the allocation of scarce resources in the context of a general secular, pluralist society, the more one will be pressed to create an answer in some procedurally fair fashion, rather than hope to discover a proper pattern for the distribution of resources to meet medical needs. However, our past has left us with the haunting and misguided hope that the answer can be discovered.

There are difficulties as well that stem from a tension within morality itself: a conflict between respecting freedom and pursuing the good. Morality as an alternative to force as the basis for the resolution of disputes focuses on the mutual respect of persons. This element of morality, which is autonomy-directed, can be summarized in the maxim, Do not do unto others what they would not have done unto themselves. In the context of secular pluralist ethics, this element has priority, in that it can more clearly be specified and justified. As a result, it sets limits to the moral authority of others to act and thus conflicts with that dimension of morality that focuses on beneficence, on achieving the good for others. This second element of morality may be summarized in the maxim, Do to others their good. The difficulty is that the achievement of the good will require the cooperation of others who may claim a right to be respected in their nonparticipation. It will require as well deciding what goods are to be achieved and how they are to be ranked. One might think here of the conflict between investing communal resources in liver and heart transplantations and providing adequate general medical care to the indigent and near indigent. The more one respects freedom, the more difficult it will be for a society to pursue a common view of the good. Members will protest that societal programs restrict their freedom of choice, either through restricting access to programs or through taxing away their disposable income.

The problem of determining whether and to what extent resources should be invested in transplantation is thus considerable. The debate must be carried on in a context in which the moral guidelines are more procedural than supplied with content. Moreover, the debate will be characterized by conflicting views of what is proper to do, as well as by difficulties in showing that there is state authority to force the participation of unwilling citizens. Within these vexing constraints societies approach the problem of allocating scarce medical resources and in particular of determining the amount of resources to be diverted to transplantation. This can be seen as a choice among possible societal insurance mechanisms. As with the difficulty of determining a safe level of pollutants, the answer with respect to the correct level of insurance will be as much created as discovered.

Insurance against the Natural and Social Lotteries

Individuals are at a disadvantage or an advantage as a result of the outcomes of two major sets of forces that can be termed the natural and social lotteries.[27,28] By the natural lottery I mean those forces of nature that lead some persons to be healthy and others to be ill and disabled through no intention or design of their own or of others. Those who win the natural lottery do not need transplantations. They live long and healthy lives and die peacefully. By the social lottery I mean the various interventions, compacts, and activities of persons that, with luck, lead to making some rich and others poor. The natural lottery surely influences the social lottery. However, the natural lottery need not conclusively determine one's social and economic power, prestige, and advantage. Thus, those who lose at the natural lottery and who are in need of heart and liver transplantation may still have won at the social lottery by having either inherited or earned sufficient funds to pay for a transplantation. Or they may have such a social advantage because their case receives sufficient publicity so that others contribute to help shoulder the costs of care.

An interest in social insurance mechanisms directed against losses at the natural and social lotteries is usually understood as an element of beneficence-directed justice. The goal is to provide the amount of coverage that is due to all persons. The problem in such societal insurance programs is to determine what coverage is due. Insofar as societies provide all citizens with a minimal protection against losses at the natural and the social lotteries, they give a concrete understanding of what is due through public funds. At issue here is whether coverage must include transplantation for those who cannot pay.

However, there are moral as well as financial limits to a society's protection of its members against such losses. First and foremost, those limits derive from the duty to respect individual choices and to recognize the limits of plausible state authority in a secular, pluralist society. If claims by society to the ownership of the resources and services of persons have limits, then there will always be private property that individuals will have at their disposal to trade for the services of others, which will create a second tier of health care for the affluent. Which is to say, the more it appears reasonable that property is owned neither totally societally nor only privately, and insofar as one recognizes limits on society's right to constrain its members, two tiers of health-care services will by right exist: those provided as a part of the minimal social guarantee to all and those provided in addition through the funds of those with an advantage in the social lottery who are interested in investing those resources in health care.

In providing a particular set of protections against losses at the social and natural lotteries, societies draw one of the most important societal distinctions—namely, between outcomes that will be socially recognized as unfortunate and unfair and those that will not be socially recognized as unfair, no matter how unfortunate they may be. The Department of Health and Human Services, for instance, in not recognizing heart transplantation as a nonexperimental procedure, removed the provision of such treatment from the social insurance policy. The plight of persons without private funds for heart transplantation, should

they need heart transplantation, would be recognized as unfortunate but not unfair.[29-31] Similarly, proposals to recognize liver transplantation for children and adults as nonexperimental are proposals to alter the socially recognized boundary between losses at the natural and social lotteries that will be understood to be unfortunate and unfair and those that will simply be lamented as unfortunate but not seen as entitling the suffering person to a claim against societal resources.[32]

The need to draw this painful line between unfortunate and unfair outcomes exists in great measure because the concerns for beneficence do not exhaust ethics. Ethics is concerned as well with respecting the freedom of individuals. Rendering to each his or her due also involves allowing individuals the freedom to determine the use of their private energies and resources. In addition, since secular pluralist arguments for the authority of peaceable states most clearly establish those societies as means for individuals peaceably to negotiate the disposition of their communally owned resources, difficulties may arise in the allocation of scarce resources to health care in general and to transplantation in particular. Societies may decide to allocate the communal resources that would have been available for liver and heart transplantation to national defense or the building of art museums and the expansion of the national park system. The general moral requirement to respect individual choice and procedurally fair societal decisions will mean that there will be a general secular, moral right for individuals to dispose of private resources, and for societies to dispose of communal resources, in ways that will be wrong from a number of moral perspectives. As a result, the line between outcomes that will count as unfortunate and those that will count as unfair will often be at variance with the moral beliefs and aspirations of particular ideological and moral communities encompassed by any large-scale secular society.

Just as one must create a standard of safety for pollutants in the work place by negotiations between management and labor and through discussions in public forums one will also need to create a particular policy for social insurance to cover losses at the natural and social lotteries. This will mean that one will not be able to discover that any particular investment in providing health care for those who cannot pay is morally obligatory. One will not be able to show that societies such as that of the United Kingdom, which do not provide America's level of access to renal dialysis for end-stage renal disease, have made a moral mistake.[33,34] Moral criticism will succeed best in examining the openness of such decisions to public discussion and control.

It is difficulties such as these that led the President's Commission for the Study of Ethical Problems in Medicine and Biomedical and Behavioral Research to construe equity in health care neither as equality in health care nor as access to whatever would benefit patients or meet their needs. The goal of equality in health care runs aground on both conceptual and moral difficulties. There is the difficulty of understanding whether equality would embrace equal amounts of health care or equal amounts of funds for health care. Since individual health needs differ widely, such interpretations of equality are fruitless. Attempting to understand equality as providing health care only from a predetermined list of services to which all would have access conflicts with the personal liberty to use private resources in the acquisition of additional care not on the list. Construing equity as providing all with any health care that would benefit them would threaten inordinately to divert resources to health care. It would conflict as well with choices to invest resources in alternative areas. Substituting "need" for "benefit" leads to similar difficulties unless one can discover, among other things, a notion of need that would not include the need to have one's life extended, albeit at considerable cost.

The commission, as a result, construed equity in health care as the provision of an "adequate level of health care." The commission defined adequate care as "enough care to achieve sufficient welfare, opportunity, information, and evidence of interpersonal concern to facilitate a reasonably full and satisfying life."[35] However, this definition runs aground on the case of children needing liver transplants and other such expensive health-care interventions required to secure any chance of achieving "a reasonably full and satisfying life." There is a tension in the commission's report between an acknowledgment that a great proportion of one's meaning of "adequate health care" must be created and a view that the lineaments of that meaning can be discovered. Thus, the commission states that "[i]n a democracy, the appropriate values to be assigned to the consequences of policies must ultimately be determined by people expressing their values through social and political processes as well as in the marketplace."[36] On the other hand, the commission states that "adequacy does require that everyone receive care that meets standards of sound medical practice."[37] The latter statement may suggest that one could discover what would constitute sound medical practice. In addition, an appeal to a notion of "excessive burdens" will not straightforwardly determine the amount of care due to individuals, since a notion of "excessiveness" requires choosing a particular hierarchy of costs and benefits.[38] Neither will an appeal to excessive burdens determine the amount of the tax burden that others should bear,[39] since there will be morally determined upper limits to taxation set by that element of property that is not communal. People, insofar as they have private property in that sense, have the secular moral right, no matter how unfeeling and uncharitable such actions may appear to others, not to aid those with excessive burdens, even if the financial burdens of those who could be taxed would not be excessive.

Rather, it would appear, following other suggestions from the commission, that "adequate care" will need to be defined by considering, among other things, professional judgments of physicians, average current use, lists of services that health-maintenance organizations and others take to be a part of decent care, as well as more general perceptions of fairness.[40] Such factors influence what is accepted generally in a society as a decent minimal or adequate level of health care. As reports considering the effects of introducing expensive new technology suggest, there is a danger that treatments may be accepted as part of "sound medical practice" before the full financial and social consequences of that acceptance are clearly understood. Much of the caution that has surrounded the development of liver and heart transplantation has been engendered by the experience with renal dialysis, which was introduced with overly optimistic judgments regarding the future costs that would be involved.

Even if, as I have argued, the concrete character of "rights to health care" is more created as an element of societal insurance programs than discovered and if the creation is properly the result of the free choice of citizens, professional and scientific bodies will need to aid in the assessment of the likely balance of costs and benefits to be embraced with the acceptance of any new form of treatment as standard treatment, such as heart and liver transplantation. A premature acceptance may lead to cost pressures on services that people will see under mature consideration to be more important. At that point it may be very difficult to withdraw the label of "standard treatment" from a technologic approach that subsequent experience shows to be too costly, given competing opportunities for the investment of resources. On the other hand, new technologic developments may offer benefits worth the cost they will entail, such as the replacement by computerized tomography of pneumoencephalography. But in any event, there is no reason to suppose that there is something intrinsically wrong with spending more than 10.5 per cent of the gross national product on health care.

Is Transplantation Special?

All investments in expensive life-saving treatment raise a question of prudence: Could the funds have been better applied elsewhere? Will the investment in expensive life-saving treatment secure an equal if not greater decrease in morbidity and mortality than an investment in improving the health care of the millions who lack health-care insurance or have only marginal coverage? If the same funds were invested in prenatal health care or the treatment of hypertension, would they secure a greater extension of life and diminution of morbidity for more people? When planning for the rational use of communal funds, it is sensible to seek to maximize access and contribution to the greatest number of people as a reasonable test of what it means to use communal resources for the common good. However, not everything done out of the common purse need be cost effective. It is unclear how one could determine the cost effectiveness of symphony orchestras or art museums. Societies have a proclivity to save the lives of identifiable individuals while failing to come to the aid of unidentified, statistical lives that could have been saved with the same or fewer resources. Any decision to provide expensive life-saving treatment out of communal funds must at least frankly acknowledge when it is not a cost-effective choice but instead a choice made because of special sympathies for those who are suffering or because of special fears that are engendered by particular diseases.

The moral framework of secular, pluralist societies in which rights to health care are more created than discovered will allow such choices as morally acceptable, even if they are less than

prudent uses of resources. It will also be morally acceptable for a society, if it pursues expensive life-saving treatment, to exclude persons who through their own choices increase the cost of care. One might think here of the question whether active alcoholics should be provided with liver transplants. There is no invidious discrimination against persons in setting a limit to coverage or in precluding coverage if the costs are increased through free choice. However, societies may decide to provide care even when the costs are incurred by free decision.

Though none of the foregoing is unique to transplantation, the issue of transplantation has the peculiarity of involving the problem not only of the allocation of monetary resources and of services but of that of organs as well. In a criticism of John Rawls' *Theory of Justice,* which theory attempts to provide a justification for a patterned distribution of resources that would redound to the benefit of the least-well-off class, Robert Nozick tests his readers' intuitions by asking whether societal rights to distribute resources would include the right to distribute organs as well.[41] He probably chose this as a test case because our bodies offer primordial examples of private property. The example is also forceful, given the traditional Western reluctance, often expressed in religious regulations, to use corpses for dissection. There is a cultural reluctance to consider parts of the body as objects for the use of persons. No less a figure than Immanuel Kant argued for a position that would appear to preclude the sale or gift of a body part to another.[42] This view of Kant's, one should note, is very close to the traditional Roman Catholic notion that one has a duty to God regarding one's self not to alter one's body except to preserve health.[43]

The concern to have a sufficient supply of organs for transplantation has expressed itself in recent political proposals and counterproposals regarding the rights of individuals to sell their organs, the provision of federal funds for the support of organ procurement, the study of the medical and legal issues that procurement may raise, and even the taking of organs from cadavers by society with the presumption of consent unless individuals have indicated the contrary.[44–49] It will be easier to show that persons have a right to determine what ought to be done with their bodies, even to the point of making donor consent decisive independently of the wishes of the family, than to show that society may presume consent. A clarification of policy, to make donor decisions definitive, would be in accord with the original intentions of the Uniform Act of Donation of Organs and would ease access to needed organs. It would not impose on people the burden of having to announce to others that they do not want their organs used for transplantation. The more one presumes that organs are not societal property, the more difficult it is to justify shifting the burden to individuals to show that they do not want their organs used. If sufficient numbers of organs are not available, it will be unfortunate, but from the point of view of general secular morality, not unfair. Free individuals will have valued other goals (e.g., having an intact body for burial) more highly than the support of transplantation. One will have encountered again one of the recurring limitations on establishing and effecting a general consensus regarding the ways in which society ought to respond to the unfortunate deliverances of nature.

Living with the Unfortunate, Which Is Not Unfair

Proposals for the general support of transplantation are thus restricted by various elements of the human condition. There is not simply a limitation due to finite resources, making it impossible to do all that is conceivably possible for all who might marginally benefit. There are restrictions as well that are due to the free decisions of both individuals and societies. Individuals will often decide in ways unsympathetic to transplantation programs that would involve the use of their private resources, including their organs. Insofar as one takes seriously respect for persons, one must live with the restrictions that result from numerous free choices. One may endeavor to educate, entice, and persuade people to participate. However, free societies are characterized by the commitment to live with the tragedies that result from the decisions of free individuals not to participate in the beneficent endeavors of others. There are then also the restrictions due to the inability to give a plausible account of state authority that would allow the imposition of a concrete view of the good life. Secular, pluralist societies are more neutral moral frameworks for negotiation and creation of ways to use their common resources than modes for discovering the proper purpose for those resources. If societies freely decide to give a low priority to transplantation and invest instead in generally improving health care for the indigent in the hope

of doing greater good, there will be an important sense in which they have acted within their right, even if from particular moral perspectives that may seem wrongheaded.

These reflections on the human condition suggest that we will need in the future to learn to live with the fact that some may receive expensive life-saving treatment while others do not, because some have the luck of access to the media, the attention of a political leader, or sufficient funds to purchase care in their own right. The differences in need, both medical and financial, must be recognized as unfortunate. They are properly the objects of charitable response. However, it must be understood that though unfortunate circumstances are always grounds for praiseworthy charity, they do not always provide grounds, by that fact, for redrawing the line between the circumstances we will count as unfortunate but not unfair and those we will count as unfortunate and unfair. To live with circumstances we must acknowledge as unfortunate but not unfair is the destiny of finite men and women who have neither the financial nor moral resources of gods and goddesses. We must also recognize the role of these important conceptual and moral issues in the fashioning of what will count as reasonable and necessary care, safe and efficacious procedures, nonexperimental treatment, or standard medical care. Though we are not gods and goddesses, we do participate in creating the fabric of these "facts."

References

1. Engelhardt HT Jr, Caplan AL, eds. Scientific controversies. London: Cambridge University Press, (in press).

2. Newman H. Medicare program: solicitation of hospitals and medical centers to participate in a study of heart transplants. Fed Regist. January 22, 1981; 46:7072–5.

3. Copeland JG, Mammana RB, Fuller JK, Campbell DW, McAleer MJ, Sailer JA, Heart transplantation: four years' experience with conventional immunosuppression. JAMA 1984; 251:1563–6.

4. DeVries WC, Anderson JL, Joyce LD, et al. Clinical use of the total artificial heart. N Engl J Med 1984; 310:273–8.

5. Dummer JS, Hardy A, Poorsattar A, Ho M. Early infections in kidney, heart, and liver transplant recipients on cyclosporine. Transplantation 1983; 36:259–67.

6. Shunzaburo I, Byers WS, Starzl TE. Current status of hepatic transplantation. Semin Liver Dis 1983; 3:173–80.

7. Starzl TE, Iwatsuki S, Van Thiel DH, et al. Evolution of liver transplantation. Hepatology 1982; 2:614–36.

8. Van Thiel DH, Schade RR, Starzl TE, et al. Liver transplantation in adults. Hepatology 1982; 2:637–40.

9. Wessel D. Transplants increase, and so do disputes over who pays bills. Wall Street Journal. April 12, 1984; 73:1, 12.

10. Spirito TH. Letter of October 29, 1982. In: Organ transplants: hearings before the subcommittee on investigations and oversight. 98th Congress, 1st Session. Washington, D.C.: Government Printing Office, 1983:226.

11. Litos PA. Letter of October 1, 1982. In: Organ transplants: hearings before the subcommittee on investigations and oversight. 98th Congress, 1st Session. Washington, D.C.: Government Printing Office, 1983:227.

12. Fiske C, Fiske M. Statements of Charles and Marilyn Fiske, and daughter Jamie, liver transplant patient. In: Organ transplants: hearings before the subcommittee on investigations and oversight. 98th Congress, 1st Session. Washington, D.C.: Government Printing Office, 1983:212–8. [see 4].

13. Gunby P. Organ transplant improvements, demands draw increasing attention. JAMA 1984; 251:1521–3, 1527.

14. *Idem.* Media-abetted liver transplants raise questions of 'equity and decency.' JAMA 1983; 249: 1973–4, 1980–2.

15. Iglehart JK. Transplantation: the problem of limited resources. N Engl J Med 1983; 309:123–8.

16. *Idem.* The politics of transplantation. N Engl J Med 1984; 310:864–8.

17. Strauss MJ. The political history of the artificial heart. N Engl J Med 1984; 310:332–6.

18. Ad Hoc Task Force on Cardiac Replacement. Cardiac replacement: medical ethical psychological and economic implications. Washington D.C.: Government Printing Office, 1969.

19. Artificial Heart Assessment Panel. The totally implantable artificial heart. Bethesda, Md.: National Institutes of Health, 1973. (DHEW publication no. (NIH)74-191).

20. Leaf A. The MGH trustees say no to heart transplants. N Engl J Med 1980; 302:1087–8.

21. Barnes BA, Dunphy ME, Koff RS, et al. Final report of the task force on liver transplantation in Massachusetts. Boston: Blue Cross and Blue Shield, 1983.

22. Engelhardt HT Jr. Bioethics in pluralist societies. Perspect Biol Med 1982; 26:64–78.

23. *Idem.* The physician-patient relationship in a secular, pluralist society. In: Shelp EE, ed. The clinical encounter. Dordrecht, Holland: D Reidel, 1983:253–66.

24. Aristotle. Nicomachaean ethics. ix 10.1170b.

25. *Idem.* Politics. vii 4.1326b.

26. Engelhardt HT. Bioethics: an introduction and critique. New York: Oxford University Press (in press).

27. Rawls J. A theory of justice. Cambridge, Mass.: Belknap Press, 1971.

28. Nozick R. Anarchy, state, and utopia. New York: Basic Books, 1974.

29. Newman H. Exclusion of heart transplantation procedures from Medicare coverage. Fed Regist 1980; 45:52296.

30. Knox RA. Heart transplants: to pay or not to pay. Science 1980; 209:570–2, 574–5.

31. Evans RW, Anderson A, Perry B. The national heart transplantation study: an overview. Heart Transplant 1982; 2(1):85–7.

32. Consensus Conference. Liver transplantation. JAMA 1983; 250:2961–4.

33. Who shall be dialysed? Lancet 1984; 1:717.

34. Aaron HJ, Schwartz WB. The painful prescription: rationing hospital care. Washington, D.C.: Brookings Institute, 1984.

35. President's Commission for the Study of Ethical Problems in Medicine and Biomedical and Behavioral Research. Securing access to health care. Vol. 1. Washington, D.C.: Government Printing Office, 1983:20.

36. President's Commission,[35] p. 37.

37. President's Commission,[35] p. 37.

38. President's Commission,[35] p. 42–3.

39. President's Commission,[35] p. 43–6.

40. President's Commission,[35] p. 37–47.

41. Nozick R. Anarchy, state, and utopia. New York: Basic Books, 1974:206–7.

42. Kant I. Kants werke: akademie textausgabe. Vol. 6. Berlin: Walter de Gruyter, 1968:423.

43. Kelly G. Medico-moral problems. St. Louis: Catholic Hospital Association, 1958:245–52.

44. Caplan AL. Organ transplants: the costs of success. Hastings Cent Rep 1983; 13(6):23–32.

45. Kolata G. Organ shortage clouds new transplant era. Science 1983; 221:32–3.

46. Overcast TD, Evans RW, Bowen LE, Hoe MM, Livak CL. Problems in the identification of potential organ donors: misconceptions and fallacies as-

sociated with donor cards. JAMA 1984; 251:1559–62.

47. Prottas JM. Encouraging altruism: public attitudes and the marketing of organ donation. Milbank Mem Fund Q 1983; 61:278–306.

48. U.S. Congress, House. To amend the public health service act to authorize financial assistance for organ procurement organizations, and for other purposes. By: Gore A. 98th Congress, 1st Session. H. Rept. 4080. 1983.

49. U.S. Congress, Senate. To provide for the establishment of a task force on organ procurement and transplantation and an organ procurement and transplantation registry, and for other purposes. By: Hatch O. 98th Congress, 1st Session. S. Rept. 2048. 1983.

Two Tiers of Care: The Unthinkable Meets the Inevitable?

Emily Friedman, Community Programs for Affordable Health Care, The Robert Wood Johnson Foundation, Chicago

What we say we want to do, and what we actually end up doing, are usually far enough apart that the discrepancy has given rise to dozens of proverbs and hundreds of learned treatises. Within health care, perhaps no gap is as troubling as the historical tension between society's desire to ensure a single level of care for all and its continuing failure to do so. In an era of increasingly restricted resources, the question takes on a more ominous form, extending beyond modest compromises of freedom of choice to what some see as unthinkable: using patient finances to determine who shall live.

Despite programs designed to end lack of access to health care, there has never been one level of care available to all Americans. "We have always had multiple tiers of care, and that's all right," says Neal Bermas, Ph.D., national director of health care productivity, National Health Care Group, Arthur Young & Co., Los Angeles. "It's not immoral—as long as the lower tier is of acceptable quality."

Michael Bromberg, executive director of the Federation of American Hospitals (FAH), points out, "Even in countries with nationalized health systems, there are no laws that prohibit building a private hospital for people who want to pay for care outside the system. On the other hand, I am not advocating a two-tiered program where the rich have private care and others have to go to the government for care."

At the heart of the question is who ends up in which tier, and why. David Kinzer, president of the Massachusetts Hospital Association, observed in the Spring 1984 issue of *Inquiry*, "Acceptance of the idea of a two-tiered system of care seems to be gaining ground in our country, but only among those who know they will land safely in the top tier."

Who is safe in a system where triage is practiced by default is open to debate, but who will probably end up in the lower tier can easily be determined. "It will be based on who's paying for the care," says Bernard Lachner, president, Evanston (IL) Hospital Corp. "There probably will be limits on care available to those for whom the government agencies pay totally, namely, Medicaid and Medicare."

Although different levels of care have existed for generations, the idea of a separate tier of health care for the poor still rankles. Daniel Callahan, Ph.D., director of the Hastings Center,

Reprinted, with permission, from *Trustee* 1984 Nov. 37:36, 39, 40, 43, 44.
When this article was written, Ms. Friedman was senior field editor, *Hospitals* magazine, American Hospital Publishing, Inc.

Hastings-on-Hudson, NY, observes, "I distinguish between conscious, intentional rationing and inadvertent rationing. The latter has always existed. But there have been fewer examples of conscious rationing, of saying who gets what."

The California legislature's decision to end freedom of choice and limit coverage of services under Medi-Cal now constitutes one such example, but the development of tiers is taking many forms. Beverlee Myers, professor and head, division of health services, UCLA School of Public Health, says, "The PPO [preferred provider organization] movement is developing multi-tiered health care systems for the whole population. Large corporations that self-insure are increasingly using preferred provider systems to limit employee choice. The payer—the employer, or the government, in the case of the poor and elderly—decides what will be provided to or paid for by its beneficiaries/employees. We have had a multi-tiered system in the past, with different paths for the military, veterans, Native Americans, and others. Now Medicare could have its own hospitals, and Medicaid in each state could have its own hospitals. There might be different systems for different employed groups as well. Employment could soon be based on how healthy a person is. Self-insurance is, after all, the ultimate in experience rating; you get rid of those employees who use a lot of health services. As for the poor and elderly, government can be as self-interested as any corporation, and it can limit choice as well."

As Myers points out, the growing role of the market in health care is forcing the issue. As Uwe Reinhardt, Ph.D., professor of economics and public affairs, Princeton University, wrote in the Spring 1984 *Hospital Management Quarterly,* "Unfortunately, as every freshman in economics quickly learns, the one feat the Invisible Hand usually cannot achieve is the distribution of commodities on a basis other than ability to pay." Lachner of Evanston Hospital sees in this problem a threat to the market movement in health care: "The major concern is that it could reverse the competitive market direction if hospitals, physicians, and government abandoned poor people and their health care needs. But it's very important to emphasize that it's not only hospitals and physicians who have the potential for abandonment, but the government as well. The government will, in effect, determine what care will be available."

Howard Newman, partner, Memel, Jacobs, Pierno & Gersh, Washington, DC, also sees tiers of hospitals. "Those voluntary institutions that play the special role of caring for people without resources have been able to fill that role because they could cross-subsidize the costs. Their capacity to do that has diminished. Therefore, they find themselves forced to move in the direction of one of two polar extremes: an institution that operates under public auspices, or one that is explicitly organized as a for-profit enterprise. They will have to mimic one of those two kinds of organizations because the circumstances that allowed voluntary hospitals to play their unique role have become so altered that they can no longer afford to play that role."

Such a change may have already occurred for the uninsured population. Barry Passett, president, Greater Southeast Community Hospital Foundation, Inc., Washington, DC, says, "We are clearly moving toward reaffirmation of the fact that there is a public system and a private system, and that the private system does not have to take care of the uninsured. That is not a tragedy. The uninsured have already fallen through all the other cracks, and the public system was created to care for them. But it would be a tragedy if Medicare and Medicaid clients ended up, essentially without choice, in public facilities. Those programs had a different promise, and that promise would be betrayed."

The dominant method of creating tiers is the shunting—direct or indirect, intentional or inadvertent—of indigent and near-indigent patients to public hospitals. Is that such a bad thing? That depends in large part on what one thinks of public hospitals. Robert White, former head of health services for the county of Los Angeles, is far from horrified by mandated public hospital care for the poor. "We need to accept the notion that we are going to evolve into a two-tiered system—and maybe we should not fight the idea. There is no question in my mind that if the total number of dollars pumped into Medi-Cal since 1968 had been pumped exclusively into public hospitals, Medi-Cal patients would have been better served."

On the other hand, a 1984 survey of 1,000 health care professionals conducted by Arthur Andersen & Co. and the American College of Hospital Administrators found that 60 percent of respondents believe that a lower quality of care is provided by public hospitals. And, as James

Mongan, M.D., executive director, Truman Medical Center, Kansas City, MO, points out, "Having a formal, separate system for the poor would be just like having a formal, separate school system for the poor. Once public hospitals were solely for poor people, they would soon lose political support. And then we really would have a lesser track of care."

In a massive study of the concept of two tiers of care conducted for the Center for Health Services and Policy Research, Northwestern University, Evanston, IL, Walter McNerney, professor of health policy for the university's Program in Hospital and Health Services Management, offers an explanation for the perception that public hospitals are inferior. "Local government is likely to be the least able to provide adequate resources. With limited funds and the handicap of a bureaucratic environment, hospital management is often weak and there may be, as a result, inordinate inefficiency. Because the poor tend to be concentrated geographically, there are limited opportunities to develop private income, and even where location is not a major problem, the willingness of middle- and upper-class patients to use public hospital facilities is highly restrained. Further, the number of poor admitted cannot be controlled, as in some private-sector hospitals. As a result, care can be less than equal to the rest of the community and even less than a reasonable standard. The difference can be significantly more than a matter of amenities."

The question of "amenities" is part and parcel of the debate. One argument is that as long as clinical care remains comparable, two tiers of care are acceptable. "*Where* one receives one's treatment is different from the question of quality," FAH's Bromberg says. "We don't say that public housing has to be as nice as private housing; we do say that the poor should have shelter. What we have to guarantee is access to treatment." Richard Egdahl, M.D., director, Boston University Medical Center, points out, "The amenities in public hospitals, in some cases, may not be the same as in private hospitals, but certainly the care can be excellent."

But there are those who oppose discrimination in amenities. "It doesn't make a nickel's worth of difference in cost," says Donald Brennan, president, Sisters of Providence Corp., Seattle. "Also, who is to say that the needs of the individual, which are emotional and spiritual as well as physical, do not require 'amenities'? Who is to

make the judgment that one person deserves less than another? In doing that, are we not ignoring the fundamental dignity of the individual, irrespective of resources?"

But the basic question goes beyond the environment in which care is provided. If, in fact, inadequate funding undercuts the ability of public hospitals to provide care comparable to that in private hospitals, and if little money can be saved by eliminating hotel-service "frills," then the real issue is whether it is acceptable to offer a lower level of *clinical* care to the poor. Kinzer poses this problem in his *Inquiry* article: "If it meant hamburger instead of steak, and ward accommodations instead of private, and open windows instead of air conditioning, that is one thing. If it meant making it more difficult for second-tier types to get inside our hospitals, that is another thing. If it meant giving them fewer medical services, that is quite something else. And if it meant consigning all of the country's indigent to understaffed and underquipped public charity hospitals, that is something else again. If second-tier people get an explanation of what the term really means, they won't like any of the four interpretations, and least of all the last three."

Whether they like the idea or not, the real question is whether they would be harmed by its implementation. The two metaphors most often used to describe the situation are that of an overcrowded lifeboat or an airplane with different classes of passengers. Says Ronald Bayer, Ph.D., associate for policy studies at the Hastings Center, "People like to use the airplane model. But the fact is that all the passengers on the plane will land at the same airport. People receiving only 'coach' health care may not end up in the same place as those receiving better care. 'Separate but equal' simply never works." As for the "lifeboat" image, Bayer says, "People ending up in a lifeboat is an accident. Resource allocation is a matter of social decision."

When a social decision is made, as in California, the results tend to reinforce Bayer's view. In the Aug. 16 issue of the *The New England Journal of Medicine*, Nicole Lurie, M.D., and others reported on at least three former Medi-Cal patients who had been shed from the program and whose deaths were attributable to their inability to afford care. Three patients out of millions could be seen as "statistical," as opposed to "identified," lives, to use the ethicist's rubric, but the report belies claims that tiers of care do no harm. In the

Summer 1984 issue of *Health Affairs,* Robert Brook, M.D., Sc.D., and others from the Rand Corp. observe, "Economic or administrative approaches to the problems of rising medical costs will reduce expenditures for the poor and the elderly, irrespective of what they might accomplish for the rest of us. If they are pursued aggressively enough without regard to their clinical implications, they may well do more harm than good, at least for dependent or disadvantaged groups. The weakest and most vulnerable will suffer the most from purely economic or administrative mechanisms to curtail medical expenditures."

Apparently, formal tiers of care are not harmless, in either practical or ethical terms. Yet, as Charles Fried pointed out in the February 1976 *Hastings Center Report,* "As long as our society considers inequality of wealth and income . . . morally acceptable—acceptable in the sense that the system that produces these inequalities is in itself not morally suspect—it is anomalous to carve out a sector like health care and say that *there* equality must reign." What we face is not a question of whether to have them, but of how to minimize the effects of income-based tiers.

At least some guidelines are emerging. Richard Zeckhauser, Ph.D., professor of political economy, Kennedy School, Harvard University, Cambridge, MA, observes, "It may be that already within the hospital, different amounts of care are given according to the patient's insurance. But differences in discretionary care are so great that this is hard to detect. Where we can fudge, we will; in some areas it's easy, even in cancer care. With big, visible treatments like transplants, it's hard." Lachner adds, "There is still a substantial capacity, within the clinical side of hospital practice, to reduce the use of resources without compromising the quality of care. As long as that capacity allows us to further reduce the rate of increase in the cost of care, we are still a good way from having to face the issue of direct clinical triage."

Egdahl of Boston University suggests, "If it could be shown that waiting for care did not affect morbidity or mortality, but is only inconvenient, then if we were absolutely strapped, we could include that type of limitation in the two tiers, and thus avoid denying acutely needed medical or surgical care." Brennan of the Sisters of Providence supports a concept he helped to implement earlier as president of the Group Health Cooperative of Puget Sound, a Seattle-based HMO. "I do believe that there is room to

question levels of activity and the usefulness of some procedures. We should look at alternative ways of providing care—but not based on the patient's sponsorship."

Mark Siegler, M.D., director, Center for Clinical Ethics, University of Chicago-Pritzker School of Medicine, believes that "it is essential that before embarking on massive changes in health policy, one should link such changes with ongoing efforts to assess the quality of care and outcomes of care. As Alvin Tarlov, M.D., said in a lecture in 1983, 'Outcome assessments should include measures of self-care, physical activity, mobility, role fulfillment, perceived health status, mental health, disease status, expenditures, and satisfaction with service.' If one can achieve these kinds of quality of care and outcome assessments using a two-tiered health care system, and prove that the lower tier does not receive a lesser quality of care as measured by these kinds of outcome data, then it might be appropriate, and fair, to proceed with a two-tiered system. But important outcome measures may be neglected if the move to a two-tiered system is based on the narrowest of outcome standards."

In his paper "Protecting the Traditions of Clinical Medicine," to be published in the *Hastings Center Report,* Siegler also recommends, "If . . . we are willing at last to do what we have never before done in medicine, to sacrifice identified lives rather than statistical lives, *let us begin with the strongest, most intelligent, and most articulate patients.* We should not begin with the poor or the aged, the uneducated or prisoners. We should rather begin with corporate vice-presidents who need heart transplants, or assembly line workers who need root-canal treatment, or school teachers who need coronary artery bypass surgery. At least these individuals and groups can defend themselves and their interests."

There are options available, although, at the moment, one tier of care for everyone does not appear to be one of them. The question is what options will be chosen, and by whom. Obviously, more efficient and appropriate care and minimal waits for elective services are preferable to casting patients adrift. Directing patients to certain sites of care, although morally repugnant to those who favor freedom of choice, could be acceptable if the quality of care at those sites meets overall standards.

But some entity has to take charge and change the process from one of default to one of design. "We are not only dealing with social responsibility," says Bermas of Arthur Young, "we are dealing with individual morality. And community conscience and individual conscience tend to follow divergent paths. We have to look at the socioeconomic issues and transcend our own personal experiences. The debate must take place." And part of that debate must be consideration of the tradeoffs involved. Drew Altman, Ph.D., vice-president, Robert Wood Johnson Foundation, says, "Any sensible person, even while holding to the goal of the same quality of care for everyone, would take the position that some care is better than no care. For the most vulnerable, an arrangement of selected institutions of adequate quality is better than nothing. The difficulty is in the trading off of some such arrangement now against the danger that accepting it will lead us to abandon the goal of a single system that enfranchises everyone in the future."

"In the end, it comes down to a question of personal values," says Newman of Menel, Jacobs, Pierno & Gersh. "The answer is ultimately a function of society's values. And the way our society responds will be a test of how humane we are."

Part 2

The Hospital within Society: Practice

Hospital trustees, executives, medical and nursing staffs, and other care-givers sometimes must think that health care ethicists debate the presence of angels on the heads of pins while Rome—and the hospital—burns. But precisely because health care is such a personal service and because every hospital has a mission, a tradition, a history, and an institutional personality that is unlike any other, developing broad rules that will guide all hospitals in making difficult, and sometimes impossible, decisions is a prickly task.

Yet there are guideposts. Health care practitioners and the hospitals within which they work are often faced with decisions that will affect the availability of hospital services in the community. These decisions involve different levels of hospital activity. What commitment should the hospital make to those who cannot afford to pay for their health care? Should resources that could benefit the paying patient be diverted to care for the poor? Which programs should the hospital offer to all and which should be provided only on the basis of ability to pay? And what are the stakes for the hospital, for the community, and for society?

In this section, the practical consequences of such ethical decision making by hospital and health care professionals are explored. First, Emily Friedman discusses what hospitals have to lose if they fail to recognize that the unappetizing job of forcing policy in health care resource allocation has fallen to them and they have no choice but to undertake this job. Judith P. Swazey, Ph.D., and Renee C. Fox, Ph.D., recall how kidney dialysis researchers in the 1960s decided who would and who would not receive that life-saving treatment, and they tell us what lessons were learned from the agonies of those researchers. Daniel E. Singer, M.D., and his coauthors share extraordinarily valuable information about a situation in which doctors were forced to ration a scarce resource—a task physicians generally eschew.

James F. Childress, using history as well as ethics, provides a powerful and useful model for allocating health care: determining clinical need and then applying an objective selection process through which all candidates have an equal chance. The experience of one hospital in making a difficult decision about whether or not to continue spending vast sums of money on a patient who was not from that community is chronicled—and applauded—in a Miami Herald *editorial. Arthur L. Caplan argues that one way to ease pressure on a scarce resource—in this case, donor organs for transplantation—is to increase the supply of that resource through a process that respects the individual's right to privacy and self-determination while honoring the needs of society. Finally, Lois K. Christopherson chronicles how one heart transplant center developed eligibility criteria and what that process and its outcome can teach us.*

Because Someone Has to be Responsible: Duty and Dilemma for the American Hospital

Emily Friedman, Community Programs for Affordable Health Care, The Robert Wood Johnson Foundation, Chicago

Why should the American hospital, which certainly has enough to keep it busy, take on the difficult and often thankless role of seeking solutions to ethical problems in health care? Especially in an age when marketplace incentives and approaches are being stressed as the solutions to the problems that have plagued the hospital in the past, is not the ethical responsibility of the hospital an antiquated concept that has little place in today's health economy?

The answers to these questions will not cause many hospitals to cheer, because they have more to do with the facts of life than with the theoretical rubrics and elevated moral arguments that characterize many debates over ethics. For it is one thing to discuss one's moral duty in a theoretical case study; it is another to have to make decisions that will determine whether a patient lives or dies, and when. It is fine to cringe at the thought of "bottom-line health care" and to shy away from any suggestion that there might be a line at which ethics and economics cross, but it is something else again to realize that an institution cannot continue to provide care to all who ask for it because the institution no longer has the money to do so.

Because of the traditional barrier that has—perhaps rightly—separated ethical theory from hospital reality, hospital professionals today find themselves ill-equipped to confront the question of what the role of the hospital should be in the growing conflicts over care of the indigent, treatment of the terminally ill, allocation of resources, and other intractable issues.

The easy answer, of course, is that if health care is truly a competitive marketplace, then agonizing over ethical issues is somewhat inappropriate. As was observed by James and Kirk Hart at the Chaiker Abbis Invitational Forum on Hospital Governance, October 1985, business ethics sometimes seem to consist of ten ways to stay out of jail, and the phrase *business ethics* itself is viewed by some observers as a contradiction in terms.[1] So the first question is, is the hospital in the new economy subject to any ethical calling beyond what might be required of the corner grocer?

The very fact that most health care professionals will answer yes to this question illustrates the bind in which the hospital finds itself. On the one hand, the "invisible hand" of the market is said to be the determinant of the future of health care. On the other hand, when we consider the proposition that this new economy frees the hospital from any special ethical duty, most of us reject the notion out of hand. At the basis of that rejection lies the rub: *whether we wish it so or not, the hospital holds a special status in American society that carries with it both great privilege and a unique burden.*

Why is the hospital special? It's a matter of perception. The vast majority of the American public thinks the hospital is special, and in this case the perception dictates the truth. If society views an entity as a social institution, then that entity is indeed bound to follow the wishes of the society, much as it might yearn for an easier—or at least more consistent—master.

Why does American society think the hospital is special? It has to do with the peculiar economics of health in this country. Most people would agree that effective health care—that is, care that saves or improves the quality of life— is a necessity, along with food, clothing, shelter, and, in some climates, fuel. Although Americans have more of a claim on life, liberty, and the pursuit of happiness as entitlements than they do under any written statement of the right to necessities, custom has decreed that people should not go without those things we have declared to be basic to survival. To this end, we try to ensure that at least some level of those necessities is available to almost everyone. For example, we provide food stamps, food pantries, and holiday gift boxes of food to the disadvantaged. Food is seen as the most basic of the basics. During the Christmas holiday, it is a gala dinner that is offered to the homeless and the otherwise down and out, despite the fact that coats or a decent place to live would be much more useful.

Similarly, in the United States there is an extensive network of publicly owned and government-subsidized housing that is reserved for the use of low-income families. Rent controls, rent subsidization, urban homesteading, and other mechanisms have also been used by government to ensure that shelter is available to most of those who need it. Although homelessness continues to grow in a sad and silent epidemic, we have not yet come to terms with it; and so we tell ourselves that those who live on the street do so from choice, despite the fact that this is rarely true.

The availability of fuel is an interesting issue, because fuel is indeed a necessity—more so, at some times of the year, than food. Yet attempts to guarantee its availability to most or all of those who need it are not nearly as sophisticated as the efforts around food and clothing. As a result, in northern cities, every winter a few deaths are reported of people who died of exposure and cold in their own homes. Often these are people who were presumed to be protected by statutes that ban the denial of fuel during cold-weather months. However, the denials can be, and are, instituted in the spring and remain intact for the following winter. Perhaps the lack of policy attention to fuel is due to the fact that suppliers of electricity and natural gas are public utilities, and, because they are regulated, we believe that their prices are controlled to the point of making their products affordable. This was, in fact, true until very recently—and the time that has passed since has been far too short to produce a workable solution on any but the community level. Remember that it took nearly a century for Medicare to be passed, starting from the time of the first efforts to develop some kind of government health insurance program.

Clothing has never been a guaranteed necessity in the United States; in fact, a significant amount of the clothing that is available to low-income Americans is donated by more-fortunate others. The lack of regulation when it comes to garments is probably due to the fact that, as long as one's expectations are not grand, there is a large amount of cheap or even free clothing around. The market, without interference, has not priced clothing out of the reach of very many people, and as a result there has not been a perceived need for policy to guarantee either affordability or availability.

Despite these attempts to make necessities other than health care available to all who need them, whether or not they can pay, it is interesting that neither food, nor clothing, nor shelter, nor fuel has been divorced from the market. What policy has done is increase the buying power of those who face a market disadvantage, by providing direct or indirect subsidies to lower the price of the product. There has been little effort to develop a different method of distribution.

The reason for continued use of the market as a distribution mechanism has a great deal to do with why health care and the institutions that provide it are viewed as unique. For when it comes down to it, with the exception of fuel, all other necessities can be price-differentiated through product lines. The fact of the matter is that any one of a series of forms of housing, strung out along a very broad spectrum, will provide the basic service one requires of shelter. The same is true of clothing and of food. One can live without truffles, without mansions, without mink coats.

But when it comes to health care, the model breaks down. For differentiation of health care into product lines is almost impossible, if one accepts the basic demands that are made of health care: preserve or improve health, save life, maintain quality of life. If a child has biliary atresia, the most effective method, *and the only method,* of saving that child's life is through a liver transplant. It does not matter if the family only has enough money for a visit to a primary care physician; that visit will not solve the problem. An adhesive strip is not equivalent to an appendectomy, and no amount of market manipulation will make it so.

At the heart of this is that health care, unlike the other necessities, is a service, not a product, and it is a hard job indeed to break a basic service into product lines. We do not differentiate what level of fire or police service a household may receive on the basis of the amount of taxes it pays or what its income is. We do not, within the increasingly troubled context of the public schools, provide more education to one child than another—at least not as a matter of policy. In determining how necessities will be made available, Americans have left products to the mercies of a monitored market—but they have pulled services out of the market.

As a result, those services have developed unique pathways of their own. Fire, police, and educational services long ago became the province of government. So have a significant proportion of American hospitals. But other institutions that provide health care have become hybrids, with one foot in the public sector and one in the private, with the trappings of charity and the pressures of the market, with certain responsibilities prescribed by law and others mandated by private employers and insurers. These various and contrary demands have shaped the hospital into something that borders on the strange.

And the demands made on hospitals are not always realistic. Leo Greenawalt, president of the Washington State Hospital Association, has observed that employers and other payers want hospitals to behave both like charities and like businesses and that, as a result, "hospitals are tearing themselves apart because of conflicting messages." Government urges hospitals to be competitive without loosing the regulatory apron strings. The employer who jawbones for the lowest possible health insurance rates for his employees finds that the sky is the limit when the cardiac arrest in question is the one he has suffered himself. And citizens who complain about the prohibitive cost of health care lose their con-

sumerism in a blind demand for everything available when it is their children who are at risk of dying.

But there is a tradeoff. Societal demands on and expectations of hospitals have been accompanied by an exaltation of the institution, which hospitals have willingly accepted. They were traditionally viewed as "economically innocent," in the words of Carl Schramm,[2] and they were trusted without question. Part of this was innocence by association, because hospitals were where physicians worked, and physicians in American society, as they are in most societies, are shamans; they are magicians. Places where they made their magic were necessarily magical themselves. With the heavily religious base of so many hospitals firmly fixed in the public mind, the presence of the shaman-physicians, the almost mystical way in which health care was viewed in the first place, and a workforce consisting mostly of women, who have a folkloric power of their own, the uniqueness of hospitals was established early, and it is being questioned only now.

It is being questioned for many reasons: the anti-institutional legacy of the 1960s, growing concerns about affordability of health care for anyone except the very wealthy, employer/insurer suspicions about what they are getting for their money, the explosion of antiphysician sentiment, and a rebellion against the increasingly technological nature of so much health care.[3] But what hospital executives, medical staff members, and trustees must keep in mind is that *why* their hospitals are being questioned is not really the point. The point is that the special regard in which hospitals have been held represents the bulk of their long-term political and social capital—and if hospitals are failing society, *or are thought to be failing society,* there is not a bit of doubt that society will return the favor, sooner or later.

This is most easily illustrated in recent press coverage of access to health care for the poor and access to an appropriate level of care for the elderly. There is a tangled universe of factors contributing to hospitals' increasing concern about their ability to provide care to the medically indigent, as there is a complex political and fiscal superstructure that has contributed to a lower length of stay for the Medicare patient. Similarly difficult contexts surround situations involving malpractice and treatment (or nontreatment) of the permanently unconscious patient and the distressed newborn. But press coverage does not probe these snarls. Instead, the hospitals are blamed for whatever goes wrong. It does not matter what the reasons are or whether the hospitals are at fault—as they sometimes are. The hospitals take the blame for the untreated low-income child, the neonate whose fate becomes a matter of public record, the elderly patient who feels he has been pitched out into the street while still sick, and the terminally ill patient who believes she is not being allowed to die on her own terms.

Certainly some of this has to do with the decline of magic in the society overall, for which hospitals can hardly be held accountable. But the fact is that society feels its hospitals are letting it down. And that must be a concern for every hospital manager, physician, trustee, and employee. There has never been more of a need for moral leadership in American health care, and it is a poor time indeed for hospitals to be perceived as not being up to the job.

So the reason that ethical behavior and ethical leadership is incumbent upon hospitals is that, first, this is what is expected of them. Second, they will be blamed for whatever happens, so it would behoove them to try to influence the course of events. Third, on the assumption that hospitals believe that their special place in society is worth the trials that accompany it, their best hope of preserving it is in acting ethically and trying to inspire others to do the same. Fourth, on a purely pragmatic level, there are simply no other candidates for the job.

Policymakers, traditionally, have been as enthusiastic about making explicit policy that might deal someone out as they have been about catching rattlesnakes barehanded. The public, content with its belief that the hospitals and the various payment programs have been taking care of everything, have not wanted to be aware of any suffering that might be going on; when such awareness does develop, Americans feel compelled to do something. Obviously, then, they have not discerned a problem.

Physicians are in some ways much better candidates for ethical leadership than are hospitals, which are conservative, slow, and given to tripping over their own trunks when they try to move fast. But physicians face an ethical dilemma of their own—if it is their job to advocate everything for their patients that might be of some help, how can they become involved in issues of resource allocation, termination of treatment, and the like? Whether or not this stance is defensible,

or advisable, in today's health economy is a matter of some conjecture; but as of now, it is not physicians' feet that are being held to the fire.

It would appear, then, that either hospitals will have to push for consideration of ethical dilemmas and the development of solutions or no one will. And it is unlikely that inaction will work as a strategy, for the reasons I have already outlined. It will work to the disadvantage of hospitals and, in all probability, to the disadvantage of society as well. It will certainly work to the disadvantage of individual patients. Patients need protection, and if the hospital to which they have turned for help does not act as their guardian, who will? Furthermore, in a society that increasingly believes that its hospitals are, in the aggregate, not as valuable and trustworthy as they once were, the scorned or abused patient can be unforgiving indeed—as a plaintiff, as a voter, and as a member of the community that ultimately will decide the hospital's fate.

Therefore, unappetizing as the menu is, hospitals would be well advised to involve themselves in what are shaping up to be the ethical issues of this decade and probably the next as well. Internally, their approach must involve administration, employees, medical staff, and trustees. Externally, they must develop cooperative forums with and within their communities and avoid the trap of dictating what should happen because they know more. Health care providers have always known more than others about health care; that's why they are the individual and institutional shamans. But they have been expected by their communities to behave morally in exchange for that information monopoly. It's about time they started to honor that bargain.

Among the issues that hospitals must help solve are the following:

Care of vulnerable populations. This used to be simply the issue of the medically indigent, who at 30 to 35 million are not an insignificant population; and to them must be added the more than 20 million Medicaid clients, the 6 million low-income Medicare clients, and the very old and very sick, all of whom are at risk of losing access to health care under the new payment conservatism. These are the populations to which some theorists say health care must be rationed; yet it is they who need health care the most. If hospitals have a duty to protect the patient, that duty extends to the potential patient who, without intervention, may never get as far as the hospital.

Appropriate care of the terminally ill. Although it is carelessly (and dangerously) being cast as an economic issue, this is actually a civil rights issue. It is at this point beyond question that the competent patient has the right to choose or refuse treatment options; custom, case law, and rationality all tell us that. Yet health care providers find it hard to let go of the traditional paternalism that has challenged patients' self-determination. It is necessary that hospitals learn to understand that one of the key quality-of-life issues is quality of death, and hospitals must work to educate their medical and nursing staffs about the need to accept patients' decisions at the close of their lives.

Use of exotic technology. One of the issues that is perhaps hardest for hospitals and physicians to accept is that somewhere along the line the endless American fascination with health care technology has turned, in some instances, to revulsion. Once technology was no longer always curative, but became instead the "halfway technology" of Lewis Thomas's classic phrase[4]—treatments that could prevent death but could not restore quality of life—our passion for it waned. Now there are few guideposts for those who wrestle with when and how to use artificial organs, transplantation, chemotherapy and radiation therapy, provision of vital substances to the comatose, and pharmaceuticals that can be as life-threatening as the conditions to which they are applied.

Furthermore, with cost an issue and insurers no longer willing to pay for whatever comes down the line, the question of access is raised. Should expensive, rare treatments be distributed on the basis of ability to pay? Should income overshadow clinical need? If not, who will pay for the care of the poor? In the case of some very costly technologies, almost everyone could become the poor. What then? Earlier in this essay I suggested that there may well be a line where economics and ethics cross; that line will likely be defined in the use of under-reimbursed, expensive technological care.

Undercare and overcare. One of the ironies of the revolution in payment systems is that market incentives are not always a perfect match for health care. One artifact of that mismatch is that some populations must worry about whether they are being provided with marginal, unnecessary, or even dangerous health care while others are being denied even basic care that they demon-

strably need. An ever-growing body of research is documenting both sides of this equation, and although many payers seem interested in eliminating overcare, it is being left to physicians and hospitals to wage the battle against undercare. It is a battle they must win, for the stakes are high.

Resource allocation. Although economics are driving much health care, there are many questions about who gets what that lie beyond the reach of finance. With only a few hundred donor hearts realistically available in a given year and tens of thousands of candidates for heart transplantation, how should the hearts be distributed? If individuals who can afford to do so wish to purchase a treatment that is seen as a luxury or of little clinical value, is it fair to deny it to them? Is there anything wrong with luxury cosmetic surgery centers proliferating in a country where the mortality rate among nonwhite infants is twice that of whites?

How health care resources should be configured and allocated is a continuing conundrum in the United States, even in the absence of economic constraint or incentive. But the strain caused by lack of policy is starting to show, and unless hospitals force development of policy, it is likely that they will have to make the decisions. If we complain about hospital cost shifting because it represents a private taxing power that was never consciously granted to hospitals, it should give us pause that we may end up asking them to decide, without guidance, who should live.

These are the issues today; but there will be more. At the end of the black-comedy film *The Hospital* (1971), there is a little vignette that tells us all we need to know about why hospitals are duty-bound to exercise ethical leadership. After a series of calamities, the hospital is the subject of a strike by house staff and a sit-in by an unhappy community group. A patient has just murdered several employees. The administrator is in tears in the parking lot, and the chief of surgery is surveying the scene with nearly suicidal depression. A young woman is urging the surgeon to run off to Mexico with her and leave the hospital to the chaotic fate into which it is rapidly sinking. He refuses; puzzled, she asks why. "Because someone has to be responsible," he responds, and, bloody but unbowed, he takes the administrator in hand and marches back into the maelstrom.

In health care, it is the hospital that will be found responsible. The difference will be in whether the hospital sought that responsibility with courage and leadership, or whether it came by it through cowardice and default. And somewhere in that process, the future of the American hospital will be determined.

References

1. Hart, J., and Hart, K. Healthcare ethics: a community hospital is not a business. Discussion paper, Chaiker Abbis Invitational Forum on Hospital Governance. Toronto, Ontario, Canada, Oct. 25, 1985.

2. Schramm, C. Can we solve the hospital cost problem in our democracy? *New Eng. J. Med.* 1984 Sept. 13. 311:729.

3. Friedman, E. What's eroding the hospital's image? *Hospitals.* 1985 Sept. 16. 59:76.

4. Thomas, Lewis. *The Lives of a Cell.* New York City: The Viking Press, 1974.

Social and Ethical Problems in the Treatment of End-Stage Renal Disease Patients

Renee C. Fox, Ph.D., Department of Sociology, University of Pennsylvania, Philadelphia
Judith P. Swazey, Ph.D., The Acadia Institute, Bar Harbor, ME
Elizabeth M. Cameron, R.N., Transplant Department, Hospital of the University of Pennsylvania, Philadelphia

Dialysis and the Allocation of Scarce Resources

How a society, or its constituent parts, can most justly or fairly distribute its limited resources is an ancient question that has long been grappled with in philosophical and political arenas.[1] In medical care, the starkest form of widespread decisions that must be made about the allocation of scarce resources is framed by the question, "Who shall live when not all can live?" This question, as Childress observed over a decade ago, "is hardly new," but it "has been urgently forced upon us by the dramatic use of artificial internal organs and organ transplantation."[2]

The intertwined social, ethical, and political issues concerning the allocation of scarce, potentially life-saving medical resources that are paradigmatically embedded in the history of chronic dialysis have fallen into two phases. In phase one, from the inception of chronic dialysis in 1960 to the passage of Public Law 92-603 in 1972, the central issues turned around the classic "lifeboat ethic" dilemma of deciding who lives and who dies when not all lives can be saved. Since the mid-1970s, with funding for the treatment of end-stage renal disease provided by Medicare and the concomitant expansion of dialysis capabilities, attention has gradually focused on two other clusters of allocation questions: the expenditure of large sums of public monies for a costly mode of long-term, palliative treatment like dialysis in relation to other health care needs; and even more difficult questions about who should decide whether and how to withhold or terminate such forms of treatment.

Allocating Dialysis before Public Law 92-603

The development of the Scribner shunt in 1960, making possible chronic dialysis as an alternative or adjunct to the then nascent procedure of renal transplantation, rapidly created a classic problem of what philosophers term distributive justice.[3] Given a large population of patients with end-stage renal disease relative to a limited dialysis capability—including funds, machines, hospital beds, and medical personnel—and the great expense of chronic treatment, who should receive

Excerpted and reprinted, with permission, from Narins, Robert G., editor. *Controversies in Nephrology and Hypertension.* New York: Churchill Livingstone, 1984. pp. 58–63.
Preparation of Dr. Fox's and Dr. Swazey's portions of this chapter was supported by a grant from the James Picker Foundation Program on the Human Qualities of Medicine.

dialysis, who should make such decisions, and what criteria should be used?

Throughout the 1960s, individual physicians, patient selection committees, and hospitals thus were forced to deal with the medical-moral dilemma of selecting a limited number of medically eligible candidates to receive dialysis, knowing that those patients not chosen would soon die unless a transplant was possible. The type of decision that recurrently had to be made—what many involved ruefully called "playing God"—was as follows: This month our hospital's dialysis unit has space for one new dialysis patient, but there are four medically eligible candidates. How do we select the recipient? Those responsible for allocating dialysis used a variety of selection methods, which were based on one or more of six principles of social justice that can be used to provide a moral basis for distributing scarce resources.

1. A *meritarian* concept of social justice allocates limited goods or resources to individuals on the basis of their merits or deserts. Merits or deserts, in turn, can be defined by the distributors—for example, a dialysis selection committee—in many ways, such as a person's conduct, achievement, or contributions to society.

2. A *needs* principle seeks to justly allocate a limited resource such as dialysis according to the essential needs of individuals, leaving for further definition the question of what constitutes "essential needs."

3. An *ability* principle distributes a scarce resource on the basis of various criteria concerning an individual's ability. For example, in a fee-for-service system ability to pay can be the determinant of who receives care, and a selection committee thus could narrow a pool of dialysis candidates by eliminating those who cannot afford to pay for treatment.

4. A principle of *compensatory justice* would distribute resources to those who have previously suffered social wrongs that deprived them of those resources, such as a lack of access to medical care because of a low socioeconomic status. (This is the principle of social justice underlying Medicaid insurance.)

5. A *utilitarian "ethometrics"* principle seeks to provide the greatest benefit or good for the greatest number of persons. This is the principle behind quantitative cost-benefit analyses

for the provision of various forms of health care, which often founder in efforts to define what variables should constitute the "greatest good"—for example, economic, personal, social—and to quantitatively calculate noneconomic "goods" such as health status.

6. An *egalitarian* principle of social justice, in American society, is often viewed as the most morally acceptable way to distribute scarce resources. There are, however, many ways to formulate egalitarian principles, and it is seldom easy to specify just what is meant by them and consequently how one should act on them. In the arena of medical care, for example, many hold that we should "provide similar treatment for similar cases," which then leads to a panorama of questions about how one defines "similar treatment" and "similar cases." During the 1960s, a number of dialysis facilities selected patients by random lottery, believing that this form of egalitarian distribution was the fairest, most neutral way of determining who might live when not all could live.

As this brief discussion of the principles of social justice underlying the allocation of dialysis during the 1960s suggests, the need to make such decisions involves a host of complex, painful medical, moral, and social issues. None involved in selecting dialysis recipients welcomed their task, or were comfortable with the selection methods they adopted. All felt there was no really good way to make such decisions; rather, they sought to find what they felt was the "least worst" selection method.

Public Law 92-603 and Its Implications

The magnitude of the problems posed both by chronic renal disease and the limited availability of treatment capabilities were recognized by the federal government in the mid-1960s with the formation of a Committee on Chronic Kidney Disease. Their report, issued in 1967, drew public attention to the fact that "until capability meets demand agonizing decisions concerning patient selection are inevitable at both the local and national level." "Approximately 5,000 patients with chronic uremia died in fiscal year 1967 because of lack of adequate treatment facilities," the Committee reported, "and by 1973 . . . a minimum of 24,000 additional medically suitable patients will have died without the opportunity for treatment by chronic dialysis or transplantation."[4]

To meet the "psychological, ethical, and political problems" created by the scarcity of treatment capabilities, particularly dialysis, the Committee recommended the establishment of a federally funded treatment program for end-stage renal disease. But its estimated cost—$800 million to $1 billion for the first 6 years—was viewed by Congress as prohibitively expensive.

Between 1967 and 1972 the number of patients receiving dialysis and transplantation increased and the costs of the procedures decreased, particularly with the advent of home dialysis programs in the late 1960s. Treatment capabilities, however, still fell far short of demand, and pressures mounted for a federal response to the economics of scarcity. As analyzed most fully by Rettig, the passage of PL 92-603, the 1972 Social Security Amendment Act, was a watershed in the provision of chronic dialysis.[5] Public law 92-603 included provisions extending Medicare insurance coverage to virtually all patients with end-stage renal disease, giving them what is perhaps their most distinguishing characteristic: They became the first, and thus far only, victims of catastrophic illness singled out for special coverage of their treatment costs by the federal government.

By largely removing the financial barriers to the provision and receipt of dialysis that created the majority of the allocation issues of the 1960s, the federal government in effect became the new "gatekeeper" of this treatment. The government's assumption of this complex role has had profound effects on the delivery of dialysis and raises a series of critical issues that extend far beyond the confines of this therapy alone.

One cluster of issues generated by the passage of PL 92-603 involves the why and how of macro-level policy decisions about the allocation of public funds within the health-care segment of the federal budget. Why renal disease should have been singled out for special coverage, and the implications of this action for the federal financing of other catastrophic illness and for the provision of a broader-based form of national health insurance are two interrelated sociopolitical and moral questions that have been debated for the past decade.

A related series of issues concern the effects of PL 92-603 upon the provision of dialysis services. Data on treatment patterns before and after 1972 have generated debate about the extent to which lowering or removing financial barriers does, in fact, resolve problems of equity of access to treatment. The data, as various analysts have emphasized, are still sparse and subject to varied interpretations. It is clear that the number of patients entering end-stage renal disease programs since 1972 is vastly greater than the estimates provided in 1967 by the Committee on Chronic Kidney Disease. Analyses of cross-national differences in the prevalance rate of dialysis treatment (home and facility) per million population show that the United States rate is more than 50 per cent higher than in any Western European nation.[34] Data also indicate wide variability in the treatment prevalence rate within the United States.

As Prottas et al. point out, "variations in the prevalence of a treatment modality can be explained in three ways: (1) differences in treatment choices made by medical practitioners; (2) differences in public policy decisions affecting the availability of treatment options; and (3) differences in the incidence of the underlying illnesses, reflecting, among other things, demographic differences in the compared populations."[6] With respect to interstate differences in dialysis treatment rates in the United States, for example, some analysts have found a socioeconomic explanation, attributing the differential rates primarily to the effects of higher treatment rates in areas where the "medical industrial complex" of proprietary dialysis centers are located.[7,8] An alternative analysis of the same data, however, points to basic epidemiological differences in the incidence of end-stage renal disease, and attributes geographic differences in rates of new referrals for dialysis primarily to age and racial characteristics of various populations that may also underlie the causes of this disease.[9] A similar interpretation has also been given to the marked differences in cross-national treatment prevalence rates: "About 50 percent of the difference . . . between [the] American experience and the European maximum can be attributed to differences in the black/white composition of the populations. Most of the remaining difference in rates appears to be due to European policies that prohibit or severely limit access to dialysis by elderly and those potential patients with significant medical complications."[6]

In 1982, some 60,000 United States citizens were receiving dialysis at an estimated cost of $1.8 billion. Many charges and countercharges have been levied about the percentage of this cost—which is far in excess of initial estimates—attributable to fiscal management, ranging from inadequate federal and local institutional controls to fraud.[10,11] But beyond these familiar, recurring problems of responsible management—which are hardly unique to the provision of dialysis—the end-stage renal disease provisions of PL 92-603 embody a rapidly escalating value conflict in our society.

There is a widely shared value in our society that all citizens have a "right" to health care, which should not be abridged by lack of financial resources. Efforts to act on the belief that health care is a right which society, through its government, has a reciprocal responsibility to meet by providing services that are available, accessible, and affordable appear to be on a collision course with escalating concerns about the costs of such care. As "cost containment" becomes a dominant theme in health policy arenas, and the "ethics of cost containment" a leitmotif in biomedical ethics, as people reexamine the "costs and benefits" of chronic dialysis and consider the implications of new technologies such as the first permanent artificial heart implant in December 1982, we hear recurrent and increasingly impassioned references to the same kind of allocation of scarce resources' dilemmas that were generated by the development of chronic dialysis in 1960.

If questions and decisions about the allocation of scarce resources are to be dealt with in more than economic terms, as we would argue they inescapably must be, it is appropriate to end this section by raising questions about the noneconomic effects of PL 92-603 on the recipients and providers of chronic dialysis. As we think back to the intertwined medical, social, and moral issues that surrounded dialysis in the 1960s, such as patient selection, the stresses on physicians and nurses, and the quality of life issues posed for and by dialysis patients, it seems to us that those involved in dialysis in the 1980s are confronted by many of the same problems as their predecessors, albeit sometimes more refined, subtle, and varied forms.

For end-stage renal disease patients, their families, and those who care for them, the option of dialysis continues to pose fundamental value questions that pivot around the "quality of life" issues that are not unique to this mode of treatment but which it frames with special clarity. In the early years of Seattle's dialysis program, one of its physicians reflected that

Doctors now find themselves able from

time to time to enter a gray, limbo-like area where they are able to prolong life without, however, being able to cure the disease or heal the injury . . . The first great anxiety, then, that one faces in approaching the question of hemodialysis is whether from the patient's point of view the whole procedure will turn out to be a blessing or merely a labored and painful hanging on to life."[12]

Though seldom made with equanimity, decisions not to initiate treatment are a facet of their work well known to medical professionals. Faced with the allocation pressures of the 1960s, the selection procedures for dialysis frequently used "medical eligibility" criteria as a first screen, to rule out candidates who, in the clinical judgment of their physician-gatekeepers, would fare so poorly on dialysis that it was not deemed in their best interests to initiate treatment. The financial relief afforded by PL 92-603 made it possible to abandon the use of other, more onerous selection criteria, such as those based on psychosocial judgments about merit or need. At the same time, in part as an understandable reaction against the "playing God" choices they had had to make, physicians also moved away from exercising more medically traditional biomedical critera as well. For they felt that, as expressed by one nephrologist in 1977, "with payment guaranteed under Social Security, there is no way—morally—to turn anyone down anymore."[13]

For medical professionals and others concerned with end-stage renal disease and its treatment, medical-moral questions about whether all candidates *should* receive dialysis now that it is available and affordable are accompanied by concerns about the medical, psychological, and social course of many of their patients. Three major changes in the dialysis population that have occurred since 1972 are increased percentages of patients who are older, of a lower socioeconomic status, or sicker compared to the more selective population of recipients in the 1960s.[14] Not surprisingly, therefore, recent studies of clinical outcomes of chronic dialysis "suggest that a larger proportion of dialysis patients than previously suspected are severely debilitated . . . any discussion of benefits should consider concurrent morbidity and the degree of occupational and physical rehabilitation, as well as the duration of extended life currently being achieved.[14]

These concerns, in turn, have raised afresh,

and on a larger scale, the same intense questions about the quality of life and about decisions to stop treatment that providers and patients and their families have grappled with since chronic dialysis became technologically possible. "Who shall live when not all can live?" "Should all those who can be kept alive live?" These are two faces of the moral and social dilemmas contained in the phrase, "the allocation of scarce resources," that will be increasingly troublesome in a world of finite resources and growing technological capacities in medicine.

References

1. 20th century? N Engl J Med 305:280, 1981. Kintzel J, Silberman H, Cameron EM: Care of the patient with renal failure. In Kintzel KD: Advanced Concepts in Clinical Nursing. 2nd Ed. J. P. Lippincott, Philadelphia, 1977, p 582.

2. Landsman M: The patient with chronic renal failure: A marginal man. Ann Intern Med 82:268, 1975.

3. Swazey JP: The Scribner dialysis shunt: ramifications of a clinical-technological innovation. In Abernathy WJ, Sheldon A, Prahalad CK, Eds: The Management of Health Care. Ballinger Publishing Co., Cambridge, MA, 1974, p. 229.

4. Gottschalk CW: Report of the Committee on Chronic Kidney Disease. Washington, DC: U.S. Government Printing Office.

5. Rettig RA: Valuing lives: the policy debate on patient care financing for victims of end-stage renal disease. Rand Corporation, Washington, D.C., 1976.

6. Prottas JM, Segal M, Sapolsky HM: Cross-national differences in dialysis rates. University Health Policy Consortium DP-39, November 1981.

7. Relman AS: Race and end-stage renal disease. N Engl J Med 306:1290, 1982.

8. Relman AS, Rennie D: Treatment of end-stage renal disease: free but not equal. N Engl J Med 303:996, 1980.

9. Rostand SF, Kirk KA, Rutsky EA, et al: Racial differences in the treatment for end-stage renal disease. N Engl J Med 306:1276, 1982.

10. Prottas JM, Sapolsky HM: Administrative problems in the end-stage renal disease program. University Health Policy Consortium PA-5, November 1981.

11. Robinson D: Kidney dialysis: A taxpayers' nightmare. Readers Digest, October 1982, p. 149.

12. Norton CE: Chronic hemodialysis as a medical and social experiment. Ann Intern Med 66:1267, 1967.

13. McLaughlin L: Self-care dialysis center planned in Boston. Boston Globe, May 18, 1977, p. 50.

14. Gutman RA, Stead WW, Robinson RR: Physical activity and employment status of patients on maintenance dialysis. N Eng J Med 304:309, 1981.

Rationing Intensive Care—Physician Responses to a Resource Shortage

Daniel E. Singer, M.D., Medical Practices Evaluation Unit, Department of Medicine, Massachusetts General Hospital, Boston
Phyllis L. Carr, M.D., Department of Medicine, Boston City Hospital, Boston
Albert G. Mulley, M.D., M.P.P., and **George E. Thibault, M.D.,** both Medical Practices Evaluation Unit, Department of Medicine, Massachusetts General Hospital, Boston

From 1960 to 1980, American health-care expenditures rose an average of 11.7 per cent per year, more rapidly than any other sector of the economy. As a result, the percentage of the gross national product spent on medical care rose from 5.2 per cent in 1960 ($26.9 billion) to 9.4 per cent in 1980 ($247.2 billion).[1] During this period, physician decision making was insulated from cost considerations by the prevailing pattern of third-party reimbursement. It remained possible for American physicians to expend health-care resources on individual patients without constraint so long as there was any hope of benefit.[2,3] The current increased awareness of resource limitations, however, has elicited a variety of strategies for containment of medical costs. One approach would simply limit the supply of health-care resources available to physicians in the hope that they would then allocate these scarce resources more efficiently. In the United States, this has been a largely theoretical strategy.[4] As a result, physician responses to such resource constraints and their consequent health effects have not been studied.

Beginning in July 1981, a shortage of intensive-care-unit nurses at Massachusetts General Hospital produced a severe curtailment in the operational bed capacity of the medical-intensive-care unit. This provided the unusual opportunity to study changes in physician behavior caused by a serious limitation in a highly used, extremely costly resource—medical intensive care. In this study, we have addressed the following questions: Do physicians systematically alter their priorities for ICU admission and transfer when ICU resources become scarce? If so, what are these changes in priorities? and Are there adverse medical consequences of these rationing decisions?

Methods

The ICU Setting
The ICU we studied is an 18-bed combined medical-intensive-care and coronary-care unit. All patients admitted since July 17, 1977, have been included in a computer-based data bank that has

Reprinted, with permission, from *The New England Journal of Medicine* 1983 Nov. 10. 309(19):1155–1160.
Supported by the John A. Hartford Foundation and the Robert Wood-Johnson Foundation.
Drs. Mulley and Singer are Henry J. Kaiser Family Foundation Faculty Scholars in General Internal Medicine. During this study, Dr. Carr was a Henry J. Kaiser Fellow in General Internal Medicine at the Massachusetts General Hospital.

facilitated the detailed description of case mix, interventions, and outcomes.[5]

From 1978 through 1980, the ICU capacity was uniformly 18 beds. Because of a shortage in nursing personnel beginning in July 1981, ICU capacity decreased to between 8 and 14 beds. This reduction in capacity preserved nurse-to-patient ratios.

Physicians' Options in Responding to Decreased ICU Resources

The options available to physicians confronted with unchanged patient volume and case mix but decreased ICU bed availability were as follows: (1) longer queues and waiting times could be allowed in the referral area—usually the emergency ward; (2) potential ICU patients could be transferred to neighboring hospitals for intensive care; (3) intensive care could be completely withheld from some potential ICU patients by sending them directly to the general medical wards; and (4) the amount of intensive care allocated to some patients could be decreased by admitting them to the ICU but transferring them to the wards after shorter ICU stays. The first two options required rationing decisions that were less explicit than did Options 3 and 4. By examining changes in ICU case mix, lengths of stay, and level of diagnostic and therapeutic intervention, we were able to determine the extent to which physicians discriminatingly exercised Options 3 and 4. Furthermore, we could infer which patient and disease characteristics were considered important by physicians in assessing the need for intensive care and in rationing ICU resources.

Data Collection

The following variables were analyzed for each patient: age, sex, admission and discharge diagnoses, number of readmissions to the ICU after initial discharge, ICU and hospital lengths of stay, ICU and hospital mortality rates, place of residence before and after ICU admission, and number of major interventions. Endotracheal intubation, cardioversion, cardiopulmonary resuscitation, pulmonary-artery line placement, arterial line placement, emergency pacemaker insertion, peritoneal dialysis, hemodialysis, and transfusion of six or more units of blood were considered major interventions.

Most of our comparisons were between the period of greatest constraint, July through December 1981 (hereafter referred to as "1981"), with the most recent comparable period of full capacity, July through December 1980 (hereafter referred to as "1980"). In addition, severity of illness, and rate of confirmed myocardial infarction were analyzed as a function of bed capacity rather than of time period. In these latter analyses, admissions from January and February 1982 were added to increase the amount of data on the relatively higher bed capacities of 12 and 14. Data from 1980 provided the results for the 18-bed capacity.

The emergency-ward log was used to identify patients with chest pain who were admitted directly to the wards. For these patients, individual patient records were reviewed to determine whether the patient had a myocardial infarction or a complication prompting subsequent admission to the ICU, or died. Three records (of 47) of such patients in 1980 and 3 (of 122) in 1981 could not be traced. These patients were excluded from the analysis. ICU occupancy was the proportion of operational bed-days occupied by patients over the six-month period. Availability was the proportion of days when one or more beds were open at the midnight census.

Statistical Analysis

P values for comparisons between 1980 and 1981 were generated by the paired t-test or Wilcoxon signed-rank test for comparisons between continuous variables and by the chi-square test for proportions. For the comparison of the number of interventions per patient, the method for analyzing incidence-density data was applied.[6] Tests of linear trend used the method of Armitage.[7] For the number of interventions per patient, this test of trend was adapted for a Poisson distribution. The confidence-interval calculation used Miettinen's test-based method.[8]

The sensitivity of physicians' diagnoses of myocardial infarction among patients with chest pain who were admitted to the hospital is measured by the proportion of patients with subsequently confirmed myocardial infarction who were admitted to the ICU. Specificity is measured by the proportion of patients with chest pain without subsequently confirmed myocardial infarction who were admitted directly to the general medical wards. Physician diagnostic accuracy in the assignment of patients with chest pain is determined by adding the number of patients with subsequently confirmed myocardial infarction who were admitted to the ICU, to the number of patients without subsequently confirmed myocardial infarction who were admitted to the wards and dividing by the total number of patients with chest pain.

Results

The Resource Constraint

Between 1980 and 1981 the occupancy rate (the average percentage of usable beds occupied) increased from 77 to 90 percent, whereas bed availability (the percentage of time during which at least one ICU bed was available) decreased from 95 to 55 percent. These restrictions forced physicians to reduce the number of ICU admissions (Table 1). Some patients who in previous years would have received ICU care were excluded from such care in 1981. The bases of these rationing decisions are explored below.

Rationing by Severity of Illness

In the ICU, one broad measure of severity of illness is the average number of major interventions per patient. This increased from 0.49 in 1980 to 0.61 in 1981 ($P < 0.01$). A somewhat different measure is the proportion of patients who received at least one major intervention. This rose as well, from 0.33 (240 of 734) in 1980 to 0.39 (225 of 570) in 1981 ($P < 0.001$).

A limited number of clinical problems accounts for the admission of a majority of patients to the medical ICU (Table 2). Each category has an associated clinical feature that provides a reasonable measure of severity of illness. Among patients admitted with precordial pain, the rate of confirmed myocardial infarction increased in 1981. Among patients with cardiac or pulmonary respiratory distress, the percentage requiring intubation increased from 34 per cent in 1980 to 43 per cent in 1981. Among patients with coma, the rate of intubation also rose from 51 per cent

Table 2. Severity of Illness in Patients Admitted to the ICU before (1980) and during (1981) the Bed Shortage, according to Clinical Subgroup

Clinical Subgroup*	1980†	1981†	Significance
Precordial pain			
% of all ICU admissions	34	36	
% of patients with precordial pain who sustained MI	31 (77/248)	43 (88/203)	P < 0.01
Respiratory distress			
% of all ICU admissions	17	18	
% of patients with respiratory distress who were intubated	34 (46/132)	43 (44/102)	0.25 > P > 0.10
Coma (including drug overdose)			
% of all ICU admissions	6.3	5.9	
% of patients with coma who were intubated	51 (24/47)	71 (24/34)	0.10 > P > 0.05
Gastrointestinal bleeding			
% of all ICU admissions	3.0	3.5	
% of patients with gastrointestinal bleeding needing transfusion of ≥ 6 units	36 (8/22)	50 (10/20)	0.5 > P > 0.25

*Categories are mutually exclusive and represent the primary admitting diagnosis. ICU denotes intensive-care unit, and MI myocardial infraction.

†July through December of 1980 and July through December of 1981.

in 1980 to 71 per cent in 1981. Similarly, among patients admitted for gastrointestinal bleeding, the percentage requiring a transfusion of six or more units of blood increased from 36 to 50 per cent. Although these differences were not consistently significant statistically, they all followed a similar trend toward increasing severity of illness among patients admitted to the ICU in 1981.

Finally, we can view severity of illness (measured by the average number of interventions per patient) as a function of bed capacity (Fig. 1). Increased operational bed capacity was associated with admission to the ICU of patients who were less severely ill. The low number of interventions per patient when capacity reached 14 beds may indicate that physicians conditioned to shortages rapidly readjusted their ICU admission criteria as bed capacity re-expanded.

Patients with Chest Pain

Physicians' rationing strategies were revealed in their responses to patients who presented with chest pain suggestive of myocardial infarction. These patients are usually admitted to the ICU because of the risk of major complications rather than because of the actual complications themselves. The purpose of ICU admission in such

Table 1. Effects of the Decrease in Intensive-Care-Unit (ICU) Bed Capacity

	July through December 1980	July through December 1981
Average daily bed capacity (range)	18 (18)	11.4 (8 to 14)*
ICU admissions per month	122	95†
Average occupancy (%)	77	90*
Average bed availability (%)	95	55*

*$p < 0.001$ as compared with the value for 1980.
†$p < 0.05$ as compared with the value for 1980.

Figure 1. The Severity of Illness of Patients Admitted to the Intensive-Care Unit (ICU) during Periods of Different ICU Bed Capacity (Measured by Number of Interventions per Patient) ($P < 0.01$ by Test of Trend).

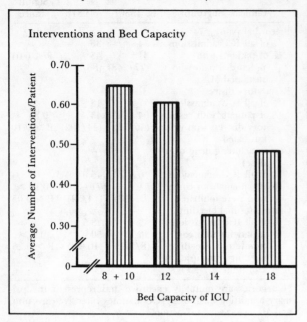

Interventions are defined in Methods. Bed Capacities of 8 and 10 are combined because of the relatively few days with a bed capacity of 8 (only 13 days).

cases is to permit intensive monitoring for incipient complications and then the rapid initiation of therapy if needed. The percentage of patients admitted to the hospital with chest pain who were admitted to the ICU fell from 85 per cent in 1980 (248 of 292) to 63 per cent in 1981 (203 of 322) ($P < 0.001$) (Table 3). As physicians became more selective in admitting patients with chest pain to the ICU, the proportion of patients admitted to the unit who actually sustained a myocardial infarction increased from 31 to 43 per cent ($P < 0.01$). This increase was accompanied by an increase in the rate of myocardial infarction among patients with chest pain who were admitted directly to the wards: 4.5 per cent in 1980, as compared with 8.4 per cent in 1981 ($P > 0.10$). Physicians increased the specificity of their ICU admission decisions (from 20 to 49 per cent) with a smaller decrease in sensitivity (from 97 to 90 per cent). Overall, physician diagnostic accuracy in these patients with chest pain increased from 41 per cent in 1980 to 62 per cent in 1981 ($P < 0.001$).

When these data were analyzed according to bed capacity, the same pattern was seen in greater detail (Fig. 2). When the operational capacity was 18 beds, 31 per cent of the patients with chest pain who were admitted to the ICU sustained a myocardial infarction. This figure rose to 45 per cent at lower bed capacities ($P < 0.05$ by test of trend).

We used subsequent transfer from the general medical wards to the ICU as a gross measure of morbidity. Nine of the patients with chest pain (three with myocardial infarction and six without) who were sent first to the wards in 1981 subsequently required ICU admission, as compared with one (with myocardial infarction) in 1980. However, none of the patients with chest pain

Table 3. Physicians' Decisions about ICU Admission in Patients with Chest Pain before (1980) and during (1981) the Bed Shortage

| | Myocardial Infarction | Admitted to | |
		ICU	General Wards
1980*	Yes	77	2
	No	171	42
		248	44
1981*	Yes	88	10
	No	115	109
		203	119

*1980 and 1981 refer to July through December of each year.

Figure 2. The Proportion of Patients with Precordial Pain Admitted to the ICU Who Actually Sustained a Myocardial Infarction (MI), Plotted as a Function of Bed Capacity ($P < 0.05$ by Test of Trend).

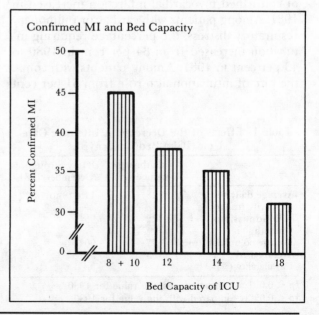

who required subsequent ICU admission died. Mortality among patients with chest pain who were admitted directly to the wards was similar in both years—2 of 44 (4.5 per cent) in 1980 as compared with 3 of 119 (2.5 per cent) in 1981 (90 per cent confidence interval for the difference in rates, −7 per cent to +3 per cent). None of the patients who died had a myocardial infarction, and none had been transferred to the ICU before death. Four of the five (including all three in 1981) were clearly perceived by their physicians as having end-stage disease that would not benefit from further therapeutic interventions.

Decreased Length of Stay

In addition to maintaining stricter criteria for ICU admission, physicians can further ration intensive care by transferring patients after shorter lengths of stay. Our data reveal that this in fact occurred. The mean length of stay in the ICU among all patients admitted to the unit fell from 3.5 days in 1980 to 3.3 days in 1981 (not significant). Because the distribution of lengths of stay was skewed, it may be better analyzed as a dichotomous variable. The proportion of patients transferred out of the ICU in less than three days was 55 per cent in 1980 and rose to 61 per cent in 1981 ($P < 0.05$, Table 4). The difference was statistically more evident among patients who were admitted primarily for monitoring—i.e., who did not receive any major interventions; 77 per cent in 1981 were transferred out in less than three days as compared with 67 per cent in 1980 ($P < 0.01$). However, even among those requiring major interventions, the trend was toward earlier transfer: 37 per cent in less than three days in 1981 versus 30 per cent in 1980 ($P < 0.10$). The decrease in ICU length of stay did not result in measurable severe medical consequences. There

was a small increase, from 6 to 8 per cent ($P < 0.10$), in complications after transfer from the ICU that led to an increase in readmission to the unit. Mortality both during and after ICU stay was constant at 10 per cent and 5 per cent, respectively, in both years.

Nonsurvivors

A controversial approach to rationing would be to withdraw care from hopelessly ill patients. Any consistent tactic of this sort should be reflected in a decreased ICU length of stay for nonsurvivors. For all patients admitted to the ICU who eventually died during the hospitalization, the mean ICU length of stay was 6.1 days in 1980 and rose to 6.2 days in 1981. The proportion of such patients whose ICU stay was less than three days was 42 per cent in both years. In contrast, 64 per cent of survivors in 1981 were transferred out of the ICU in less than three days, as compared with 57 per cent in 1980 ($P < 0.05$, Table 4). Among patients who died after ICU transfer, nine died within three days of transfer in 1980, as compared with 11 in 1981.

Other Potential Bases for Rationing

Although physicians systematically chose the more severely ill patients for admission to the ICU in 1981, there was no apparent age discrimination. The mean age was virtually the same in both years (62 vs. 61), and there was no change in the percentage of patients older than 80 or 90. However, fewer patients were admitted from other chronic-care facilities, such as nursing homes—2 per cent in 1981, and 4 per cent in 1980 ($P < 0.10$)—suggesting that physicians may have considered social or functional criteria in their admission policy.

Discussion

In recent years, rising costs have forced a review of health-care policy to identify strategies for more efficient care. Among the strategies that have been considered is some form of planned rationing of health services[3]—that is, some limitation in the use of a potentially beneficial resource because of cost.

There are two broad strategies for rationing healthcare resources. Limits can simply be set on the resources available for health care (primary rationing), or in addition, detailed regulations for the distribution of health services for individual patients can be established (secondary ration-

Table 4. Percentages of Patients Staying in the ICU for Less than Three Days before (1980) and during (1981) the Bed Shortage*

	1980 %	1981 %	Significance
All patients	55	61	$P < 0.05$
Patients primarily being monitored	67	77	$P < 0.01$
Patients who received major interventions	30	37	$0.10 > P > 0.05$
ICU patients who died in the hospital	42	42	
ICU patients who survived to hospital discharge	57	64	$P < 0.05$

*1980 and 1981 refer to July through December of each year.

ing).[3,9] The former policy has the advantage of distancing the administrative agent from the many thorny decisions about health-care distribution and dispersing the responsibility for these decisions among numerous physicians and patients.[10]

The curtailment of services due to a shortage of nurses in our study ICU provided the unusual opportunity to assess physician responses to limits on primary resources. In effect, the nursing shortage produced a model of primary rationing. The decrease in the number of operational ICU beds produced a marked decrease in the bed-availability rate and an overall fall in the number of ICU admissions of 22 per cent. Physicians could have responded by simply restricting ICU admissions on a first-come-first-served basis while preserving previous thresholds for admission and length of stay. Instead, without explicit administrative rules guiding use of the ICU, physicians were able to adjust their ICU admission and discharge decisions to achieve more efficient use of the scarcer resources.

The nature of the change in physician priorities was perhaps best revealed in the subgroup of patients admitted with chest pain suggestive of myocardial infarction. Such patients constitute 35 per cent of all admissions to our medical ICU and are the major subgroup of patients admitted to coronary-care units. Although such patients are routinely admitted to coronary-care units, many are not severely ill at the time of admission. In essence, two levels of monitoring are applied to these patients. The first is the repeated testing in the ICU to determine whether they are sustaining a myocardial infarction. If they are not, they are at very low risk for short-term complications.[11] The second is the monitoring of those who have in fact had a myocardial infarction. Most of these patients also have an uncomplicated course; relatively few have complications that are reversible only by ICU care. Some clinicians have suggested that even this second level of monitoring is excessive, that intensive care is not necessary for apparently uncomplicated myocardial infarction.[12] A more widely accepted view is that the first level of monitoring should be applied more selectively—that is, that fewer patients without myocardial infarctions should be admitted to the ICU. Indeed, several statistical algorithms have been developed to help achieve this goal.[13,14] Under the pressure of bed constraints and without using any explicit algorithm, physicians in our study successfully increased the accuracy of their ICU-admission decisions. They increased the percentage of patients admitted to the ICU with chest pain who had myocardial infarctions by 12 per cent, while increasing the percentage of patients with myocardial infarctions who were admitted directly to ward care by only 4 per cent. None of the patients with myocardial infarction who were admitted directly to the wards died. Although deaths did occur among patients with chest pain who were sent first to the wards, they appeared to be the result of terminal chronic conditions. The number of such deaths was similar in both 1980 and 1981.

Monitoring is also the principal function of intensive care during the final day or two before transfer to the general medical floor. This period of observation assures the physician that the patient's condition is stable. It can be shortened to allow more patients admission to the ICU. By shortening it, physicians accept the greater risk involved in observing patients outside the ICU. In return they can accommodate new patients with illness that is more acute. We had expected that shortening of the length of stay in the ICU would be applied more selectively to the group of patients who were less severely ill. In fact, the ICU length of stay was shortened in all patients, including the severely ill (those requiring major interventions).

The dominant strategy that physicians used to cope with decreased bed availability in the ICU was to restrict its use for monitoring purposes. Although this strategy may be intuitively appealing, it is worth noting that it is not necessarily the optimal use of the ICU. There are patients with manifest critical illness who are admitted to ICUs whose outcomes are not affected by intensive care. Conversely, there are patients who are admitted solely for monitoring in whom complications develop that are reversed only because they are in an ICU. The problem is that physicians cannot feel certain about the marginal benefit of ICU care for any patient. As a result, they appear to ration ICU beds on the basis of immediate need rather than of ultimate benefit. This approach appears to extend to the care of the dying patient. Among patients admitted to the ICU who subsequently die, there are some whose fate seems unavoidable well before their actual death. We attempted to determine whether physicians withdrew ICU care from these hopelessly ill patients during the period of limited ICU resources. Although we could not specifically identify such patients among our study population, we could make some inferences from our data. If earlier withdrawal of care from dying patients generally occurred, then the length of stay of dying patients in the ICU should have decreased. In fact, in contrast to the shortening of length of stay seen among surviving patients, the length of stay in the ICU of patients who died in the hospital remained the same. Physicians appeared to be reluctant to conserve resources by withdrawing care from acutely ill patients even when the anticipated benefit of that care was vanishingly small.

In sum, physicians responded to decreased ICU resources by curtailing the monitoring function of the ICU. Our data suggest that this strategy led to little or no increase in measurable adverse medical consequences. What was initially perceived as a clear sacrifice of patient care evolved to become a more efficient, although perhaps not optimal, allocation of scarce ICU resources. It is uncertain whether our results can be generalized to apply to ICUs in other hospitals. Comparisons among hospitals are confounded by differences in severity of illness. However, monitoring or observation as the main indication for intensive care is widespread among both medical and nonmedical ICUs.[15] More sparing use of this monitoring function should produce increased efficiency in intensive care.

Our results suggest that moderate resource limitations can encourage more efficient use of intensive care. However, these results should not be viewed as a blanket endorsement of primary rationing of healthcare resources. Simply to restrict resources like ICU beds without providing guidelines for their use is to flirt with two potential dangers. The first is that physicians may not know which patients will benefit most by ICU care. Their triage decisions would be greatly assisted by the availability of rules for assessing a patient's risk on a daily basis. The formulation of such rules for patients in the ICU is currently an area of active research.[16] The second danger is that the allocation of resources may be inequitable. In the absence of explicit guidelines, socioeconomic status and other nonmedical features may affect allocation decisions.[3,9,10,17,18] Any attempt to apply a policy of primary rationing must carefully consider these problems of information and equity.

The authors are indebted to G. Octo Barnett, M.D., and Susan A. Stickler of the Laboratory of Computer Science, Massachusetts General Hospital, for their steadfast support with data management and analysis; to Patricia A. Kelleher, R.N., for research assistance and careful review of the data; to Dr. E. Francis Cook for statistical advice; to Carol A. Scola and Corinne L. CaraDonna for assistance in the preparation of the manuscript; and to Drs. Britain W. Nicholson and Carol L. Smith for critical review of the original manuscript.

References

1. Health, United States: 1981. Hyattsville, Md.: Public Health Service, 1981. (DHHS publication no. (PHS)82-1232).

2. Russell LB. Technology in hospitals. Washington D.C.: The Brookings Institution, 1979.

3. Fuchs VR. The growing demand for medical care. N Engl J Med 1968; 279:190–5.

4. Mechanic D. Approaches to controlling the costs of medical care: shortrange and long-range alternatives. N Engl J Med 1978; 298:249–54.

5. Thibault GE, Mulley AG, Barnett GO, et al. Medical intensive care: indications, interventions, and outcomes. N Engl J Med 1980; 302:938–42.

6. Kleinbaum DG, Kupper LL, Morgenstern H. Epidemiologic research: principles and quantitative methods. Belmont, Calif.: Lifetime Learning Publications, 1982:283–311.

7. Armitage P. Statistical methods in medical research. New York: John Wiley, 1971:363.

8. Rothman KJ, Boice JD Jr. Epidemiologic analysis with a programmable calculator. Washington, D.C.: Department of Health, Education, and Welfare, 1979:11. (DHEW publication no. (NIH)79-1649).

9. Calabresi G, Bobbitt P. Tragic choices. New York: WW Norton, 1978.

10. Blumstein J. Rationing medical resources: a constitutional, legal, and policy analysis. Texas Law Rev 1981; 59:1345–400.

11. Mulley AG, Thibault GE, Hughes RA, Barnett GO, Reder VA, Sherman EL. The course of patients with suspected myocardial infarction: the identification of low-risk patients for early transfer from intensive care. N Engl J Med 1980; 302:943–8.

12. Hill JD, Hampton JR, Mitchell JRA. A randomised trial of home-versus-hospital management for patients with suspected myocardial infarction. Lancet 1978; 1:837–41.

13. Pozen MW, D'Agostino RB, Mitchell JB, et al. The usefulness of a predictive instrument to reduce inappropriate admissions to the coronary care unit. Ann Intern Med 1980; 92:238–42.

14. Goldman L, Weinberg M, Weisberg M, et al. A computer-derived protocol to aid in the diagnosis of emergency room patients with acute chest pain. N Engl J Med 1982; 307:588–96.

15. Knaus WA, Wagner DP, Draper EA, Lawrence DE, Zimmerman JE. The range of intensive care services today. JAMA 1981; 246:2711–6.

16. Madsen EB, Hougaard P, Gilpin E, Pedersen A. The length of hospitalization after acute myocardial infarction determined by risk calculation. Circulation 1983; 68:9–16.

17. Mechanic D. The growth of medical technology and bureaucracy: implications for medical care. Milbank Mem Fund Q 1977; 55:61–78.

18. Mulley AG. The allocation of resources for medical intensive care. In: Securing access to health care. Vol. 3. Washington, D.C.: The President's Commission for the Study of Ethical Problems in Medicine and Biomedical and Behavioral Research, 1983:285–311.

Who Shall Live When Not All Can Live?

James F. Childress, Ph.D., Departments of Religious Studies and Medical Education, University of Virginia, Charlottesville

Who shall live when not all can live? Although this question has been urgently forced upon us by the dramatic use of artificial internal organs and organ transplantations, it is hardly new. George Bernard Shaw dealt with it in *The Doctor's Dilemma:*

Sir Patrick: Well, Mr. Savior of Lives: which is it to be? that honest decent man Blenkinsop, or that rotten blackguard of an artist, eh?
Ridgeon: It's not an easy case to judge, is it? Blenkinsop's an honest decent man; but is he any use? Dubedat's a rotten blackguard; but he's a genuine source of pretty and pleasant and good things.
Sir Patrick: What will he be a source of for that poor innocent wife of his, when she finds him out?
Ridgeon: That's true. Her life will be a hell.
Sir Patrick: And tell me this. Suppose you had this choice put before you: either to go through life and find all the pictures bad but all the men and women good, or go through life and find all the pictures good and all the men and women rotten. Which would you choose?[1]

A significant example of the distribution of scarce medical resources is seen in the use of penicillin shortly after its discovery. Military officers had to determine which soldiers would be treated—those with venereal disease or those wounded in combat.[2] In many respects such decisions have become routine in medical circles. Day after day physicians and others make judgments and decisions "about allocations of medical care to various segments of our population, to various types of hospitalized patients, and to specific individuals,"[3] for example, whether mental illness or cancer will receive the higher proportion of available funds. Nevertheless, the dramatic forms of "Scarce Life-Saving Medical Resources" (hereafter abbreviated as SLMR) such as hemodialysis and kidney and heart transplants have compelled us to examine the moral questions that have been concealed in many routine decisions. I shall not attempt in this chapter to show how a resolution of SLMR cases can help us in the more routine ones that do not involve a conflict of life with life. Rather I shall develop an argument for a particular method of determining who shall live when not all can live. No conclusions are implied about criteria and procedures for determining who shall receive med-

Reprinted, with permission, from *Soundings* 1970 Winter. 53:339–355.

ical resources that are not directly related to the preservation of life (e.g., corneal transplants) or about standards for allocating money and time for studying and treating certain diseases.

Just as current SLMR decisions are not totally discontinuous with other medical decisions, so we must ask whether some other cases might, at least by analogy, help us develop the needed criteria and procedures. Some have looked at the principles at work in our responses to abortion, euthanasia, and artificial insemination.[4] Usually they have concluded that these cases do not cast light on the selection of patients for artificial and transplanted organs. The reason is evident: in abortion, euthanasia, and artificial insemination, there is no conflict of life with life for limited but indispensable resources (with the possible exception of therapeutic abortion). In current SLMR decisions, such a conflict is inescapable, and it makes them morally perplexing and fascinating. If analogous cases are to be found, I think that we shall locate them in moral conflict situations.

Analogous Conflict Situations

An especially interesting and pertinent one is *U.S. v. Holmes.*[5] In 1841 an American ship, the *William Brown*, which was near Newfoundland on a trip from Liverpool to Philadelphia, struck an iceberg. The crew and half the passengers were able to escape in the two available vessels. One of these, a longboat, carrying too many passengers and leaking seriously, began to founder in the turbulent sea after about twenty-four hours. In a desperate attempt to keep it from sinking, the crew threw overboard fourteen men. Two sisters of one of the men either jumped overboard to join their brother in death or instructed the crew to throw them over. The criteria for determining who should live were "not to part man and wife, and not to throw over any woman." Several hours later the others were rescued. Returning to Philadelphia, most of the crew disappeared, but one, Holmes, who had acted upon orders from the mate, was indicted, tried, and convicted on the charge of "unlawful homicide."

We are interested in this case from a moral rather than a legal standpoint, and there are several possible responses to and judgments about it. The judge contended that lots should have been cast, for in such conflict situations, there is no other procedure "so consonant both to humanity and to justice." Counsel for Holmes, on the other hand, maintained that the "sailors adopted the only principle of selection which was possible in an emergency like theirs,—a principle more humane than lots."

Another version of selection might extend and systematize the maxims of the sailors in the direction of "utility"; those are saved who will contribute to the greatest good for the greatest number. Yet another possible option is defended by Edmond Cahn in *The Moral Decision.* He argues that in this case we encounter the "morals of the last days." By this phrase he indicates that an apocalyptic crisis renders totally irrelevant the normal differences between individuals. He continues,

> In a strait of this extremity, all men are reduced—or raised, as one may choose to denominate it—to members of the genus, mere congeners and nothing else. Truly and literally, all were "in the same boat," and thus none could be saved separately from the others. I am driven to conclude that otherwise—that is, if none sacrifice themselves of free will to spare the others—they must all wait and die together. For where all have become congeners, pure and simple, no one can save himself by killing another.[6]

Cahn's answer to the question "who shall live when not all can live" is "none" unless the voluntary sacrifice by some persons permits it.

Few would deny the importance of Cahn's approach, although many, including this writer, would suggest that it is relevant mainly as an affirmation of an elevated and, indeed, heroic or saintly morality that one hopes would find expression in the voluntary actions of many persons trapped in "borderline" situations involving a conflict of life with life. It is a maximal demand that some moral principles impose on the individual in the recognition that self-preservation is not a good that is to be defended at all costs. The absence of this saintly or heroic morality should not mean, however, that everyone perishes. Without making survival an absolute value and without justifying all means to achieve it, we can maintain that simply letting everyone die is irresponsible. This charge can be supported from several different standpoints, including society at large as well as the individuals involved. Among a group of self-interested individuals, none of whom volunteers to relinquish his life, there may be better and worse ways of determining who shall survive. One task of social ethics, whether religious or philosophical, is to propose relatively just institutional arrangements within which self-interested and biased men can live. The question then becomes: which set of arrangements—which criteria and procedures of selection—is most satisfactory in view of the human condition (man's limited altruism and inclination to seek his own good) and the conflicting values that are to be realized?

There are several significant differences between the *Holmes* and SLMR cases, a major one being that the former involves *direct* killing of another person, while the latter involve only *permitting* a person to die when it is not possible to save all. Furthermore, in extreme situations such as *Holmes,* the restraints of civilization have been stripped away, and something approximating a state of nature prevails, in which life is "solitary, poor, nasty, brutish and short." The state of nature does not mean that moral standards are irrelevant and that might should prevail, but it does suggest that much of the matrix that normally supports morality has been removed. Also, the necessary but unfortunate decisions about who shall live and die are made by men who are existentially and personally involved in the outcome. Their survival too is at stake. Even though the institutional role of sailors seems to require greater sacrificial actions, there is obviously no assurance that they will adequately assess the number of sailors required to man the vessel or that they will impartially and objectively weigh the common good at stake. As the judge insisted in his defense of casting lots in the *Holmes* case: "In no other than this [casting lots] or some like way are those having equal rights put upon an equal footing, and in no other way is it possible to guard against partiality and oppression, violence, and conflict." This difference should not be exaggerated, since self-interest, professional pride, and the like obviously affect the outcome of many medical decisions. Nor do the remaining differences cancel *Holmes's* instructiveness.

Criteria of Selection for SLMR

Which set of arrangements should be adopted for SLMR? Two questions are involved: Which standards and criteria should be used? and, Who should make the decision? The first question is basic, since the debate about implementation, e.g., whether by a lay committee or physician, makes little progress until the criteria are determined.

We need two sets of criteria, which will be applied at two different stages in the selection of recipients of SLMR. First, medical criteria should be used to exclude those who are not "medically acceptable." Second, from this group of "medically acceptable" applicants, the final selection can be made. Occasionally in current American medical practice, the first stage is omitted, but such an omission is unwarranted. Ethical and social responsibility would seem to require distributing these SLMR only to those who have some reasonable prospect of responding to the treatment. Furthermore, in transplants such medical tests as tissue and blood typing are necessary, although they are hardly fully developed.

"Medical acceptability" is not as easily determined as many nonphysicians assume, since there is considerable debate in medical circles about the relevant factors (e.g., age and complicating diseases). Although ethicists can contribute little or nothing to this debate, two proposals may be in order. First, "medical acceptability" should be used only to determine the group from which the final selection will be made, and the attempt to establish fine degrees of prospective response to treatment should be avoided. Medical criteria, then, would exclude some applicants but would not serve as a basis of comparison between those who pass the first stage. For example, if two applicants for dialysis were medically acceptable, the physicians would *not* choose the one with the *better* medical prospects. Final selection would be made on other grounds. Second, psychological and environmental factors should be kept to an absolute minimum and should be considered only when they are without doubt critically related to medical acceptability (e.g., the inability to cope with the requirements of dialysis, which might lead to suicide).[7]

The most significant moral questions emerge when we turn to the final selection. Once the pool of medically acceptable applicants has been defined and still the number is larger than the resources, what other criteria should be used? How should the final selection be made? First, I shall examine some of the difficulties that stem from efforts to make the final selection in terms of social value; these difficulties raise serious doubts about the feasibility and justifiability of the utilitarian approach. Then I shall consider the possible justification for random selection or chance.

Occasionally criteria of social worth focus on past contributions, but most often they are primarily future-oriented. The patient's potential and probable contribution to the society is stressed, although this obviously cannot be abstracted from his present web of relationships (e.g., dependents) and occupational activities (e.g., nuclear physicist). Indeed, the magnitude of his contribution to society (as an abstraction) is measured in terms of these social roles, relations, and functions. Enough has already been said to suggest the tremendous range of factors that affect social value or worth. (I am excluding from consideration the question of the ability to pay, because most of the people involved have to secure funds from other sources, public or private, anyway. Legislation in 1972 provided payment for most persons who need kidney dialysis or transplantation.) Here we encounter the first major difficulty of this approach: How do we determine the relevant criteria of social value?

The difficulties of quantifying various social needs are only too obvious. How does one quantify and compare the needs of the spirit (e.g., education, art, religion), political life, economic activity, technological development? Joseph Fletcher suggests that "some day we may learn how to 'quantify' or 'mathematicate' or 'computerize' the value problem in selection, in the same careful and thorough way that diagnosis has been."[8] I am not convinced that we can ever quantify values, or that we should attempt to do so. But even if the various social and human needs, in principle, could be quantified, how do we determine how much weight we will give to each one? Which will have priority in case of conflict? Or even more basically, in the light of which values and principles do we recognize social "needs"?

One possible way of determining the values that should be emphasized in selection has been proposed by Leo Shatin.[9] He insists that our medical decisions about allocating resources are already based on an unconscious scale of values (usually dominated by material worth). Since there is really no way of escaping this, we should be self-conscious and critical about it. How should we proceed? He recommends that we discover the values that most people in our society hold and then use them as criteria for distributing SLMR. These values can be discovered by attitude or opinion surveys. Presumably if 51 percent in this testing period put a greater premium on military needs than technological development, military men would have a greater claim on our SLMR than experimental researchers. But valuations of what is significant change, and the student revolutionary who was denied SLMR in 1970 might be celebrated in 1990 as the greatest American hero since George Washington.

Shatin presumably is seeking criteria that could be applied nationally, but at the present, regional and local as well as individual prejudices tincture the criteria of social value that are used in selection. Nowhere is this more evident than in the deliberations and decisions of the anonymous selection committee of the Seattle Artificial Kidney Center, where such factors as church membership and Scout leadership have been deemed significant for determining who shall live.[10] As two critics conclude after examining these criteria and procedures, they rule out "creative nonconformists, who rub the bourgeoisie the wrong way but who historically have contributed so much to the making of America. The Pacific Northwest is no place for a Henry David Thoreau with bad kidneys."[11]

Closely connected to this first problem of determining social value is a second one. Not only is it difficult if not impossible to reach agreement on social value, but it is also rarely easy to predict what our needs will be in a few years and what the consequences of present actions will be. Furthermore it is difficult to predict which persons will fulfill their potential function in society. Admissions committees in colleges and universities experience the frustrations of predicting realization of potential. For these reasons, as someone has indicated, God might be a utilitarian, but we cannot be. We simply lack the capacity to predict very accurately the consequences which we then must evaluate. Our incapacity is never more evident than when we think in societal terms.

Other difficulties make us even less confident that such an approach to SLMR is advisable. Many critics raise the specter of abuse, but this should not be overemphasized. The fundamental difficulty appears on another level: the utilitarian approach would in effect reduce the person to his social role, relations, and functions. Ultimately it dulls and perhaps even eliminates the sense of the person's transcendence, his dignity as a person that cannot be reduced to his past or future contribution to society. It is not at all clear that we are willing to live with these implications of utilitarian selection. Wilhelm Kolff, who invented the artificial kidney, has asked: "Do we really subscribe to the principle that social standing should determine selection? Do we allow patients to be treated with dialysis only when they are married, go to church, have children, have a job, a good income and give to the Community Chest?"[12]

The German theologian Helmut Thielicke contends that any search for "objective criteria" for selection is already a capitulation to the utilitarian point of view which violates man's dignity.[13] The solution is not to let all die, but to recognize that SLMR cases are "borderline situations" which inevitably involve guilt. The agent, however, can have courage and freedom (which, for Thielicke, come from justification by faith) and can

> go ahead anyway and seek for criteria for deciding the question of life or death in the matter of the artificial kidney. Since these criteria are . . . questionable, necessarily alien to the meaning of human existence, the decision to which they lead can be little more than that arrived at by casting lots.[14]

The resulting criteria, he suggests, will probably be very similar to those already employed in American medical practice.

He is most concerned to preserve a certain *attitude* or *disposition* in SLMR—the sense of guilt that arises when man's dignity is violated. With this sense of guilt, the agent remains "sound and healthy where it really counts."[15] Thielicke uses man's dignity only as a judgmental, critical, and negative standard. It only tells us how all selection criteria and procedures (and even the refusal to act) implicate us in the ambiguity of the human condition and its metaphysical guilt. This approach is consistent with his view of the task of theological ethics: "to teach us how to understand and endure—not 'solve'—the borderline situation."[16] But ethics, I would contend, can help us discern the factors and norms in whose light relative, discriminate judgments can be made. Even if all actions in SLMR should involve guilt, some may preserve human dignity to a greater extent than others. Thielicke recognizes that a decision based on any criteria is "little more than that arrived at by casting lots." But perhaps selection by chance would come the closest to embodying the moral and nonmoral values that we are trying to maintain (including a sense of man's dignity).

The Values of Random Selection

My proposal is that we use some form of randomness or chance (either natural, such as "first come, first served," or artificial, such as a lottery) to determine who shall be saved. Many reject randomness as a surrender to nonrationality when responsible and rational judgments can and must be made. Edmond Cahn criticizes "Holmes' judge" who recommended the casting of lots because, as Cahn puts it, "the crisis involves stakes too high for gambling and responsibilities too deep for destiny."[17] Similarly, other critics see randomness as a surrender to "non-human" forces which necessarily vitiates human values. Sometimes these values are identified with the process of decision-making (e.g., it is important to have persons rather than impersonal forces determining who shall live). Sometimes they are identified with the outcome of the process (e.g., the features such as creativity and fullness of being that make human life what it is are to be considered and respected in the decision). Regarding the former, it must be admitted that the use of chance seems cold and impersonal. But presumably the defenders of utilitarian criteria in SLMR want to make their application as objective and impersonal as possible so that subjective bias does not determine who shall live.

Such criticisms, however, ignore the moral and nonmoral values that might be supported by selection by randomness or chance. A more important criticism is that the procedure that I develop draws the relevant moral context too narrowly. That context, so the argument might run, includes the society and its future and not merely the individual with his illness and claim upon SLMR. But my contention is that the values and principles at work in the narrower context may well take precedence over those operative in the broader context, both because of their weight and significance and because of the weaknesses of selection in terms of social worth. As Paul Freund rightly insists, "The more nearly total is the estimate to be made of an individual, and the more nearly the consequence determines life and death, the more unfit the judgment becomes for human reckoning. . . . Randomness as a moral principle deserves serious study."[18] Serious study would, I think, point toward its implementation in certain conflict situations, primarily because it preserves a significant degree of *personal dignity* by providing *equality* of opportunity. Thus it cannot be dismissed as a "nonrational" and "non-human" procedure without an inquiry into the reasons, including human values, which might justify it. Paul Ramsey stresses this point about the *Holmes* case:

> Instead of fixing our attention upon

"gambling" as the solution—with all the frivolous and often corrupt associations the word raises in our minds—we should think rather of *equality* of opportunity as the ethical substance of the relations of those individuals to one another that might have been guarded and expressed by casting lots.[19]

The individual's personal and transcendent dignity, which on the utilitarian approach would be submerged in his social role and function, can be protected and witnessed to by a recognition of his equal right to be saved. Such a right is best preserved by procedures which establish equality of opportunity. Thus selection by chance more closely approximates the requirements established by human dignity than does utilitarian calculation. It is not infallibly just, but it is preferable to the alternatives of letting all die or saving only those who have the greatest social responsibilities and potential contribution.

This argument can be extended by examining values other than individual dignity and equality of opportunity. Another basic value in the medical sphere is the relationship of trust between physician and patient. Which selection criteria are most in accord with this relationship of trust? Which will maintain, extend, and deepen it? My contention is that selection by randomness or chance is preferable from this standpoint too.

Trust, which is inextricably bound to respect for human dignity, is an attitude of expectation about another. It is not simply the expectation that another will perform a particular act, but more specifically that another will act toward him in certain ways—which will respect him as a person. As Charles Fried writes:

Although trust has to do with reliance on a disposition of another person, it is reliance on a disposition of a special sort: the disposition to act morally, to deal fairly with others, to live up to one's undertakings, and so on. Thus to trust another is first of all to expect him to accept the principle of morality in his dealings with you, to respect your status as a person, your personality.[20]

This trust cannot be preserved in life-and-death situations when a person expects decisions about him to be made in terms of his social worth, for such decisions violate his status as a person. An applicant rejected on grounds of inadequacy in social value or virtue would have reason for feeling that his "trust" had been betrayed. Indeed, the sense that one is being viewed not as an end in himself but as a means in medical progress or the achievement of a greater social good is incompatible with attitudes and relationships of trust. We recognize this in the billboard which was erected after the first heart transplants: "Drive Carefully. Christiaan Barnard Is Watching You." The relationship of trust between the physician and patient is not only an instrumental value in the sense of being an important factor in the patient's treatment. It is also to be endorsed because of its intrinsic worth as a relationship.

Thus the related values of individual dignity and trust are best maintained in selection by chance. But other factors also buttress the argument for this approach. Which criteria and procedures would men agree upon? We have to suppose a hypothetical situation in which several men are going to determine for themselves and their families the criteria and procedures by which they would want to be admitted to and excluded from SLMR if the need arose.[21] We need to assume two restrictions and then ask which set of criteria and procedures would be chosen as the most rational and, indeed, the fairest. The restrictions are these: (1) The men are *self-interested*. They are interested in their own welfare (and that of members of their families), and this, of course, includes survival. Basically, they are not motivated by altruism. (2) Furthermore, they are *ignorant* of their own talents, abilities, potential, and probable contribution to the social good. They do not know how they would fare in a competitive situation, e.g., the competition for SLMR in terms of social contribution. Under these conditions which institution would be chosen—letting all die, utilitarian selection, or the use of chance? Which would seem the most rational? the fairest? By which set of criteria would they want to be included in or excluded from the list of those who will be saved? The rational choice in this setting (assuming self-interest and ignorance of one's competitive success) would be random selection or chance since this alone provides equality of opportunity. A possible response is that one would prefer to take a "risk" and therefore choose the utilitarian approach. But I think not, especially since I added that the participants in this hypothetical situation are choosing for their children as well as for themselves; random selection or chance could be more easily justified to the children. It would make more sense for men who are self-interested but uncertain about their relative contribution to society to elect a set of criteria that would build in equality of opportunity. They would consider selection by chance as relatively just and fair.[22]

An important psychological point supplements earlier arguments for using chance or random selection. The psychological stress and strain among those who are rejected would be greater if the rejection is based on insufficient social worth than if it is based on chance. Obviously stress and strain cannot be eliminated in these borderline situations, but they would almost certainly be increased by the opprobrium of being judged relatively "unfit" by society's agents using society's values. Nicholas Rescher makes this point very effectively:

> a recourse to chance would doubtless make matters easier for the rejected patients and those who have a specific interest in him. It would surely be quite hard for them to accept his exclusion by relatively mechanical application of objective criteria in whose implementation subjective judgment is involved. But the circumstances of life have conditioned us to accept the workings of chance and to tolerate the element of luck (good or bad): human life is an inherently contingent process. Nobody, after all, has an absolute right to ELT [Exotic Lifesaving Therapy]—but most of us would feel that we have "every bit as much right" to it as anyone else in significantly similar circumstances.[23]

Although it is seldom recognized as such, selection by chance is already in operation in practically every dialysis unit. I am not aware of any unit that removes some of its patients from kidney machines in order to make room for later applicants who are better qualified in terms of social worth. Furthermore, very few people would recommend it. Indeed, few would even consider removing a person from a kidney machine on the grounds that a person better qualified *medically* had just applied. In a discussion of the treatment of chronic renal failure by dialysis at the University of Virginia Hospital Renal Unit from November 15, 1965 to November 15, 1966, Dr. Harry Abram writes: "Thirteen patients sought treatment but were not considered because the program had reached its limit of nine patients."[24]

Thus, in practice and theory, natural chance is accepted, at least within certain limits.

My proposal is that we extend this principle (first come, first served) to determine who among the medically acceptable patients shall live or that we utilize artificial chance such as a lottery or randomness. "First come, first served" would be more feasible than a lottery since the applicants make their claims over a period of time rather than as a group at one time. This procedure would be in accord with at least one principle in our present practices and with our sense of individual dignity, trust, and fairness. Its significance in relation to these values can be underlined by asking how the decision can be justified to the rejected applicant. Of course, one easy way of avoiding this task is to maintain the traditional cloak of secrecy, which works to a great extent because patients are often not aware that they are being considered for SLMR in addition to the usual treatment. But whether public justification is instituted or not is not the significant question; it is rather what reasons for rejection would be most acceptable to the unsuccessful applicant. My contention is that rejection can be accepted more readily if equality of opportunity, fairness, and trust are preserved, and that they are best preserved by randomness or chance.

This proposal has yet another advantage since it would eliminate the need for a committee to examine applicants in terms of their social value. This onerous responsibility can be avoided.

Finally, there is a possible indirect consequence of widespread use of random selection which is interesting to ponder, although I do *not* adduce it as a good reason for adopting random selection. It can be argued, as Professor Mason Willrich of the University of Virginia Law School has suggested, that SLMR cases would practically disappear if these scarce resources were distributed randomly rather than on social worth grounds. Scarcity would no longer be a problem because the holders of economic and political power would make certain that they would not be excluded by a random selection procedure; hence they would help to redirect public priorities or establish private funding so that life-saving medical treatment would be widely and perhaps universally available.

In the framework that I have delineated, are the decrees of chance to be taken without exception? If we recognize exceptions, would we not open Pandora's box again just after we had succeeded in getting it closed? The direction of my argument has been against any exceptions, and I would defend this as the proper way to go. But let me indicate one possible way of admitting exceptions, while at the same time circumscribing them so narrowly that they would be very rare indeed.

An obvious advantage of the utilitarian approach is that occasionally circumstances arise that make it necessary to say that one man is practically indispensable for a society in view of a particular set of problems it faces (e.g., the president when the nation is waging a war for survival). Certainly the argument to this point has stressed that the burden of proof would fall on those who think that the social danger in this instance is so great that they simply cannot abide by the outcome of a lottery or a first come, first served policy. Also, the reason must be negative rather than positive; that is, we depart from chance in this instance not because we want to take advantage of this person's potential contribution to the improvement of our society, but because his immediate loss would possibly (even probably) be disastrous (again, the president in a grave national emergency). Finally, social value (in the negative sense) should be used as a standard of exception in dialysis, for example, only if it would provide a reason strong enough to warrant removing another person from a kidney machine if all machines were taken. Assuming this strong reluctance to remove anyone once the commitment has been made to him, we would be willing to put this patient ahead of another applicant for a vacant machine only if we would be willing (in circumstances in which all machines are being used) to vacate a machine by removing someone from it. These restrictions would make an exception almost impossible.

While I do not recommend this procedure of recognizing exceptions, I think that one can defend it while accepting my general thesis about selection by randomness or chance. If it is used, a lay committee (perhaps advisory, perhaps even stronger) would be called upon to deal with the alleged exceptions, since the doctors or others would in effect be appealing the outcome of chance (either natural or artificial). This lay committee would determine whether this patient was so indispensable at this time and place that he had to be saved even by sacrificing the values preserved by random selection. It would make it quite clear that exception is warranted, if at all, only as the "lesser of two evils." Such a defense would be recognized only rarely, if ever, pri-

marily because chance and randomness preserve so many important moral and nonmoral values in SLMR cases.[25]

Notes

1. George Bernard Shaw, *The Doctor's Dilemma* (New York, 1941), pp. 132–33.

2. Henry K. Beecher, "Scarce Resources and Medical Advancement," *Daedalus* (Spring 1969), 279–80.

3. Leo Shatin, "Medical Care and the Social Worth of a Man," *American Journal of Orthopsychiatry*, 36 (1967), 97.

4. Harry S. Abram and Walter Wadlington, "Selection of Patients for Artificial and Transplanted Organs," *Annals of Internal Medicine*, 69 (September 1968), 615–20.

5. *United States v. Holmes*, 26 Fed. Cas. 360 (C.C.E.D. Pa. 1842). All references are to the text of the trial as reprinted in Philip E. Davis, ed., *Moral Duty and Legal Responsibility: A Philosophical-Legal Casebook* (New York, 1966), pp. 102–18.

6. *The Moral Decision* (Bloomington, Ind., 1955), p. 71.

7. For a discussion of the higher suicide rate among dialysis patients than among the general population and an interpretation of some of the factors at work, see H. S. Abram, G. L. Moore, and F. B. Westervelt, "Suicidal Behavior in Chronic Dialysis Patients," *American Journal of Psychiatry*, 127 (1971): 1119–1204. This study shows that even "if one does not include death through not following the regimen the incidence of suicide is still more than 100 times the normal population."

8. Joseph Fletcher, "Donor Nephrectomies and Moral Responsibility," *Journal of the American Medical Women's Association*, 23 (December 1968), 1090.

9. Leo Shatin, pp. 96–101.

10. For a discussion of the Seattle selection committee, see Shana Alexander, "They Decide Who Lives, Who Dies," *Life*, 53 (November 9, 1962), 102. For an examination of general selection practices in dialysis see "Scarce Medical Resources," *Columbia Law Review* 69:620 (1969) and Abram and Wadlington.

11. David Sanders and Jesse Dukeminier, Jr., "Medical Advance and Legal Lag: Hemodialysis and Kidney Transplantation," *UCLA Law Review* 15:367 (1968), 378.

12. "Letters and Comments," *Annals of Internal Medicine*, 61 (August 1964), 360. Dr. G. E. Schreiner contends that "if you really believe in the right of society to make decisions on medical availability on these criteria you should be logical and say that when a man stops going to church or is divorced or loses his job, he ought to be removed from the programme and somebody else who fulfills these criteria substituted. Obviously no one faces up to

this logical consequence" (G. E. W. Wolstenholme and Maeve O'Connor, eds. *Ethics in Medical Progress: With Special Reference to Transplantation*, A Ciba Foundation Symposium [Boston, 1966], p. 127).

13. Helmut Thielicke, "The Doctor as Judge of Who Shall Live and Who Shall Die," *Who Shall Live?* ed. by Kenneth Vaux (Philadelphia, 1970), p. 172.

14. Ibid., pp. 173–74.

15. Ibid., p. 173.

16. Thielicke, *Theological Ethics*, Vol. I, *Foundations* (Philadelphia, 1966), p. 602.

17. Cahn, op. cit., p. 71.

18. Paul Freund, "Introduction," *Daedalus* (Spring 1969), xiii.

19. Paul Ramsey, *Nine Modern Moralists* (Englewood Cliffs, N.J., 1962), p. 245.

20. Charles Fried, "Privacy," in *Law, Reason, and Justice*, ed. by Graham Hughes (New York, 1969), p. 52.

21. My argument is greatly dependent on John Rawls's version of justice as fairness, which is a reinterpretation of social contract theory. Rawls, however, would probably not apply his ideas to "borderline situations." See "Distributive Justice: Some Addenda," *Natural Law Forum*, 13 (1968), 53. For Rawls's general theory, see "Justice as Fairness," *Philosophy, Politics and Society* (Second Series), ed. by Peter Laslett and W. G. Runciman (Oxford, 1962), pp. 132–57 and *A Theory of Justice* (Cambridge, Mass., 1971).

22. Occasionally someone contends that random selection may reward vice. Leo Shatin (op. cit., p. 100) insists that random selection "would reward socially disvalued qualities by giving their bearers the same special medical care opportunities as those received by the bearers of socially valued qualities. Personally I do not favor such a method." Obviously society must engender certain qualities in its members, but not all of its institutions must be devoted to that purpose. Furthermore, there are strong reasons, I have contended, for exempting SLMR from that sort of function.

23. Nicholas Rescher, "The Allocation of Exotic Medical Lifesaving Therapy," *Ethics*, 79 (April 1969), 184. He defends random selection's use only after utilitarian and other judgments have been made. If there are no "major disparities" in terms of utility, etc., in the second stage of selection, then final selection could be made randomly. He fails to give attention to the moral values that random selection might preserve.

24. Harry S. Abram, M.D., "The Psychiatrist, the Treatment of Chronic Renal Failure, and the Prolongation of Life: II," *American Journal of Psychiatry* 126: 157–67 (1969), 158.

25. I read a draft of this paper in a seminar on "Social Implications of Advances in Biomedical Science and Technology: Artificial and Transplanted Internal Organs," sponsored by the Center for the Study of Science, Technology, and Public Policy of the University of Virginia, Spring 1970. I am indebted to the participants in that seminar, and especially to its leaders, Mason Willrich, Professor of Law, and Dr. Harry Abram, Associate Professor of Psychiatry, for criticisms which helped me to sharpen these ideas. Good discussions of the legal questions raised by selection (e.g., equal protection of the law and due process) which I have not considered can be found in "Scarce Medical Resources," *Columbia Law Review*, 69:620 (1969); "Patient Selection for Artificial and Transplanted Organs," *Harvard Law Review*, 82:1322 (1969); and Sanders and Dukeminier, op. cit.

Annotated Bibliography

Blackstone, William R.: "On Health Care as a Legal Right: An Exploration of Legal and Moral Grounds," *Georgia Law Review* 10 (1976), pp. 391–418. Blackstone examines a number of legal and moral positions which can be used to argue for or against some kind of right to health care. He argues in favor of a public, socialized, or nationalized health system.

Ehrenreich, Barbara and John: "Health Care and Social Control," *Social Policy* 5 (May/June 1974), pp. 26–40. In this radical critique of the American health care system, the Ehrenreichs provide a historical and critical analysis of the ways in which our medical system functions as an instrument of social control.

Enthoven, Alain C.: "Consumer-Choice Health Plan," *The New England Journal of Medicine* 298 (Mar. 23, 1978), pp. 650–658 and (Mar. 30, 1978), pp. 709–720. The subtitles of this two-part article indicate its subject matter: (Part I) "Inflation and Inequity in Health Care Today: Alternatives for Cost Control and an Analysis of Proposals for National Health Insurance." (Part II) "A National-Health Insurance Proposal Based on Regulated Competition in the Private Sector."

Fein, Rashi: "On Achieving Access and Equity in Health Care," *Milbank Memorial Fund Quarterly* 50 (October 1972), pp. 157–190. Fein provides a historical and critical analysis of some of the economic criteria used to set a value on human life and to allocate medical resources.

Feinberg, Joel: *Social Philosophy* (Englewood Cliffs, N.J.: Prentice-Hall, 1973), chap 7. In this chapter, titled "Social Justice," Feinberg discusses in some detail the formal and material principles of justice.

Freedman, Benjamin: "The Case for Medical Care, Inefficient or Not," *Hastings Center Report* 7 (April 1977) pp. 31–39. Freedman concentrates on the following public policy issue: Should allocation for preventive medicine take priority over allocation for medical care? He examines the *ethical costs* of giving priority to preventive medicine and argues that a "relative primacy" should be given to medical care.

Fuchs, Victor R.: *Who Shall Live?: Health, Economics, and Social Choice* (New York: Basic Books, 1974). Fuchs surveys some important aspects of the American health system, e.g., physicians and hospitals, the system of drug manufacture and distribution, and payment and insurance plans. He relates all this to what the data reveal about our health needs. Fuchs concludes that heredity, life-style, and environment have more impact on individual health than the money spent on medical care.

Illich, Ivan: *Medical Nemesis* (New York: Pantheon, 1976). Illich's book is an extended criticism of our "misguided overreliance" on health care professionals. He attacks the "medical establishment" which he sees as a threat to health and as responsible for numerous iatrogenic ills. According to Illich, health care in our society can be improved only if individuals take the responsibility for their own health away from the professionals. He criticizes national healthcare schemes whose purpose is to increase the provision of treatment. Such programs, he maintains, will further diminish the individual's responsibility for his or her own health.

"Patient Selection for Artificial and Transplanted Organs," *Harvard Law Review* 82 (1969), pp. 1322–1342. This article contains four sections: (I) a brief survey of scientific developments in artificial organs and transplantation; (II) a survey of the practices in patient selection which were current when the article was written; (III) an examination of the competing values which should govern the selection process; and (IV) a consideration of some of the constitutional issues involved and recommendations regarding substantive and procedural measures for a fair system of allocation.

Rexed, Bror, and Daniel Juda: "Planning for Scarcity in Sweden: An Interview with Bror Rexed," *Hastings Center Report* 7 (June 1977) pp. 5–7. Bror Rexed is the Director General of the Swedish National Board of Health. In this interview Rexed discusses the social impact of the Arab oil embargo of 1973. The interview is especially interesting in relation to this chapter because it shows the kind of public policy decisions regarding the provision of medical care which can only be made and implemented in a society in which the whole medical system is under government control.

Sparer, Edward V.: "The Legal Right to Health Care: Public Policy and Equal Access," *Hastings Center Report* 6 (October 1976), pp. 39–47. Sparer is concerned with the "legal" right to medical care. He examines the legal rights we do have in regard to medical care and various public policy decisions regarding the right to medical care, e.g., decisions regarding Medicare and Medicaid. He concludes with a list of recommendations whose purpose is to promote the achievement of a broad public right to good medical care.

Steiner, Hillel: "The Just Provision of Health Care: A Reply to Elizabeth Telfer," *Journal of Medical Ethics* 2 (1976), pp. 185–189. Steiner examines the four positions offered by Elizabeth Telfer in the article reprinted in this chapter. He criticizes Telfer, and argues for a fifth position which incorporates the important elements of Telfer's two extreme positions—the laissez faire and *pure* socialist approaches to health care delivery. A brief reply by Telfer follows Steiner's article.

Veatch, Robert M., and Roy Branson, eds.: *Ethics and Health Policy* (Cambridge, Mass.: Ballinger, 1976). Included in this collection of articles are several dealing with justice and health care delivery. Those interested in John Rawls' theory of distributive justice will be especially interested in the article by Ronald M. Green, "Health Care and Justice in Contract Theory Perspective."

℞ For Reason

It is indisputable that, in the absence of policy to guide them, health care providers often must make resource-allocation decisions as best they can. James M. Jackson Memorial Hospital, the public-general teaching hospital in Dade County, Florida, which includes the cities of Miami and Miami Beach, was faced with a particularly difficult decision in 1982. It is often argued that implicit, private, behind-the-scenes decision making is easier for providers, because the glare of publicity can make them seem heartless or immoral when their decisions come to light. In this case, however, Jackson gained editorial support from the area's largest newspaper, because the decision it made was perceived as fair by the community. It offers an argument for a more explicit approach to provider decision making when the stakes are high.

The hammer of treatable lethal illness dropped onto the anvil of Dade County's crushing burden of medical care for indigents last week. Pitiably, a handsome Argentine engineering student named Daniel Ramirez was caught by the blow.

Mr. Ramirez has no kidneys. He hopes that county-owned Jackson Memorial Hospital will find a donor for him. He also has no money to cover the $40,000 that he already owes JMH or to pay the $30,000 that a needed second transplant would cost. The hospital accordingly dropped him from its waiting-donor list pending payment of the $70,000 total. His own government in Buenos Aires has spent $80,000 for treatment, including a previous unsuccessful transplant, and says it can spend no more.

This case tests the boundaries both of generosity and of fiscal responsibility. The conscience of most Dade residents would dictate that the young man should receive treatment that could save his life. But the sense of reason in those same Dade taxpayers must conclude that hospital officials are correct in refusing to provide further treatment for a nonresident without payment.

If anyone bears responsibility for the young Argentine's medical bills, it is his own government. Jackson is a county facility supported by local property taxes. It cannot permit its location adjacent to the Caribbean and the attraction of its bilingual ambience to make it the treatment center of last resort for the indigents of Central and South America. Cannot, should not, and must not.

Mr. Ramirez's government was able at least to provide the first $80,000 for care that unfortunately proved unsuccessful. That contribution reflects Argentina's relative wealth. Imagine how many potential dialysis and transplant patients there must be among the millions of destitute citizens of Haiti, Bolivia, Brazil, and Honduras. Can Jackson accept the burden of providing unlimited treatment to any of those unfortunates who can raise air fare to Miami?

No, of course not. The hard truth is that

An editorial reprinted, with permission, from *The Miami Herald* 1982 Friday, Dec. 3.

people in those countries die every day for lack of medical care that is routine in any U.S. city. Diarrhea kills babies. Tuberculosis kills adults. Bacterial disease kills young and old alike.

The taxpayers of Dade County cannot save them all, much as they might wish it possible. Lines must be drawn. JMH officials properly drew it in front of a foreign national who already has received $40,000 worth of care at Dade's expense. They made the only responsible decision available to them.

Ethical and Policy Issues in the Procurement of Cadaver Organs for Transplantation

Arthur L. Caplan, The Hastings Center, Hastings-on-Hudson, New York

In the past few years there has been a dramatic rise in the demand for organs for transplantation. Advances in surgical techniques, tissue typing, and the development of powerful immunosuppressive drugs, such as cyclosporine, has made it possible to transplant both a larger number and an increasing variety of organs. Among organs and tissues currently being transplanted from cadavers are kidneys, hearts, lungs, livers, bone marrow, skin, corneas, and pancreases.

Although some of these procedures are still experimental, graft and recipient survival rates for transplantations have shown steady improvement during the past decade.[1,2] Many centers report five-year graft survival rates of 60 per cent among patients who have received kidneys from cadavers. More than 95 per cent of those who receive corneas from cadavers have their sight restored. Moreover, recent survival rates for heart transplantation are approaching 50 per cent at five years.

This remarkable progress in the field of organ transplantation raises numerous moral and policy problems for the medical profession and the general public. Who ought to pay the high costs associated with these procedures? What rate of survival justifies the labeling of a procedure as therapeutic, and who should be responsible for making such determinations? When the number of organs is insufficient to meet the demand, what policies should be instituted to help increase the availability of these precious tissues?

It is the last question that, in many ways, is the most disturbing of all. The large gap that exists between the available supply and the demand for organs for transplantation has been well documented. The Centers for Disease Control has estimated that no more than 15 per cent of the 20,000 persons who might serve as organ donors actually do so.[3]

The gap between supply and demand with respect to organ transplantation is not only large but growing in proportion to the rapid advances being made in this area. Nationwide, between 6000 and 10,000 people are being maintained on either hemodialysis or peritoneal dialysis while awaiting a kidney transplant[3]; nearly 4000 are estimated to be in need of corneal transplants. Indeed, the public has grown all too familiar with televised pleas for a liver, heart, or other tissue to save the life of a relative or friend.

The potential demand for organs is much greater than present levels may indicate. For ex-

Reprinted, with permission, from *The New England Journal of Medicine* 1984 Oct. 11. 311(15): 981–983.

ample, the majority of liver transplantations are performed in children with congenital defects. However, if liver transplantation should prove to be an effective therapeutic option for adults with cirrhosis of the liver, then tens of thousands of persons might be potential recipients. Similar projections can be made for transplantations involving the heart, lungs, and pancreas.[2,4]

Given the current and potential future demand for cadaver organs, there may be no way to avoid the problem of rationing for many forms of transplantation. Nonetheless, it would appear to be both ethically and medically sensible to examine current public policy with respect to the procurement of organs for transplantation, to determine whether legal or regulatory changes might be effected that would help maximize the supply of tissues available to those in need.

For the past 15 years this country has been committed to a policy of what might best be termed "voluntarism" in the procurement of tissues for transplantation.[5] As transplantation of certain tissues between genetically related family members became possible during the early 1960s, it soon became evident that physicians required both legal and moral guidance in developing procedures to procure tissue for this purpose.

Since many of the organs used for transplantation during this period were procured from living donors, legal authorities and the courts tended to stress the importance of voluntary consent in the procurement process. There was an understandable concern that family members, particularly those who were minors or had diminished mental capacities, were at some risk of being coerced to make donations against their will. Various court cases recognized the legal right of a person to give consent to the transplantation of tissue as long as he or she was both free from coercion and well informed about the risks and benefits of the procedure. Courts even gave children and the retarded the right to donate in the belief that they might suffer greatly from the loss of a sibling or other family member.

When the prospects for the transplantation of tissues from cadaver donors improved during the late 1960s, public policy was modified in order to encourage this form of donation. In 1968 the Uniform Anatomical Gift Act was enacted, which recognized the legal status of donor cards and "living wills," as well as the authority of the next of kin to make a donation in a situation in which the deceased had not indicated any opposition to donation.

Free choice and voluntarism played key parts in the moral and legal arguments that surrounded the passage of this legislation. Proponents of donor cards, donor statements on driver's licenses, and other forms of living wills argued that a system of cadaver organ procurement built on voluntarism would promote socially desirable virtues, such as altruism, and at the same time, protect the rights of persons who might, for various reasons, oppose the procurement of tissues from cadavers.

As noted above, this system has been only partially successful in securing organs for transplantation. In the light of the fact that the demand for cadaver organs is likely to increase, the time has come for a reexamination of current public policy regarding the procurement of such organs.

Although many of those involved in organ procurement are making heroic efforts to increase the supply of organs from cadaver donors, there are a number of factors that severely inhibit the ability of the present system to take advantage of the supply of tissues potentially available from cadavers. Both economic and legal fears impede the present system of voluntary donation.[5,7] Moreover, there is a real danger that unless something is done to improve the efficacy of the voluntary system, advocates of a free-market solution will attempt to create a for-profit system to meet the large demand for organs.[6]

Among the factors that diminish the effectiveness of the current voluntaristic approach to cadaver donation are the lack of trust on the part of physicians and hospital administrators in the legal authority of donor cards, the failure of the public to sign and carry donor cards, the failure of hospital personnel to locate donor cards, and most important, the failure of physicians and nurses to inquire about the possibility of organ donation in the absence of a written directive on the part of the deceased.[7]

There would appear to be a number of incentives that work against the efficacy of the current voluntaristic policy in obtaining cadaver organs. First of all, many people simply find the subject of death and organ donation upsetting and distasteful. Although surveys show that the public is willing to support organ donation,[8] it is difficult to transform willingness into concrete realization on a donor card or driver's license.

Secondly, most physicians and nurses do not want to inquire about organ donation. The highly emotional circumstances under which such requests are made make it uncomfortable for both families and medical personnel to communicate about the subject of donation. Moreover, at least some health professionals doubt that family members are able to give informed, voluntary consent in the context of the sudden death of a loved one.[5]

Finally, many hospitals fear adverse legal and financial consequences from their involvement with organ procurement. Many hospital administrators refuse to allow their staff to become involved with a procedure that carries some risk of legal complications and no promise of financial return.

Current federal policy is aimed at improving the present system by centralizing the collection of information concerning donors and recipients and by encouraging further efforts at public and professional education.[2,9] However, these efforts are not likely to prove useful in improving the supply of organs available from cadaver sources, since they do not address the major factors hindering the efficacy of the current system.

There is a public-policy option available at both the federal and state levels, however, that might increase the supply of organs available from cadavers. Legislation could be enacted that would require a routine inquiry of available family members as part of the existing procedures in each state for discontinuing life-support measures in hopeless situations. Such a law would mandate that no one on a respirator who might serve as an organ donor could be declared legally dead (assuming that the medical requirements for such a declaration had been met) until a request for donation had been made of any available next of kin or legal proxy. The request would have to be made by a physician, nurse, or physician's assistant with no connection to the determination of the actual occurrence of death, in order to assure the public that declarations of death would be made without regard to the need to obtain organs for transplantation. If family members or guardians were not available, organs could be removed only if a donor card or other similar legal document existed.

A policy of "required request" directly addresses the major obstacles in procuring cadaver organs for transplantation. Such a policy requires that hospital personnel routinely consider the need for transplantable tissues. It ensures that the burden of decisions concerning donation is equitably allocated among all families whose relatives might serve as organ donors. A policy of routine required request standardizes the process of routine inquiring about organ donation in such a way that it lessens the psychological burden on both health professionals and family members at a time of great stress and emotional upheaval. Moreover, it removes the option not to inquire, which is often chosen under the present system because of fears concerning legal and financial consequences. Finally, a policy of required request preserves the right of individuals to refuse consent, since voluntary choice remains the ethical foundation on which organ donation rests.

The benefits to society in terms of an increase in the supply of cadaver organs for transplantation would appear to outweigh the loss of clinical freedom inherent in a required-request policy for cadaver organ donation. In view of the desperate needs of those who are now awaiting organs and the large number of persons who will be able to benefit from transplantation in the years to come, the loss of this freedom would seem to be a small price to pay.

References

1. Van Thiel DH, Schade RR, Starzl TE. After 20 years, liver transplantation comes of age. Ann Intern Med 1983; 99:854–6.

2. Iglehart JK. Transplantation: the problem of limited resources. N Engl J Med 1983; 309:123–8.

3. Kolata G. Organ shortage clouds new transplant era. Science 1983; 221:32–3.

4. Final report of the task force on liver transplantation in Massachusetts. Prepared for the Department of Public Health, State of Massachusetts, 1983.

5. Caplan AL. Organ transplants: the costs of success. Hastings Cent Rep 1983; 13(6):23–32.

6. Chapman DE. Retailing human organs under the Uniform Commercial Code. John Marshall Law Rev 1983; 16:393–417.

7. Overcast TD, Evans RW, Bowen LE, Hoe MM, Livak CL. Problems in the identification of potential organ donors. JAMA 1984; 251:1559–62.

8. The Gallup Organization. Attitudes and opinions of the American public towards kidney donations. Prepared for the National Kidney Foundation, Washington, D.C. 1983., (GO 8305).

9. Koop CE. Increasing the supply of solid organs for transplantation. Public Health Rep 1983; 98:566–72.

Heart Transplants

Lois K. Christopherson, M.S.W., M.S., Stanford University Clinic, Stanford University Medical School, Stanford

In December 1967 Christiaan Barnard of the Union of South Africa performed the first heart transplant in a human. The next year became known in newspaper headlines as the "Year of the Transplant," as sixty-four transplant teams in twenty-two countries performed 101 operations. The ease with which transplantation could be accomplished surgically was deceptive; by the fall of 1970, few of the recipients were still alive. Most transplant teams had established either a formal or a de factor moratorium on the procedure.

Only two American transplant groups regularly performed this operation during much of the 1970s—the transplant team at Stanford Medical Center headed by Norman Shumway and Edward Stinson, and the transplant group at the Medical College of Virginia under the leadership of Richard Lower. A decade of laboratory research by leaders of each of these teams preceded the decision to begin cardiac transplantation in human subjects. As a result, these teams acquired a greater knowledge of techniques for dealing with the serious problems of infection and rejection and achieved survival rates that ex-

ceeded those of other, less experienced centers.

During the past few years, perhaps because of the continuing research and success of the Stanford and Virginia transplant groups, interest in cardiac transplant technology has revived. Surgeons who were trained in cardiac transplantation at Stanford have established two programs—at New York's Downstate Medical Center and at the University of Arizona Health Sciences Center. Other programs, conspicuous more for the lack of fanfare they have attracted, have been started in medical centers where the availability of specialists, including representatives of immunology and infectious disease as well as cardiac surgery and cardiology, offers hope that the techniques and results of the Stanford group can be replicated or bettered.

In at least one instance, at Massachusetts General Hospital, the request of appropriate chiefs of service for permission to initiate a transplant program was denied after careful consideration by the hospital's Board of Trustees. They cited as reasons the extensive resources that a transplant program would require, the impact of the diversion of these resources on other patients the

Reprinted, with permission, from the author and *The Hastings Center Report* 1982 Feb. 12:18–21.
Supported in part by the James Picker Foundation Program on the Human Qualities of Medicine and by NIH grant number HL 13108.

hospital serves, and the current status of cardiac transplant research and its therapeutic effectiveness, particularly the problem of tissue rejection.[1]

Cardiac transplantation raises a host of ethical issues. In its most restrictive definition, cardiac transplant surgery involves the removal of a still viable, unimpaired vital organ from the body of a "neurologically dead" donor and the placement of that organ in the chest of a recipient whose own heart has been removed, who has been judged to have little hope of greater than six months' survival without a new heart, and whose chances for extended survival even with the surgery are statistically much improved but still unpredictable.

If the analysis is broadened beyond specific organ transfer, however, still other issues are raised. These include allocation of scarce resources (the time and energy of highly skilled professionals as well as the costs of the research and medical care); the basis of selection of the relatively few patients who will have the opportunity to benefit from the procedure (or, in a darker view, be experimented upon); the complexities of informed consent when a patient is simultaneously told by a physician that he or she is dying and that the transplant is the only operation that might extend life; and the question of whether medical care, in its most innovative forms, should be funded or guaranteed by the government for all or for specifically identified patients, or whether access can be limited by the ability to pay, either directly or through third-party payers.

Cardiac Transplantation Today

Between January 1968 and May 1981, 208 patients received one or more heart transplants at Stanford. Seventy-five of these recipients are currently alive for periods of time ranging from two months to eleven and one-half years; an additional forty-seven survived more than one year and thirteen more than four years with a transplanted heart but are now dead.

Figure 1 illustrates current probabilities for survival after cardiac transplantation using Stanford's recipient data and actuarial methods. Sixty-five percent of the patients transplanted since 1974 have survived one year, and between 40 percent and 45 percent have survived or are projected to survive for at least five years. The curve

Figure 1. Stanford Cardiac Transplantation

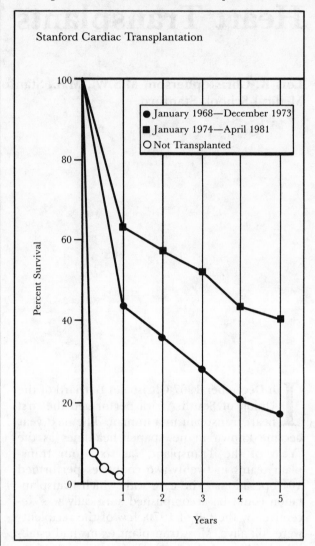

illustrating the death rate for those who were selected as recipients but for whom a donor heart was not found in time shows how severely ill they were; more than 90 percent died within three months of selection.

Quality of life is more difficult to measure because the concept includes subjective as well as objective parameters. However, approximately 85 percent of the recipients surviving longer than one year have returned to full-time employment or schooling or have resumed comparable avocational and family activities. The remainder are disabled primarily from the side effects of immuno-suppressant drugs, the most common of which are decalcification of bones and secondary infection.

Recipient Selection

To be considered as a Stanford transplant recipient, a patient must meet the following medical and psychosocial criteria:

• The patient must have New York Heart Association Class IV cardiac disability (essentially a bed-to-chair existence) and/or have an estimated life expectancy of less than six months. Other major organ systems must be free from disease, and the patient can have no infections and no recent history of pulmonary embolism.

• There must be strong family support for the patient and for further discussion of the transplant procedure, as well as a history of good compliance with medical instructions. The patient's and family's ability to understand the risks and limitations as well as the possible benefits of the procedure and to give informed consent (or refusal) are important. Although clinical research grant funds help pay for post-transplant hospitalization, other expenses for travel and living away from home as well as pre-transplant hospitalization must be met by third-party payers, the patient and family, or community fund-raising.

• Most centers have set an upper age limit of approximately fifty years, because excessive morbidity and mortality rates for older recipients are very high. A history of psychiatric illness or substance abuse usually counts against transplantation.

Recipient selection raises two kinds of ethical problems, one having to do with the selection process during the clinical research phase and the second relating to the many additional questions that may well be raised if the procedure becomes increasingly successful.

Currently accepted selection criteria[2] have been designed to ensure both that the patient has a critical medical need for the graft, with no alternate medical or surgical means of achieving greater survival, and that the procedure has a reasonable chance of successful outcome given the current state of transplant technology. Transplant teams active during much of the 1970s gave a high priority to identifying selection criteria and making them even more rigorous. Those who were convinced of the potential therapeutic benefit of the operation sought not only to improve the procedure and its follow-up care, but also to define as precisely as possible those who were most likely to be helped.

Not everyone was satisfied with the criteria developed during the clinical research phase of cardiac transplantation. Patients who were turned down, for example, because they were infected or were diabetics requiring insulin were occasionally perceived as having been denied their "one chance at life, no matter how small." Patients who were rejected primarily because of psychosocial factors, say, a young adult whose medical compliance was poor and who was estranged from family and friends, could arouse similar indignation. "You mean to tell me you don't have families that can adopt and take care of someone like this poor young man? He's had a terrible life, and now you are going to let him die because of it."

Even within medical centers where transplants were performed, perceptions of the selection process appeared occasionally to be influenced by perceptions of the value of transplantation itself. Staff members who saw the procedure as valuable and effective were more likely to believe that recipients were selected from well-educated and financially comfortable groups. Those who were particularly aware of the procedure's limitations and uncertainties were more likely to suspect that transplantation was performed disproportionately on the poor and unsophisticated.

Here are some questions that must be raised regarding recipient selection during the clinical research phase of transplantation: is it reasonable or fair that transplantation should be restricted to those who are judged to have the greatest probability of surviving the procedure? To what extent must the restrictions be documented by experience to support their inclusion as selection criteria? Almost all the Stanford criteria are the result of one or more memorably unsuccessful outcomes in patients who would today not be accepted as recipients. Yet one or two failures may not form the basis for a criterion. Furthermore, the morbidity and mortality experienced by a particularly large subgroup (e.g., recipients over age fifty) is so high that the restriction probably should have been enforced sooner or more rigorously.

Who should make decisions about recipient selection? The Stanford selection group includes a cardiologist, clinical social worker, and cardiac surgeon, all of whom have been associated with the transplant group since its beginning and all of whom have significant responsibility for direct patient care. Continuity and accountability, inherent in this system, are helpful to patient selection. Continuing care of the recipient provides immediate feedback regarding the wisdom of any given choice, and colleagues have consistently felt free to assess the performance of the selection group. The temptation of accepting more recipients than could be transplanted in a given period of time is countered by the first-hand knowledge that patients will be offered hope— only to die.

Looking to the future, the questions of patient selection will increase dramatically. As the procedure becomes more successful, it will move from experimentation into the realm of clinical practice; research restrictions and the accompanying outside surveillance by site visitors and funding agencies will apply to a smaller proportion of the patient population. Physicians who do not now recommend transplantation will increasingly do so both because they will be more confident that it may be helpful and because of the legal ramifications if they fail to discuss a potentially beneficial procedure with a dying patient. Patients and families who have been unwilling to consider the upheaval of moving to the east or west coast for as long as a year with no certainty of obtaining a transplant may well request priority when transplantation is performed in a regional medical center or state university hospital.

There is already some evidence that the pressure of referrals is causing transplant groups to consider criteria other than expected outcomes for limiting patients. For some the possibility of specializing by age is appealing, for example, limiting transplants to children or adolescents. Others, especially tax-funded state university hospitals, may have to establish preference for state residents.

At some point during the coming decade, the demand for cardiac transplants by those likely to benefit will almost certainly exceed both the number of transplants that hospitals can perform and the number of appropriate donor hearts. The gatekeeping function can be delegated by conscious decision or default to each transplant team and the parent hospital. Or it can be assumed by a broader cross-section of society—from the constituents of a given medical center to the federal government.

Costs and Scarce Resources

Questions of recipient selection are unavoidably interwoven with questions of payment. The federal government has been the primary source of

funding for research and development at some centers and has often met through clinical research monies the costs of post-transplant medical care not covered by third-party payers. Payment for hospitalization required prior to transplantation has been made, variously, by insurance plans, Medicaid, or patients and families but has also posed the greatest hurdle for some potential recipients. Whether transplantation is a covered service or an exclusion (usually because it is deemed "experimental") varies among insurance companies (and policies), as well as from state to state.

It is not unusual for a patient to discover that insurance or Medicaid will cover required hospitalization until death but will not pay for costs related in any fashion to the one procedure that might extend life. Even if transplant-related coverage is available, the patient and family may lack the personal resources or the community fundraising support needed to meet the costs of travel to a distant transplant center and living expenses for as long as a year. The transplant centers involved have borne the stigma of "letting people die because they can't pay." This burden has been a serious consideration for hospitals contemplating a transplant program. A typical argument runs: "We can't take a loss on transplantation without endangering the quality of other programs. The repercussions if we take only those who can pay may be greater than we want to face." Additionally, those hospitals equipped to begin transplantation are already likely to have high occupancy rates for their intensive care units, high costs for the purchase and maintenance of sophisticated medical equipment, and an acute awareness of the shortage of highly trained nurses and technical staff. Transplant consideration includes not only direct costs or losses but also the costs of diverting scarce resources from other valued programs.

Data from the Stanford transplant experience give some information about the cost of an average transplant hospitalization and also highlight the difficulties encountered in making future predictions. The records of twenty-seven patients transplanted from May 1978 to April 1979 indicate an average hospital and ancillary services bill of $110,023 (in 1980 dollars). In individual cases, however, these costs have ranged from $35,000 to $140,000. The final bills of eleven patients recently transplanted using a new immunosuppressant drug (Cyclosporin A) that reduces the incidence of infection reveal a drop in average cost to $65,662. If the early results with Cyclosporin are maintained, transplant groups will achieve equal or improved recipient survival while lowering unit costs of care.

Whatever the costs, the underlying questions remain the same: is the ability to pay for the transplant a fair, or an unfair but necessary, requirement? If the answer is no, which it almost always is on first response, who should pay for the costs? Given the extensive national attention to containment of health care costs and competing demands for limited dollars, few medical centers would be willing or able to develop a transplant program if a local subsidy were required.

Some insurance policies exclude transplantation; others provide payment but, of course, only to the limits of a holder's coverage. While improved transplant results may well make it more difficult for a policy to exclude transplantation as an "experimental" procedure, the costs and length of hospitalization will still in effect exclude people with limited policies.

The governmental role in payment for cardiac replacement has two aspects: first, should persons who are already covered by Medicare and/or Medicaid receive full transplant coverage? Does state control over Medicaid eligibility and costs include the right to deny transplantation to a patient because of his or her place of residence? Should the Health Care Financing Administration (HCFA), which is currently reviewing cardiac transplantation, approve future coverage for those who are on Medicare? Second, should payment for virtually all cardiac transplants be guaranteed by the federal government through special Medicare coverage similar to that now provided for dialysis and renal transplant patients? If that did occur, would present criteria for the selection of patients be continued or tightened, or would it become much more difficult to turn away high-risk recipients? What would be the implications for the obviously limited supply of appropriate donor hearts? Given the likely continuing geographic maldistribution of transplant centers, would the government link payment for travel and living costs with Medicare coverage to ensure equal access to all patients? What are the opportunity costs of full government payment for cardiac transplantation?

A participant in a recent meeting protested, "Transplantation doesn't have anything to do with health care costs. It has to do with saving lives!"

Of course, that is an understandable reaction when someone you care about is dying, but social indignation over economic barriers to health care has not been matched by a willingness to assume the costs for those who are otherwise excluded.

Organ Donation

Transplanting vital organs or tissue from one human being to another has become generally accepted during the past two decades. Most major religious groups have seen the goal of transplantation as the preservation or extension of life and have supported both organ donation and organ receipt. The flood of letters that warned heart transplant surgeons in the early 1970s of their eternal place on God's blacklist has slowed to one every few months. Even small fundamentalist groups have begun to accept the procedure as it takes on a personal meaning for them. I remember with particular poignancy the long hours of prayer—and the subsequent revelation from God that transplantation was part of His plan—that preceded one religious group's decision that a dying member could undergo cardiac replacement.

Organ procurement centers have been established in major cities and form the lifeline for most renal and cardiac transplant programs. Neurologists and neurosurgeons in agreement with the concept of brain death have worked individually with transplant groups; the staffs of a few emergency rooms, usually under the leadership of a key nurse or physician, have begun to think of organ donation when a critically brain injured person is admitted.

The limitations of such a system, however, are considerable. Only twenty-seven states have laws defining death as a function of brain activity, and these statutes vary considerably. Funding for organ procurement groups, whose staff members also perform public and professional teaching functions, is usually obtained in competition with a variety of other public needs and agencies. Efforts of groups such as the National Kidney Foundation are highly effective in publicizing the general need for donor organs but have limited impact on the day-to-day needs of the large number of dialysis patients who would prefer renal transplantation. Approximately one of four patients awaiting a donor heart dies before one becomes available, and the proportion might be greater if existing programs were enlarged without concurrent attention to donor supply.

No technology is presently available to provide hemodialysis-type life support for end-stage cardiac patients for more than a few days. Even with anticipated improvements in cardiac support systems, it is likely that quality of life and independence from constant medical surveillance will depend, for any given patient, upon obtaining a new heart.

Most cardiac donors are young adults who were in excellent health until an unexpected and unpredictable event, such as as a motor vehicle accident, suicide, murder, or intracranial bleed caused brain death. Families are forced to face simultaneously the sudden loss of a loved one and the horror of the trauma itself. In the midst of such circumstances hundreds of families decide each year that they want to donate one or more of the victim's organs. Countless others do not, for reasons ranging from denial of the death to inability to think about the surgical invasion of the body. In many instances organ donation simply does not come to mind until months after the death. Even then family members may be unsure what course of action they might have chosen had donation been discussed with them at the time. With a few dramatic exceptions, most organ transplant groups have been willing to engage in public education about the need for organ donation but not in specific patient-oriented appeals for a donor heart or in direct persuasive appeals to a potential donor family. Even when the deceased was carrying an apparently valid donor card, the wishes of surviving family members, if they were opposed to donation, have been given precedence. Costs related to organ procurement have often been paid by recipients or their insurance, but there has been no known instance in which additional payment was made for a donor organ.

The care and thoughtfulness with which organ donation has generally taken place during the past two decades ought not obscure the questions that may need to be faced or reevaluated if demand continues to grow and supply to be limited. Protection for donors and donor families requires that parameters of brain death be sufficiently defined and agreed upon by neurologists and neurosurgeons. The question of whose wishes take precedence, those of a dead youth carrying an organ donor card or those of the surviving family, may sooner or later require not only further ethical discussion but also legal tests, either because family members are divided over the decision to donate or because a transplant center decides to confront the issue.

Even if it is generally accepted that no payment will be made for donor organs, the question does occasionally arise in the form of funeral and burial costs, and more subtle negotiations—or misunderstandings—are not uncommon. I recently received a call from a distressed donor parent who felt that we had broken our promise to bring the donor family and recipient together within a month of the transplant. The "promise" had been conveyed to the family by a television reporter who also wanted to film the meeting. The family was helped to understand that such get-togethers were not routinely scheduled, and they were also sensitive to the recipient's wish for anonymity.

Under only slightly changed circumstances, however, the desire to obtain a needed donor heart might lead well-meaning health care professionals to assure a grief-stricken family that they could see a loved one "live on" through continued contact with the recipient. The need for a heart might make payment of donor accident expenses an obvious and "kindly" step for a financially comfortable recipient family. Most donor families have the remarkable capacity to offer without recompense or recognition a genuine gift of life. But that does not eliminate the need to further examine the circumstances under which donation takes place and to formulate guidelines that will provide maximum protection for all parties involved in the valued exchange.

One of the pioneers in renal transplantation surgery, Dr. Roy Cohn, wrote in 1967, "Thanks to years of experimentation, human organs . . . can now be transplanted. Much medical research remains, but the problems which now loom largest are economic, legal, and moral."[3] His observation is appropriate not only for cardiac transplantation but also for many other areas of medical research and innovation. The transplantation experience may serve as an example, or a cautionary tale.

Notes

1. *New England Journal of Medicine.* 1980, May 8.

2. The *Federal Register of January 22, 1981,* contains a request for hospitals and medical centers to participate in a study of cardiac transplantation. Institutions that wish to apply for inclusion in the study must adhere to the detailed set of recipient selection criteria outlined in the publication and briefly summarized here.

3. *Stanford Today.* 1976 Winter.

Part 3

The Patient within the Hospital: Theory

Parallel with, but separate from, the hospital's interrelationship with society and the community it serves is the hospital's interaction with the patient within its walls. This relationship is every bit as problematic as the hospital's community experience, and in some ways it is even more so, because every patient is different. Indeed, the fluid nature of illness and debility is such that rules to govern the fragile bargains that must be struck between patient and provider are hard to come by.

Ethics has a rubric that points out the differentiation between the identified *life and the* statistical *life, that is, the distinctions we draw between the faceless mass of people who will never be known to us and the individual person whom we know and care about, whose fate is of personal interest. Richard Zeckhauser, Ph.D., professor at the John F. Kennedy School of Government, Harvard University, has pointed out that it is* statistical *lives that are always at risk because we do not have a personal relationship with them. He explains that we do not willingly vote for funds to erect safety barriers on the highway, because we do not know if we will personally benefit from such barriers. Preventive health services are the constant victims of such discrimination, because if a preventive act or program works, we will never know whose life was saved by it. After all, which image seduces the American imagination: a frail child trembling on the brink of death because she needs an organ transplant, or a healthy child to whom we can point and say, "See? He doesn't have smallpox." American society heavily emphasizes the named, individual life when it comes to resources and attention.*

And when that named, individual life belongs to a hospital patient, how the hospital does, or does not, treat the patient can lead all concerned into an ethical thicket. In this section, some means of establishing who has a right to what are examined. Leon R. Kass, M.D., Ph.D., explores the conflicts faced by physicians in hospitals when it comes to appropriate care for patients, especially the severely and terminally ill, and what ethical aid is available. Franz J. Ingelfinger, M.D., discusses providers' putative arrogance, its limits and its benefits. Sidney H. Wanzer, M.D., and his coauthors, in a still-controversial article, offer parameters for appropriate care for the hopelessly ill. George J. Annas, J.D., M.P.H., and Joan E. Densberger, M.P.H., provide a comprehensive review of what constitutes competence and the competent patient's rights.

Paul B. Hofmann summarizes the findings of the American Hospital Association's Special Committee on Biomedical Ethics, which try to balance conflicting value systems with the central right of the patient to choose, or reject, treatment options. Finally, three pieces address one partial solution to many in-hospital ethical quandaries: the institutional ethics committee (IEC). Alexander M. Capron, L.L.B., discusses IECs in the context of the law; Richard A. McCormick, S.J., discusses IECs' potential for problem solving as well as problem creation; and Sister Corrine Bayley and Ronald E. Cranford, M.D., summarize what has been learned by hospitals' limited but rich experience with IECs to this point.

Ethical Dilemmas in the Care of the Ill

Leon R. Kass, M.D., Ph.D., College and Committee on Social Thought, University of Chicago, Chicago

1. What Is the Physician's Service?

How should one speak to physicians about ethical dilemmas in the care of the ill? Experienced physicians certainly need no introduction to the subject. They regularly confront concrete, troublesome, and often poignant dilemmas in their day-to-day practice. Their ability to face these dilemmas is unlikely to be improved by exposure to the remote and scholarly ethical argumentation practiced by academic "ethicists." Exhortations to be good and sermons to avoid evil, while perhaps useful on some occasions, are usually too simplistic to touch either the troublesome questions or the questionable practices. Discussions of shocking and bizarre cases usually do little to illuminate the myriad ordinary practical difficulties. How does one usefully speak to medical practitioners about ethical matters?

In more than ten years of discussing questions of medical ethics with physicians, I have been impressed by their reluctance to generalize the principles of their conduct. They counter philosophical argument of principles with anecdotal accounts of cases. "Every case is altogether unique," they frequently insist. For several years, I must confess, I was impatient with this approach. It seemed to me then that my physician interlocutors were either too lazy or thoughtless to articulate the tacit premises of their conduct (premises that seemed, to me at least, readily accessible through analysis of their cases) or else too frightened to subject those premises to careful scrutiny and criticism. Moreover, it just is not true that the ethical aspects of each case are in *every* respect unique, any more than are the medical aspects. Why not seek the same clarity and precision in thinking about medical ethics that we seek about disease, which, after all, also manifests itself only in particular cases, each in some sense unique?

This article might be said to be a reflection on this question and on the peculiar antipathy of physicians toward formal and abstract ethical reasoning. I have come in large measure to appreciate the practitioners' point of view. Indeed, I increasingly believe that the attempt to replace

Reprinted with permission from the author and from the *Journal of the American Medical Association* 1980 Part 1. Oct. 17, 244 (16):1811–1816; Part 2. Oct. 24/31. 244(17):1946–1949.

Based on a lecture given at the 13th Annual Medical Symposium, "Controversies in Internal Medicine," presented by the Southern California Permanente Medical Group and Kaiser Foundation Hospitals, Los Angeles, Oct. 5, 1979.

the often inarticulate yet prudent judgments of discerning physicians with explicit rules or procedures will not lead to better decisions. It is an old story—easily verified by living in a university—that there is no necessary connection between sophistication in ethical argumentation and good conduct.

Yet the superiority of trusting in the prudence or discernment of the practitioner in *specific* cases presupposes that the practitioner understands *in general* what his practice is and what it is for. To contribute to such general reflection on the nature of medicine, I shall here consider certain general and unavoidable perplexities regarding the physician's proper business, rather than the more usually discussed specific ethical dilemmas, e.g., abortion, confidentiality, or the allocation of scarce resources. I begin with some general observations about ethics and medicine.

Some General Remarks about Ethics and Medicine

"What is an ethical dilemma?" What makes an ethical dilemma ethical? Identifying an ethical dilemma is sometimes as difficult as resolving it, as the following story makes clear.

A shabbily dressed elderly man has come to consult the professor of philosophy with a question about business ethics. "Me and my partner, we have a confectionary store in the Bronx. Last week in comes a young man, very distracted, probably in love, asks for a package of cigarettes. Staring dreamily at the ceiling, he puts down a $10 bill, takes his cigarettes and starts out of the store, leaving his change on the counter. Now, Professor, comes a question, business ethics. Should I or should I not tell my partner?"

Identifying ethical dilemmas depends not only on the perceived presence or absence of relationships that may give rise to obligations of honesty or justice. Even more does it depend on our perceptions and opinions about human nature and the nature of morality. For some of us, morality is primarily conceived of in terms of right and wrong, good and evil, purity and sin, and issues forth in rules designed to guide but primarily to restrain wayward humanity, seen as destined toward the bad in the absence of such restraints. For others, morality is primarily conceived of in terms of benefits and harms, and issues forth in calculations aimed at optimizing pleasure, safety, and comfort, and minimizing

pain, danger, and disease, mankind being seen as already correctly disposed by nature toward the former and away from the latter. Still others talk the moral language of rights and correlative duties, a morality that issues forth in procedural and institutional arrangements that seek to maintain and extend a precarious individual autonomy, threatened by the fact that everyone is assumed to be at best selfishly indifferent to the good of unrelated others. Finally, others talk not of sins, costs and benefits, or rights, but of virtue and vice, of the dispositions or stands of human beings regarding fear or bodily pleasure, or wealth or honor, an approach to ethics that emphasizes character rather than rules of conduct and that seeks to nourish by habituation in good deeds the latent, yet otherwise feeble, human tendency toward goodness, thought to be present in most human beings.

I bother you about these different approaches to ethics—the approaches that emphasize (1) moral rules of thou shalts and shalt nots, (2) calculations of benefits and harms, (3) procedures to protect freedom and autonomy, and (4) the cultivation of fine character—for two reasons. First, because it is important to recognize that the very formulation and definition of ethical problems is itself subject to broad variation and debate, indeed, about extremely fundamental matters. Second—and this is my underlying thesis, to which I will return briefly later—I suspect that some of the difficulties medicine now faces stem from the fact that the profession's traditional perception of the ethical universe differs sharply from the prevailing American culture on this very matter. Medicine, long a profession of cultivated gentlemen, and always a profession of action, has relied largely on the character of physicians and their esteemed virtues of tact, gentleness, gravity, patience, modesty, justice, humanity, and, above all, prudence or practical wisdom to cope with the myriad human situations they would encounter in practice. Though there have been codes of ethics for physicians—something like rules of conduct—these have not until recently been thought desirable or necessary for regulating the behavior of the well-intentioned and well-brought-up practitioner, who must in any case be allowed to exercise the prudent judgment of the man on the spot that practice requires and for which rules cannot be given.

In contrast, the ethos of our community has different sources: the great religious traditions, with their commandments and rules, some embodied also in our criminal law; the Anglo-American libertarian tradition, with its freedoms and rights, and, to protect these liberties, institutional arrangements meant to supply the defect of the want of better motives; and the utilitarian tradition of comfort and safety, fueled by technological progress, which strives to make life less poor, nasty, brutish, and short. If this thesis is correct, then it is small wonder that medicine should find itself somewhat at odds with the broader community even in the formulation of what constitutes an ethical dilemma, let alone what one should do about it. Physicians who have long taken for granted their benevolent intentions toward their patients and prided themselves on their ability to judge the just-right thing to do in the circumstances will not see the need for, and understandably will bridle at, the proposals of moralists and legislators to establish fixed rules of conduct, of economists and health policy planners who want to convert everything into cost-effectiveness data, or of lawyers and patient advocates who insist on establishing a patient bill of rights or laying down an explicit contract between the so-called consumers and providers of health services. The profession jealously and, I think, by and large justifiably, guards its own view of its professional responsibility, and, more important, its own ability to discern, describe, and face its ethical dilemmas.

Yet, however reasonable it is to see medicine as an autonomous profession, with its own ethical views and practices, it cannot be denied that individual physicians are members of the broader community and the institution of medicine is subject to law and enmeshed in the broader social matrix. It is the dilemmas caused by these external relations that I want to consider next, as I turn to the first of the three larger perplexities I wish to consider.

Whom Does the Doctor Serve?

Whom does the doctor serve? He serves his patients: the ill, the diseased, the dying, and also the worried-well who might be ill, diseased, or dying. This is a truism and has been so since the beginning of medicine. The Oath of Hippocrates states: "I will apply dietetic measures for the benefit of the sick according to my ability and judgment; I will keep them from harm and injustice," and, again, "Whatever houses I may visit, I will come for the benefit of the sick."

Yet, this is not the last word. There are, and

have always been, other potential beneficiaries of the physician's services. And I do not mean only the physician himself, whose self-interest is notoriously not always congruent with those of his patients, whether in matters of time or money. The patient's family, other unrelated patients, community institutions such as schools or corporations, and the broader sociopolitical community sometimes bid for, or lay claim to, the physician's services and attention. Sometimes the service demanded conflicts with the physician's service to individual patients.

This is not a new problem. Since antiquity physicians attached to armies on the battlefield have served to maximize the army's fighting strength. Today, triage medicine is justifiably practiced in battle, where the overarching purpose of the common defense and community survival justifies overriding the usual presumption to help those most in need in favor of restoring those most able to fight. In peacetime, for reasons of public health and safety, physicians are legally obliged to report cases of venereal disease or gunshot wounds, and, if the Tarasoff decision in California establishes a precedent, may be not only permitted but required to violate patient confidentiality to inform other people who may be at risk for serious harm from potentially homicidal maniacs. In practices that have not received the critical ethical scrutiny they deserve, psychiatrists now serve as officers of the court in civil commitment proceedings, and many physicians are in the employ of businesses or athletic teams, often, at best, with divided loyalties, and sometimes, in fact, undertreating or mistreating employees or athletes for the sake of the organization's purpose. The rise of family medicine and family psychiatry has acknowledged that the well-being of families is intimately connected with that of the ill, thus overcoming a sometimes unfortunate exaggeration of the focus on ailing persons, as when, e.g., psychiatrists encourage patients to undertake or continue extramarital affairs, indifferent to the effects on the patient's spouse and children.

Though the problem of divided loyalty is old, it has been greatly exacerbated in recent years, and threatens to become much worse, for several related reasons. First, there are changes in the character of medical care. Some fruits of technological progress, such as renal dialysis or transplantation or the intensive care units, raise explicit questions of patient selection for services in short supply, often placing a physician in a bind between loyalty to one patient and another or between loyalty to patient and institutional policy. Second, the enormous costs of medical care, in large measure the result of its technological sophistication, have meant new roles for third parties. What insurance companies will pay for often determines what patients will receive, and this frequently means unnecessary hospitalizations and other measures not clearly in the patient's best interests. The actuarial and statistical approach that necessarily governs the practices and policies of third parties is frequently at cross purposes with the best treatment or procedure for a given patient with special needs or problems. Third, and probably most important, is the massive role of the federal government, in its hospital building programs, Medicare and Medicaid, kidney machine legislation, health maintenance organizations (HMOs) and Professional Standards Review Organizations (PSROs), human experimentation committees, food and drug regulations, and equal opportunity employment regulations, and other species of intervention too numerous to mention. Finally, there is the rise of the public health movement, with its focus on whole populations rather than the individually ill, a focus supported also by the statistically inclined cost-effectiveness orientation of our leading health economists and policy makers.

One conclusion is obvious. The physician's attempt to benefit sick patients is constrained and shaped decisively on all sides by many non-medical considerations. The individual doctor-patient relationship occurs in institutional settings and under ruling practices that have little whatsoever to do with the needs of the individually ill, and the powerful interests of these larger organizations, from hospitals to the US Department of Health and Human Services, in many cases take precedence. Looking to the future, we can expect this tendency to increase—not just in medicine, but in education and many other activities—and some have called on us to abandon our preference for individual attention and opt for what one thoughtful physician has called "statistical compassion."

What are physicians to think about all this? Can the medical profession retain its integrity if it abandons its patient-centered orientation? The American medical profession has traditionally said no. Yet there are signs of change, to me at least, disturbing signs of change. The text of the new proposed Code of Medical Ethics under consideration by the American Medical Association is much more ambiguous on this subject than one might wish. Only one of the seven proposed articles deals with the physician's primary business, namely, patient care, and moreover, strange to say, it makes no mention of the patient: "A physician shall be dedicated to providing medically competent service with compassion and respect for human dignity."[1] Competent service to whom and for whose benefit? And why not "respect for the dignity of his patients" or even "of human persons," rather than the more abstract "respect for human dignity"? The other provisions occasionally speak of the patient, but their themes are the physician's relationship to the profession; the law; rights; learning and consulting and informing the public; the physician's freedom "to choose whom to serve"; and his responsibilities as a member of society. Surprisingly, there is nothing in the proposed code equal to the shiningly clear statement of the World Medical Association's 1948 Declaration of Geneva: "The health of my patient will be my first consideration."[2]

Now there is no question but that medicine cannot be a simply autonomous profession. In truth, it never has been. As Aristotle long ago observed, the political is most authoritative and architectonic; politics, i.e., the ruling laws, institutions, and customs of a regime, "ordains which of the sciences are to be in the cities . . . and legislates as to what people shall do and what things they shall refrain from doing."[3] Moreover, as health has become a major public business—now 8% of our gross national product is spent on health care—it is to be expected and even welcomed that the political community as a whole, at its various levels, deliberate about how best to promote the nation's health, given that resources will always be limited. The allocation of scarce resources has always been ultimately a political matter, here and elsewhere, to be resolved by the political process—even when that political process decided that government not interfere in a free-market allocation. Medicine may seek to influence the outcome of political deliberation, and no doubt we would have better health policies if our health planners were more intimately familiar with the actual practice of medicine in hospital, home, and examining room. But the ruling character of the political must be conceded, even if with fear and trembling.

The crucial question lies elsewhere: Can these broad social and political considerations be allowed to enter within the bounds of the doctor-patient relationship? Here, perhaps, lies the greatest threat to the traditional ethic of the profession: the intrusion of the political or societal perspective into the day-to-day care of single patients.

In a recent article in *The Hastings Center Report*,[4] a physician and a philosophy professor discussed a case that turned on whether an elderly woman, with a recurrent episode of severe respiratory failure, previously successfully treated, should again be treated with a respirator, a decision to treat requiring that she occupy the last bed in the intensive care unit. The young physician wrote not only to oppose treatment but also to oppose leaving the decision either to the patient and her family or to the physician:

> Although Mrs. A's family has the right to refuse the ICU [intensive care unit] transfer and respirator, they do not have the right to demand it. Self-determination with regard to medical care is one thing, but a just allocation of scarce resources is another. The first right belongs to the patient, but the second is a claim which society makes upon the use of its health care resources.
>
> Shall the physician decide? This would be an odd way to decide such questions (although in fact many are decided by physicians). Physicians, like families, have vested interests in some patients compared to others. And little in their educational background qualifies them as experts *in the just allocation of scarce life-saving medical resources* (emphasis added).

But the proper question before the physician was not one of just allocation of medical resources (though it might have become one if he had two patients both of whom needed the last bed). The question was whether his patient needed help and whether she could benefit from the treatment—and never mind if it meant filling the empty last bed in the ICU, which, after all, is there to be used. The questions of distributive justice have their place, say, in the decision to build or expand the ICU. But once the facility is available, these considerations are irrelevant to the physician's judgment that therapy will be beneficial, and should not prevent his offering it to the patient if the patient is willing. Within the broader limits set by social and institutional policy, the physician must practice unswervingly the virtues of loyalty and fidelity to his patient.

This is no mere sentimentality or moralizing.

The principles involved are easy to state. They go to the very heart of the medical activity. Loyalty to the patient must be paramount, first, because the mysterious activity of healing depends on trust and confidence, which trust is lodged by the vulnerable and dependent patient with the physician, in the very act of submitting to his care. (By the way, would it not be unethical to undermine or betray such trust, even were it not indispensable for the healing activity?) One who is ill submits to the care of the healer in the expectation that the healer will care for his well-being as much as he does himself and that the healer will pursue it to the best of his ability. Even more fundamentally, the legitimate claim for individual patient-centered medicine can *never* be obliterated, even come the revolution, for the obvious, but sometimes forgotten, reason that illness almost always happens to bodies, and nothing is more individuating and private than body. My pain, my weakness, my illness—unlike my thoughts on these matters—are absolutely unsharable. Even the socialization of medicine could not socialize the radically private property of body. An ultimately individualistic orientation is necessarily constitutive for the healing profession under any political order.

What Does the Doctor Serve?

Having established provisionally that the physician serves first and most the patient, we face the second perplexity: *What* about the patient is served by the physician? The dilemma may be put this way: Does the physician serve the patient's *needs* or his *desires* and *wishes*? Or again, does the physician serve the patient's *good* or his *rights*? Can it be simply true, without qualification, that the good physician is the *servant* of the *patient*?

Let me illustrate with some examples. When cosmetic surgeons lift faces, inflate bosoms, and straighten noses, are they serving needs or desires? When the obstetrician agrees to determine the sex of the unborn child by amniocentesis and abort fetuses of the unwanted gender, does he serve need or desire? When the internist gives in to a mother's request to tranquilize her teenaged daughter's anxiety before her first cello recital, does he serve need or wish? And what of the psychiatrist who has sexual relations with his patients in the office as part of his treatment of frigidity?

Honoring so-called patient rights may also conflict with serving the patient's good. It is now claimed that patients have a right to know the whole truth about their diagnosis and treatment, including an account, in detail, of all possible complications and untoward consequences of proposed therapies. There is said to be a right of access to medical records, a right to refuse treatment as well as a right to obtain treatment (especially for persons involuntarily committed for mental illness), a right to health care, a right to determine the fate of one's body, even a right to die or to be mercifully killed. Some of these claims seem to me to be dubious, while others touch on important matters that could be accommodated without resorting to the uncompromising and contentious talk of "rights." But be that as it may, the main point here is that physicians increasingly face the uncomfortable choice of either risking harm to patients by catering to their rights or risking suit from patients by ignoring their rights to serve their good.

One suspects that these difficulties and tensions will increase, for they seem to be related to powerful tendencies of modern life. The increasingly sophisticated means for intervening in the human body and mind have also produced new ends for the use of biomedical technique. And it has been noted often that the triumph of technique, fueled initially by rather modest and unexceptionable goals, itself gives rise to an inflation and proliferation of desires, which in turn breed the further growth of technology needed for their satisfaction. This is especially true under conditions of great freedom and prosperity, in cultures such as our own that esteem comfort and safety, and in which a highly literate and demanding populace comes to expect a technical solution to all life's difficulties.

The swelling of demands and desires for goods and services is paralleled by the rising stress on personal autonomy, in the face of declining influence of the authority of tradition and traditional authorities and often a frank attack on *all* authority, including that of the professions, medicine among them.

There is no doubt that physicians will have to make their peace with these tendencies requiring them to serve patient desires and respect patient rights. The AMA's proposed new Code of Medical Ethics has, perhaps unwittingly, made clear concessions in that direction. It says, for instance, that "A physician shall be dedicated to providing medically competent service" (not "competent *medical* service") without specifying anywhere in the code the end to be served by medical competence. Indeed, the word "health" occurs in the code only twice, both times as an adjective in the phrase "other health professionals." The code also says that "A physician shall respect the rights of patients" without specifying what rights patients are deemed to have and who will determine them. It would be most instructive, if we had time, to compare the understanding of the doctor-patient relation implied by the notion "respect the *rights* of the patient" with the more traditional understanding implied by the Hippocratic Oath's "I will keep them from *harm* and *injustice*," the former emphasizing the patient's autonomy, prerogatives, and rights, the latter, the patient's neediness and the over-arching norms of good and of right; the former presupposing a physician who needs to be exhorted not to violate his patients, the latter presupposing a benevolent healer who must keep the oft intemperate patient from violating himself.

But the medical profession should be wary of conceding too much in making its peace. For, as with the first perplexity, there are some fundamental matters at stake, matters that again strike at the heart of the healing relation. If we could recover a deeper understanding of this relation and of the art of medicine generally, we might be more alert to the dangers that threaten it. One danger is contained in the pressures to treat medicine not as an art or a profession that is practiced, but as a technical service that is delivered, like auto repair or plumbing—in this case, a service "provided" by physicians or by the "health care delivery system" and "consumed" by patients. This new understanding shifts the focus to the buying and selling—to the relation of exchange—and away from the mysterious activity of healing and the crucial and incomparable interpersonal bonds of the healing relation, far beyond what the psychiatrists call transference and counter-transference.

Many in the so-called consumer movement, not particularly sensitive to fine distinctions, would replace an understanding of the healing relationship founded on ideas of covenant, vocation, philanthropy, fidelity and trust, or devotion to the art with a new view: a relation of contract, with explicitly defined items contracted for exchange. Such a notion both presupposes a lack of trust and further exacerbates it, thus interfering with the healing relation. Indeed, it simply misunderstands and hence denies the essence of the healing activity, which depends on hope and confidence, care and trust, no less than on technique. It is an activity whose nature and effectiveness are shrouded in mystery, and whose outcome is always uncertain and so subject to the vicissitudes of conditions and circumstances as to make contractual promises unreasonable. It is an activity much like child rearing or teaching, activities also grossly misunderstood by those who would reduce these as well to a species of contract.

A second mortal danger is contained in the now-popular notion that a person has a right over his body, a right that allows him to do whatever he wants to it or with it. Civil liberatarians may applaud such a notion, as an arguably logical expansion of right of privacy, of the right to be free from unwanted or offensive touchings of one's body. But for a physician, the idea must be unacceptable. No physician worthy of the name would honor a patient's request to pluck out his eye if it offends him nor lop off a breast to improve a lady's golf swing. Medicine violates the body only to heal it. Physicians respect the integrity of body not only because and if the patient wants or allows them to. They respect and minister to bodily wholeness because they recognize, at least tacitly, what a wonderful and awe-inspiring—not to say sacred—thing the healthy living human body is. They know or should know—for they practice a profession whose very foundation presupposes—the precariousness of human life and the dependence of all good things on a well-working body, whose great powers and frailty both command respect and modesty. No physician who understands the profession should be guilty of the contempt for the body or arrogance of the will that declares "my body" to be a mere thing to be disposed of or carved up at "my will." (I commend to the reader's attention on the subject of the body the writings of Richard Selzer, MD, *Mortal Lessons* and *Confessions of a Knife.)*

Now, to be fair, one must concede that medicine has not itself been sufficiently mindful of these matters. The assertion of patient's rights and the move toward increasing patient autonomy, it must be acknowledged, are in part in response to excessive authoritarianism and mystification—even arrogance—on the part of physicians. If patients stridently insist on being treated as persons, demand that their wishes be honored, and occasionally show contempt for the body, it is perhaps because physicians have all too often shown a forgetfulness of the soul, of the human aspects of patients and patient care. Sad to say, one can even learn contempt for the body from some physicians, who in their eagerness to treat this or that abnormality forget about the well-working of the body as a whole or prescribe dangerous drugs to remedy trifling complaints. Thus, while it is true that the physician has been rightly committed more to patient good than to patient rights, to patient need than to patient wish, it is also true that physicians frequently now hold too narrow a view of need and of good, too shrunken a view of the integrity of the human organism, and almost no view at all of the riches and mysteries of the human soul. Modern science and modern medicine have not taught our culture well on most of these matters.

Can we find a way out of this perplexity regarding the doctor-patient relationship and the object of medical service, and the dilemmas it creates? Even in thought, there is no simple answer. It is not always easy to distinguish a need from a desire, or a reasonable from an unreasonable desire, or to decide which clearly reasonable desires and wishes deserve the services of a physician. Patients do have a need for respectful treatment and for by and large truthful and patient counsel, and it is good for them to take as large a role in their own health-maintenance as is possible—even if these needs and goods are not owed them because they claim them as rights. There is truth in the slogan that patients are, first of all, persons, and only secondarily patients to the physician's ministrations.

Practically speaking, there are like-wise no simple rules for balancing these considerations in deciding what to do in patient care. Certain virtues seem to be required: moderation in the physician's view of what he can and cannot accomplish, gravity before the awesome mysteries of human being, understanding of the human aspects of the lives, hopes, and fears of the ill, courage to resist unwarranted demands for pills or procedures, and prudent judgment to discern the warranted from the unwarranted. These are not the virtues of the servile. And though it is true that the physician must not seek to be a master, so also must he not stoop to be a slave.

Indeed, to close this section, it is worth reconsidering whether we have not been mistaken in the very posing of our questions: Whom and what does the physician serve? Is the doctor really a *servant?* In a way he is, providing we remember that one can serve not only people but also ideals, not only a worldly master but also a noble calling. One way of stating the conclusion of this part of my argument is to assert that the physician's loyalty to his patient must be decisively qualified by the doctor's loyalty to his art and to its norms and goals, or, again, that the doctor serves not the patient simply but, rather, the *good* of the patient. At a deeper level, one could say that in healing the human body the physician is also assisting and serving that innate power of nature that is manifested in each patient but greater than all of them, a power that all ancient peoples acknowledged in regarding medicine as a sacred or holy art. (Consider in this connection the beginning of the Hippocratic Oath, the discussion of healing in Leviticus 13 and 14, or the Greek deification of the founders of medicine.)

Yet, the language of service is also not quite right when applied to the relation between physician and patient. For service implies mastery or lordship, and the doctor is, in truth, neither a master nor a servant of the patient. With respect to the patient's body, he is a helper, a co-worker with nature and with the patient himself, in providing the ill body its proper aid. With respect to the patient as person, one of his main functions, often neglected, is to be a leader and a teacher, one who leads the activities of healing and one who teaches patients and the community about regaining and maintaining healthy functioning. The word "doctor" literally means "teacher," from the Latin verb *docere,* to teach—in this case one who teaches the wisdom and wonders of the body to patient and pupil alike.

2. What Is the Patient's Good?

In reflecting on the nature of the medical vocation, we have come via a somewhat labyrinthine path to a not very startling assertion: the doctor, by teaching and technique, through patient understanding and astute judgment, promotes the patient's good. Our third perplexity follows directly: What is the patient's good? More precisely, of the many things that are good for the patient, which is it the physician's business to promote? We are no longer asking about medicine's foreign or domestic relations, but about its very constitution: What is the purpose of medicine?

This is, in a way, a strange question to be asking, since most of the time physicians can go about unreflectively doing their proper business, tacitly if silently clear about the nature and limits of the purposes of medicine. But because new technological powers permit physicians to serve multi-ple ends, and because much of medical practice is so fragmented and specialized, there is today some confusion and uncertainty about the nature and limits of the purposes of medicine. In an article published a few years ago, "Regarding the End of Medicine and the Pursuit of Health," I suggested that this confusion was a serious cause of the malaise of American medicine. Against the growing tendency to enlarge the medical mission, I argued that health was the proper end of medicine, whereas other albeit worthy goals, such as pleasure, contentment, happiness, civil peace and order, virtue, wisdom, and truth, were false goals for the healing art. Against the narrow perspective of the high-technology, highly specialized therapy-centered predilections of recent decades, I also tried to outline a functional notion of health and argued that health, understood as the "well-working" of the organism as a whole, is not just the absence of disease, but a positive good and the proper norm for medical practice, one that implies that there is more to healing illness than curing disease. I will not repeat that part of the argument here and will trust that few physicians would deny that health is the main purpose of medicine or that some tacit notion of the norm is latent in every attempt at healing— "healing" meaning literally, "a making whole."

Instead, I want to consider a quandary that arises even if we all agree not only that health is the physician's primary business, but also on the meaning of healthiness: What to think and what to do in the face of incurable disease and unhealable illness? What good does the physician seek to promote when healthy functioning is out of the question?

To be sure, some level of healthy functioning is never out of the question, this side of death. The degree of health and departures from health form a continuum, and even people in the so-called persistent vegetative state must have healthy vegetative functions—respiration, metabolism, and excretion. But few of us would accept the preservation of such a reduced level of function as a proper *goal* for medicine, even though we sadly accept it as an unfortunate and unforeseen *result* of treatment that had higher aspirations and even if we refuse actively to cause such vegetative life to cease. So the question remains, not only regarding the comatose, but also the terminally ill, the irretrievably dying, the irreversibly deteriorating—especially in mind and awareness—and the otherwise anguished and miserable: What should medicine's goal be for them?

To be sure, easing of pain and relief of suffering, along with supporting and comforting speech, are always in order, all the more so in the presence of incurable and progressive illness. Relief of suffering stands, next to health, as a crucial part of the medical goal, and medicine has always sought to comfort where it cannot heal. The real quandaries concern activities for prolongation or preservation of life. When, if ever, is it appropriate to withhold or interrupt treatments that might be life preserving or life prolonging?

This, too, is an old quandary, faced by physicians even before the modern era of antibiotics, respirators, and defibrillators, say, in decisions about whether or not to amputate a gangrenous limb in an elderly patient. But there is no doubt that such dilemmas now arise vastly more frequently and have generated a burgeoning professional and public concern. The main causes include (1) the effectiveness of life-sustaining technologies and the zeal of young physicians in their use, (2) the existence of many more "incurables" who, particularly in hospital settings, are especially impotent in expressing their wishes to be left alone, many of whom have no enduring relationship with a physician who could knowingly act on their behalf, and (3) the physician's fear of criminal and civil liability, partly in the face of ambiguity regarding the law, e.g., whether turning off a respirator is a proximate cause of death. Yet, recognizing these sources of our dilemmas in no way diminishes them. Nearly everyone agrees that the practice of intervening and prolonging has gotten out of hand in many, many cases.

How to think about this problem? I confess I find it enormously difficult. Indeed, perhaps the most important lesson to be driven home by the medical profession and to its members is just how complicated a matter this is. It simply will not yield to simple formulas such as "death with dignity," or "life is sacred," or "dispense with extraordinary means." Terms like "incurable," "dying," "terminal," and "hopeless" are notoriously vague, not to speak of "dignity." "Ordinary" and "extraordinary" sometimes mean only "customary" and "unusual," sometimes are relativized to the particular circumstances of each patient, so that what would be ordinary for one patient becomes extraordinary for another. Even the word "treatment" is ambiguous, sometimes implying effective therapy, sometimes merely naming the applied procedure or intervention.

Measures that can be said to be life preserving span a continuum from respirators and dialysis machines, through antibiotics and insulin, to intravenous glucose and water, even to food and drink. The distinction between an action and an omission, which I find useful in some cases, is neither always obvious nor obvious to all, especially if judged only from the result. There are notorious problems in discerning the patient's own judgment regarding his state of being and suffering or his desire to be treated or not. For at least these reasons, the attempt to solve these dilemmas—by generalizations embodied in rules, guidelines, or statutes, or even by court decisions—seems fraught with dangers, some of which I will indicate soon. In no other area is there a greater need for sober and prudent judgment of the man on the spot, and yet, in no other area is there more reluctance and resistance to leave matters simply to prudence. When it comes to the utter finality of the end of a life, we all long to proceed with certitude and clear conscience.

The easy way out is to adhere always to the principle "Sustain life regardless," and there is much to be said for the sentiment involved (if not for the practice), reverence for life being a constitutive yet fragile principle of decent human community. Nevertheless, it seems to me that a true reverence for life might include permitting it to end, free from further assaults on life's sanctity committed in its name. This, I submit, has been the traditional view of the medical profession, and, I might add, of Christian religious tradition [e.g., see Ramsey P: "On (Only) Caring for the Dying," in *The Patient as Person.* New Haven, Conn, Yale University Press, 1970, chap 3].

Illuminating this view is in part the recognition of human finitude. Even the most healthy human being must someday die, despite all efforts of the most competent physician. Such it is to be a mortal being, and such it is to have but extremely limited powers. Physicians need to accept these lessons no less than anyone else. If medicine takes aim at death prevention, rather than at health and relief of suffering, if it regards every death as premature, as a failure of today's medicine—but avoidable by tomorrow's—then it is tacitly asserting that its true goal is bodily immortality. Once it is put that way, it should be clear that physicians must teach themselves and their patients to make their peace with finitude. As I have argued elsewhere, physicians should try to:

Keep their eye on their main business, restoring and correcting what can be corrected and restored, always acknowledging that death will and must come, that health is a mortal good, and that as embodied beings we are fragile beings that must snap sooner or later, medicine or no medicine. To keep the strings in tune, not to stretch them out of shape attempting to make them last forever, is the doctor's primary and proper goal.[5]

Medicine has traditionally refused to make prolongation of life its goal, not only because the goal was finally unreachable, but also because it recognized that efforts in that direction often produced more harm than good—in pain and discomfort as well as anguish and anxiety. (Many have observed that anxiety about death from disease has never been higher, and it would be a hollow victory indeed if the extra time medicine provides us is squandered in worry. And of the deeper ills of a society dedicated to staying alive rather than to living well, we are but dimly aware.)

These thoughts suggest a useful beginning for thinking about the concrete cases in which healing is impossible and interventions are being contemplated. The first question should not be "Will this intervention prolong life?" but "Will this intervention increase or decrease this patient's discomfort, pain, and suffering?" The concern of the physician should be the condition of the life to be sustained and not especially its duration. This means, e.g., being willing, if the circumstances are correct, to give high doses of narcotics if needed, even at the risk of respiratory depression, or to forego resuscitation or antibiotics in the face of underlying terminal illness or severe debilitation of mind. To judge if the circumstances are correct, here and now, is the work of prudence or practical wisdom or discernment—a virtue not teachable in medical school and not replaceable by computer programs. It is the cardinal virtue of experienced and seasoned practical men.

Now, against this view there are important arguments. Some will suggest that I am urging that physicians begin to make judgments of so-called quality of life. It may be argued that such a move also invites considerations of "social worthiness" or other alien matters to contaminate medical decisions, with not only individual lives, but our very reverence for life, in jeopardy. The consideration in medicine of quality of life, it is

correctly said, was the fundamental error of the Nazi physicians. These are serious concerns, not to be taken lightly. I too am made uncomfortable by breezy talk about quality of life, and even by the terms in which the sanitized notion of "quality" is substituted for "goodness," with the attendant implication that quality is a readily measurable matter. Nevertheless, I do believe consideration of the condition of the individual patient's health, activity, and state of mind must enter these decisions, if the decision is indeed to be for the patient's good. I think one can walk between the extremes of vitalism and "quality control" and uphold in so doing the respect that life itself commands for itself. For life is to be revered not only as manifested in physiological powers, but also as these powers are organized in the form of *a life*, with its beginning, middle, and end. Thus, life can be revered not only in its preservation, but also in the manner in which we allow a given life to reach its terminus. For physicians to adhere to efforts at indefinite prolongation not only reduces them to slavish technicians without any intelligible goal, but also degrades and assaults the gravity and solemnity of a life in its close.

Fortunately, protection against the dangers of callous indifference, patient neglect, and the intrusion of alien considerations is available, if the physician assesses the patient's condition from the patient's point of view. This usually means open and frank discussion with the patient, where that is possible. Delicate questions of truth telling emerge—how much to say, and when and how—never to be settled by an inflexible adherence to principle. Even more difficult is to discern truly from the patient's words and what he actually believes and feels. In a recent article in the *New England Journal of Medicine,* Jackson and Younger[6] show how patient ambivalence, reactive depression, displacement, fear, and ignorance or family misperceptions of patient attitudes can lead astray a physician who relies too much on a verbalized request for cessation of treatment. Discerning the patient's true sentiments and outlook is, again, often a matter of tact and care and subtlety. Physicians will soon need to be sensitive in detecting pressures applied to patients because of the emerging climate of opinion that trumpets cessation of treatment, that romanticizes "death with dignity," or that trivializes death's meaning by turning dying into a management problem for death-experts called thanatologists, just as they should have been sensitive in the past to how their own bias for "prolongation regardless" also subtly manipulated patient attitudes. The physician must know each patient if he is to teach him appropriately.

To be frank, the record of the profession as a whole in its treatment of the untreatable has left many dissatisfied, and there are growing movements, from several quarters, to remove the matter from the discretion of individual physicians and to bring practice under some form of external and uniform guidelines. We shall probably see more of this in the future, and the prospect is not encouraging. Consider, e.g., the California Natural Death Act, passed in 1976.[7] This well-intentioned statute permits a person prospectively to execute a written directive to his physician to withhold or withdraw life-sustaining procedures in the event of a "terminal condition," but the operating clause indicates that such instruction is valid *only* in cases in which "death is imminent, *whether or not* such procedures are utilized" (emphasis added). In other words, the law permits the patient only to instruct the physician to desist from useless procedures, a halt that should be regarded by physicians not as a legally granted privilege but rather as a professionally based duty. By implication, the law seems to cast some doubt on whether withholding treatment under any other conditions is acceptable, or whether any patient who has not written such a directive must be assumed to desire full-scale and recurrent prolongation efforts. Could the physician decline to resuscitate a senile woman with crippling arthritis, but with no terminal illness, either with or without such a directive? Does the law silently forbid—or discourage—what it does not explicitly permit?

Or consider the Saikewicz case in Massachusetts,[8] which has been followed by a spate of other cases, brought to court by physicians who mistakenly believed that they now need a judicial directive to cease treatment if the patient is incompetent [see also Ramsey P: The Saikewicz precedent: What's good for an incompetent patient. *Hastings Cent Rep* 8:36–42, December 1978]. To be sure, they need a judicial opinion in advance if they wish to obtain immunity against possible legal action for their decision, but what are we to think of the self-understanding of the profession if it will practice only under the promise of immunity for its errors? Moreover, the risk of penalty is almost nonexistent. I believe it is still true that no American physician has been sued or prosecuted for terminating treatment of a dying patient, competent or incompetent, for whom there is no hope of cure.

Guidelines set by the profession may also needlessly tie physician's hands. A widely discussed article in the *New England Journal of Medicine,* "Orders Not to Resuscitate,"[9] proposes that orders not to resuscitate are appropriate if the disease is irreversible, the physiological status of the patient is irreparable, and death is imminent, "in the sense that in the ordinary course of events, death probably will occur within a period not exceeding two weeks." Are there no conditions of the patient other than imminent death within two weeks that could justify a refusal to defibrillate? And can a physician now no longer write orders not to resuscitate such patients?

While there are pitfalls at every turn, sure footing will not be had as a result of statutes, court decisions, or professional guidelines and regulations. Indeed, here is an area where dilemmas cannot be neatly solved but only soberly faced, where the desire for certainty and the cleanest conscience must give way to the satisfaction that a grave decision was conscientiously made, with utmost seriousness and adequate consultation, and in the interest of doing the most good and causing the least suffering to the individual patient, as that patient himself would wish. Written directives, rules, and guidelines are no substitute for sobriety, common sense, and discernment in the search for the patient's good.

Yet I would make one qualification, and propose one rule, well stated already in the Oath of Hippocrates: "I will neither give a deadly drug to anybody if asked for it, nor will I make a suggestion to this effect." There is a difference between permitting to die and directly killing, if not in the result for the patient, then certainly in understanding the activity of the agent. This age-old rule against mercy-killing by physicians, though supported by Judaism and Christianity, and by Anglo-American law, has its true roots in the very idea of the physician as healer. Hans Jonas[10] has put the matter well:

As to outright hastening death by a lethal drug, the doctor cannot fairly be asked to make any of his ministrations with this *purpose*, nor the hospital staff to connive by looking the other way if someone else provides the patient the means. The law forbids it, but more so (the law being changeable) it is prohibited by the innermost meaning of the medical vocation, which should never cast the physician in the role of a dispenser of death, even at the subject's request (p 34).

Coda

I close with a few general observations, again about ethics and medicine, as these emerge from my reflections. Though it is perhaps nothing to brag about, I know that I have said little that could help the reader solve any ethical dilemma now waiting for him in the hospital. I have chosen to concentrate on some basic elements of the profession: Who and what is the physician? What is his relation to his patient and society? What are the goals of his art? I believe that what is most needful at present is self-conscious reflection by physicians regarding themselves and the nature of their professional commitments. To be sure, through some procedures and rules, we can try to "solve" or at least cope with this and that ethical dilemma; but it is through clarity about his ends and prudence and moderation in his choice of means that a self-understanding physician is able to stand well before all dilemmas.

There is notion abroad that there is, or that there can and should be, a science of medical right and wrong or, at least, of proper decision making to which physicians can turn for expert help to solve medicine's ethical dilemmas. This is worse than an illusion. It represents a declaration of moral bankruptcy on the part of the profession, which once understood the ethical as integral to the medical, and which never supposed that the "dilemmas of caring for the ill" could be neatly solved. The call for rules, guidelines, and procedures, the convening of ethics committees, and the encouragement of statutory regulations are a search for yet one more technical solution—this time a technical *ethical* solution—for problems produced by our already foolish tendency to seek technical medical solutions for the weighty difficulties of human life. If a doctor would be a physician and not merely a body technician, he must also be a knower of souls, those of his patients and, not least, his own.

References

1. *Proceedings of the American Medical Association House of Delegates, Annual Meeting, Chicago, July 22–26, 1979.* Chicago, American Medical Association, 1979, p 245.

2. Declaration of Geneva. *World Med Assoc Bull* 1:109–111, 1949.

3. Aristotle: *Nicomachean Ethics* I. 2. 1094a28-1094b5.

4. Schiffer RM, Freedman B: The last bed in the ICU: A medical or moral decision? *Hastings Cent Rep* 7(No. 6):21–22, 1977.

5. Kass LR: Regarding the end of medicine and the pursuit of health. *Public Interest* 40:11–42, Summer 1975.

6. Jackson DL, Younger S: Patient autonomy and 'death with dignity.' *N Engl J Med* 301:404–408, 1979.

7. 'Natural Death Act,' California Health and Safety Code, AB 3060, div 7, pt I, chap 3.9, section 7185–7195, Aug 30, 1976.

8. *Superintendent of Belchertown State School et al vs Joseph Saikewicz,* 370 NE 2d 417 (SJC, Mass, 1977).

9. Rabkin MT, Gillerman G, Rice NR: Orders not to resuscitate. *N Engl J Med* 295:364–369, 1976.

10. Jonas H: The right to die. *Hastings Cent Rep* 8:31–36, August 1978.

Arrogance

Franz J. Ingelfinger, M.D.

In this George W. Gay Lecture, specifically designated as "upon medical ethics," I shall focus on three issues. The first, an example of intergroup tensions, deals with the common accusation that bioscientists are arrogant, i.e., that they are presumptuous and overweening in their attitudes, decisions, and goals; that they exhibit, in the fashionable noun of the day, hubris. I shall argue that the bioscientist may be arrogant, but no more so than any other group and perhaps just a little bit less so.

The second issue bears on the personal encounter between physician and patient: Is it marked by authoritarianism, paternalism, and domination? My answer is not only "Yes" but also that a certain measure of these characteristics is essential to good medical care. In fact, if you agree that the physician's primary function is to make the patient feel better, a certain amount of authoritarianism, paternalism, and domination are the essence of the physician's effectiveness.

Thirdly, I shall maintain that many physicians are indeed arrogant in their behavior toward patients, but in a way that is not even specifically identified by any of the dictionary definitions of the word "arrogance."

Although no learned vocation is exempt from the accusation, the professional group most often belabored for arrogance is that which uses advanced and complex technology in its thinking and doing. It is the scientist, whether in physics or in molecular biology, or even the parascientist in medicine, who is seen as making policy decisions motivated by self-interest and acting with a total disregard for broad human needs. Almost reflexly the hoary Clemenceauism is trotted out that war must be not left to the generals. Because of this societal apprehension, decision-making bodies are being created with the express purpose of limiting the influence of specifically those scientists who possess expertise relevant to the questions that must be answered. Physicians are well acquainted with the provisions of Public Law 93-641, enacted in 1974, which establishes a network of health-systems agencies. The majority of members appointed to bodies responsible for planning and implementing this system, such as area governing boards and sub-area councils, must consist of so-called consumers rather than providers of health care. The same principle is being

Reprinted, with permission, from *The New England Journal of Medicine* 1980 Dec. 25. 303(26):1507–1511.
Based on the George W. Gay Lecture, delivered by Dr. Ingelfinger at Harvard Medical School on May 5, 1977, shortly before he retired as editor of *The New England Journal of Medicine*. Dr. Ingelfinger died on March 26, 1980.

applied to even more momentous issues, such as whether arbitrary limits should be placed on mankind's search for knowledge. Thus, many maintain that the current frenetic argument about further research in recombinant DNA should be resolved by groups in which the representatives of science are not only restricted but eliminated altogether.

Indisputable reasons exist why decisions affecting society as a whole should be made by persons broadly representative of that society and not by those who might be biased, perhaps by reasons of personal gain or by entirely honorable but nevertheless unbalanced and enthusiastic intellectual commitment to a discipline. Indeed, the principle is basic in most democratic societies. Whether in Britain or the United States, it is Parliament or Congress after all, that decides how much money should be spent on various programs of biomedical research and public health.

The justness of society's control is not the issue. Nor is it deniable that many specialists in the biosciences entertain a hemianoptic view of the world. It is understandable, furthermore, that the bulk of biomedical scientists and parascientists will as a group make decisions grossly influenced by their own skills and resources. Under many a circumstance the surgeon will cut when the internist will use antibiotics. My concern is that the words "arrogant scientist" imply that the ignorant, whether lay or professional, have no such faults. But the arrogance of ignorance can be as devastating as the arrogance of expertise. Yet the arrogance of ignorance or the arrogance of the antiscientific or anti-intellectual activist is hardly ever mentioned, although it may be as flagrant as that of the most doctrinaire member of the conventional scientific establishment.

Let us start with an example of relatively low emotional intensity, that of diet. Over the years various dietary practices have been endorsed or condemned by physicians, and the popularity with the public of this or that dietary fad is an ancient but continuing phenomenon. For years doctors and public alike were convinced that the consumption of some foods aggravated or even caused peptic ulcers of the stomach or duodenum, or that other foods had salubrious effects. Harmful staples were identified as spicy, coarse, and strongly colored; those designated as beneficial were bland, smooth, and colorless. White protein such as chicken and fish was permissible, but red meats such as beef and lamb forbidden. One school of thought—indeed, both

medical and nonmedical—exercised reductionism to its ultimate: the ulcer patient was simply told to eat a white diet. Farina, potatoes, and milk, I suppose, were intended, but I always wondered if the literal minded might not also include horseradish.

The influence of superstition, mysticism, and religion on dietary beliefs is of course strong. In 1910, for example, a popular fad was Fletcherism, the practice of chewing each bite of food intensely—perhaps 30 times. The originator of the cult, Horace Fletcher, always wore white suits to emphasize the spiritual purity of his obsessive mastication. Perhaps similar occult powers enhance the appeal of the white diet in the treatment of peptic ulcer.

Nowadays we still know little about the cause and cure of peptic ulcer. Indeed, many excellent scientific studies employing the resources of modern technology have, on the one hand, increased knowledge about the nature of peptic ulcer but, on the other hand, increased the expert's recognition of how little he knows about the causes of this disorder. More knowledge has paradoxically highlighted non-knowledge. Correspondingly, the value of dietary regimens imposed, in retrospect with somewhat arbitrary ignorance, is questioned by the skepticism of scientific expertise.

Currently another dietary vogue is attracting the faithful: the overly refined, low-roughage foods of the industrialized West are said to cause diverticulosis and perhaps cancer of the large bowel, hemorrhoids, varicose veins, and calcifications of pelvic veins. Perhaps these processed foods are harmful, but the categorical endorsement of high-roughage diets impresses me as another example of an arbitrary, authoritarian pronouncement based on half-knowledge and on an unacknowledged ignorance of overall effects—in other words, somewhat arrogant. In 1952, long before Burkitt and others became interested in the effects of diet on the pathogenesis of colonic diverticula, a pathologist in Lima, Peru told me that at autopsy he could always differentiate the colon of the Spanish descendant from that of the Andean Indian. The Spanish descendant's colon, to be sure, might have diverticula, but the Indian's did not. On the other hand, the Indian characteristically had a very long colon, particularly a long and convoluted sigmoid. Because of this characteristic, Indians frequently suffered fatal volvulus of this organ. Albert Schweitzer recorded the huge prevalence of hernia in the patients he saw. So high-roughage diets may have their unfavorable as well as favorable consequences, but one would never know it from the denunciation one hears of low-roughage diets. I even suspect that mystic and moralistic forces are at work here, for obviously a high-roughage diet is a return to the natural conditions of the noble savage and the endurance of hardships, whereas the refined diet indicates an effete and self-indulgent luxury.

My dietary homilies are intended to illustrate the multifarious societal forces that underlie questionable policy decisions—in this case, policies about what to eat. The public, the doctor, the professor of physiology participated in decisions that were spun arbitrarily out of flimsy strands of evidence. Their reasoning depended on what Alvin Weinberg has called trans-science. "Many of the issues," Weinberg wrote in 1972,[1] "that arise from the interaction between science or technology and society . . . hang on the answers to questions that can be asked of science and yet *which cannot be answered by science*. I propose the term trans-scientific for these questions since, though they may arise in or around science, and can be stated in the language of science, they are unanswerable by science—that is, they transcend science."

Failure to differentiate between science and transcience, failure to recognize that a regulation or recommendation may be concocted in a vacuum of knowledge is to my mind a manifestation of the arrogance of ignorance.

I must make a distinction here: I do not assert that conclusions reached in the absence of reliable fact are per se arrogant. Such conclusions unavoidably characterize politics, science, and medicine, especially when the need for action is urgent. Arrogance enters when those reaching various decisions in the absence of adequate data fail to recognize or to admit how empty their cupboard of information is. Superior scientists or doctors, I should like to believe, are always aware of how little they know. Doubt tempers arrogance, and for this reason perhaps some bioscientists might be credited with sophrosyne rather than condemned for its opposite, hubris. (I admit I never heard of sophrosyne before I prepared for this lecture, but it has all the prerequisites for becoming a stylish word.)

Sociologists, ethicists, and others like to speak disparagingly of what they call the doctor's authoritarianism, paternalism, or domination. Such a position, I submit, is unrealistic and untenable.

The physician is a person to whom patients go because they need or think they need help. Let us assume that the physician they select is competent and compassionate. In spite of these virtues, there is usually little the physician can do physically, that is, by cutting or by a chemical manipulation, to eradicate the cause of the patient's distress. That is why epidemiologists keep pointing out—and the recent book by Thomas McKeown (*The Role of Medicine: Dream, Mirage, or Nemesis?*) is an outstanding example—that the physician's intervention has done little to prolong life or eliminate serious morbidity. The figure generally quoted—although it may be an arrogant figure in that the substantiating data are fragmentary—is that 90 per cent of the visits by patients to doctors are caused by conditions that are either self-limited or beyond the capabilities of medicine. In other words, if we assume that physicians do make patients feel better most of the time, it is chiefly because the physician can reassure the patient or give medication that is mildly palliative. Even an operation may once in a while make a patient feel better, although it does not prolong his life or eradicate the source of his problems.

If the physician is to be effective in alleviating the patient's complaints by such intangible means, it follows that the patient has to believe in the physician, that he has confidence in his advice and reassurance, and in his selection of a pill that is helpful (though not curative of the basic disorder). Intrinsic to such a belief is the patient's conviction that his physician not only can be trusted but also has some special knowledge that the patient does not possess. He needs, if the treatment is to succeed, a physician whom he invests with authoritative experience and competence. He needs a physician from whom he will accept some domination. If I am going to give up eating eggs for the rest of my life, I must be convinced, as an ovophile, that a higher authority than I will influence my eating habits. I do not want to be in the position of a shopper at the Casbah who negotiates and haggles with the physician about what is best. I want to believe that my physician is acting under higher moral principles and intellectual powers than a used-car dealer.

I'll go further than that. A physician who merely spreads an array of vendibles in front of the patient and then says, "Go ahead and choose, it's your life," is guilty of shirking his duty, if not of malpractice. The physician, to be sure, should list the alternatives and describe their pros and cons but then, instead of asking the patient to make the choice, the physician should recommend a specific course of action. He must take the responsibility, not shift it onto the shoulders of the patient. The patient may then refuse the recommendation, which is perfectly acceptable, but the physician who would not use his training and experience to recommend the specific action to a patient—or in some cases frankly admit "I don't know"—does not warrant the somewhat tarnished but still distinguished title of doctor.

Although I have subscribed for some time to the principle that the physician must be authoritarian and paternalistic to some degree, my experience as a patient has substantiated that belief in the strongest way possible. If you will forgive me for being both anecdotal and personal, let me tell you how the lack of authoritarian decision brought agony to me and my family. About a year and a half ago it was discovered that I had an adenocarcinoma, a glandular cancer, sitting astride the gastroesophageal junction. Ironically, this had been an area of the gut to which I had paid much attention in my professional career as a clinical investigator and consultant; therefore, I can hardly imagine a more informed patient. The need for surgery was indisputable if I hoped to continue to be able to swallow. But after a successful operation my real dilemmas began. The surgeon had found no visible evidence that the cancer had spread. But this proved nothing, because cancers can spread to form tiny nests of cancer elsewhere—micrometastases. The current medical practice is to assume that a patient who has had an operation for any of a variety of cancers (including the type I had) should also be given prophylactic treatment in an effort to eradicate the micrometastases before they enlarge. For this purpose both chemotherapy and radiotherapy are being used extensively. So one question was: Should I have chemotherapy, with all its side effects? And if chemotherapy, what kind? Even more debatable was the question of whether I should have radiotherapy. There is no generally acceptable evidence that residual nests of adenocarcinoma cells will respond. In addition, radiation would involve for me a number of complications, such as fibrosis of the lungs, and the possibility of a host of less frequent but nevertheless serious side effects. At that point I received from physician friends throughout the country a barrage of well-intentioned but contradictory advice. The question of prophylactic

radiotherapy was particularly moot. As a result, not only I but my wife, my son and daughter-in-law (both doctors), and other family members became increasingly confused and emotionally distraught. Finally, when the pangs of indecision had become nearly intolerable, one wise physician friend said, "What you need is a doctor." He was telling me to forget the information I already had and the information I was receiving from many quarters, and to seek instead a person who would dominate, who would tell me what to do, who would in a paternalistic manner assume responsibility for my care. When that excellent advice was followed, my family and I sensed immediate and immense relief. The incapacity of enervating worry was dispelled, and I could return to my usual anxieties, such as deciding on the fate of manuscripts or giving lectures like this.

If arrogance in the sense of paternalism and dominance is an ingredient of beneficial medical care, these qualities have to be used appropriately. To the extent that paternalism and dominance are infected by some of the other meanings of arrogance, a physician's conduct with patients is correspondingly worsened. Thus, if his paternalism is accentuated by insolence, vanity, arbitrariness, or a lack of empathy, the care he attempts to provide his patients is nullified. In other words, a physician can be beneficially arrogant, or he can be destructively arrogant.

Physicians as a class, I suspect, are probably no more vain or insolent than any other people. Some are presumptuous and condescending, others self-effacing and sympathetic. Although arrogance in some of its more nefarious meanings—vanity, insolence, and ruthlessness, for example,—cannot, I believe, be identified as a general characteristic of the medical profession, the profession as a whole is affected by a brand of arrogance subsumed under lack of empathy. Doctors for various reasons find it difficult to put themselves in the patient's place; they do not sufficiently appreciate, or perhaps do not have the time to appreciate, how the patient feels and how he reacts to the medical information and procedures to which he is exposed.

The problem, discussed to some extent in the April, 1977 issue of the *Annals of Internal Medicine,* has two components—one intellectual and to some degree ameliorable, and the other emotional and requiring for its correction the utmost in medical art. The first component is simply a matter of language. The argot of the physician has not only been ridiculed extensively but criticized as one of the devices used by the medical profession to maintain its mystique. This explanation may have held true in Molière's time, but I doubt its validity today. The profession's addiction to its vocational jargon is probably a matter of habit, difficult to dispel because of the physician's training, his incessant intercourse with other doctors, his reading of *The New England Journal of Medicine,* and his relative ineptitude with ordinary English. Whatever the reasons, physicians tend to use terms that laymen either do not understand or misinterpret. Even one of the best communicators with the public I know, Dr. Timothy Johnson, may on occasion allow the guests on his popular program, "House Call," to lapse into language more appropriate for the medical amphitheatre than the public forum. "Endometrial carcinoma" is much easier for the medical tongue than "cancer of the lining of the womb."

Many patients, to be sure, are acquainted with medical terms and use them, and it has been proposed that teaching the patient about medicine—enriching his vocabulary rather than profaning that of the doctor—might improve communication between the two parties. But do patients really understand medical words? We physicians certainly have problems with the principles and jargon of other skills, as is evident in the reproving letters I receive when we publish articles dealing with the arcane statistics or economics of medicine. Similarly, even if the patient uses words such as "myocardial infarction," does he really appreciate the spectrum of pathologic, diagnostic, prognostic, and therapeutic implications that this common expression conveys to the physician? All but the most medically sophisticated patients need to be informed, I suspect in nontechnical terms, and the physician who ignores this obligation is guilty of a form of arrogance.

Even if a physician takes pains to use appropriate language, he may still lack empathy if he is not acutely sensitive to the emotional state of the patient seeking consultation. Distraught by anxiety, fear, and perhaps suspicion, the patient hears the sound but not the meaning of words; reassurances that cancer is an unlikely diagnosis, and a barrage of tests to prove this point, may convince the patient that the opposite is true. "We shall not need another operation" is recorded in the patient's mind as "another operation." Advice that antihypertensive drugs or insulin are in order, possibly for a lifetime, may give the pa-

tient the idea of incurability. Even advice on smoking and overeating may elicit negative instead of positive results in the susceptible.

Perhaps one of the most flagrant examples of non-empathic arrogance today—an example not confined to the medical profession—is the pervasive idea that the failure of medical ministrations is the patient's fault. If he does not follow instructions and appears to disregard words of medical wisdom, the patient is labeled as non-compliant—another word in vogue. Blaming the victim is currently a popular excuse for therapeutic failure, but to me it smacks of arrogance. It is a doctor's obligation, by explanation and persuasion, to get the patient to take his medication as prescribed. If the patient fails to do so, the blame is often as much the physician's as the patient's.

It is of course easy enough for a speaker to moralize and to demand more empathy on the part of the physician. But what practical resources are available to the physician who is aware that the patient's emotional state may color and distort ordinary conversation? Getting to know the patient, his convictions and his problems, and the attitudes of his family, will of course help, but in these days of group practices, ancillary help, specialization, and mobile populations, "getting to know the patient" may be as difficult as containing medical costs. Currently popular measures to enhance medical efficiency also do not help. If a patient—whether an expectant mother, an alcoholic with early cirrhosis, or a heavy smoker with lung cancer—is first processed through a battery of questionnaires or computer terminals, then interrogated and examined by ancillary personnel, and finally seen by the doctor—to be delivered, to be subjected to liver biopsy, or to undergo pulmonary resection—that patient will not now the doctor, and vice versa. How can the doctor under such circumstances be aware of his patient's thoughts and emotions? Efficient medical practice, I fear, may not be empathic medical practice, and it fosters, if not arrogance, at least the appearance of arrogance.

In medical school, students are told about the perplexity, anxiety, and misapprehension that may affect the patient as he enters the medical-care system, and in the clinical years the fortunate and sensitive student may learn much from taking to those assigned to his supervision. But the effects of lectures and conversations are ephemeral and are no substitute for actual experience. One might suggest, of course, that only those who have been hospitalized during their adolescent or adult years be admitted to medical school. Such a practice would not only increase the number of empathic doctors; it would also permit the whole elaborate system of medical-school admissions to be jettisoned.

Reference

1. Weinberg, A. M. Science & trans-science. In: *Civilization and Science: In Conflict or Collaboration?* A Ciba Foundation Symposium. Amsterdam: Elsevier Press, 1972, pp. 105–22.

The Physician's Responsibility toward Hopelessly Ill Patients

Sidney H. Wanzer, M.D., and S. James Adelstein, M.D., both Harvard Medical School, Boston

Ronald E. Cranford, M.D., Neurological Intensive Care Unit, Hennepin County Medical Center, Minneapolis

Daniel D. Federman, M.D., Harvard Medical School, Boston

Edward D. Hook, M.D., University of Virginia Medical Center, Charlottesville, VA

Charles G. Moertel, M.D., Department of Oncology, Mayo Clinic and Medical School, Rochester, MN

Peter Safar, M.D., Resuscitation Research Center, University of Pittsburgh Medical School, Pittsburgh

Alan Stone, M.D., Harvard Law School, Cambridge, MA

Helen B. Taussig, M.D., Johns Hopkins University School of Medicine, Baltimore

Jan van Evs, Ph.D., M.D., Department of Pediatrics, University of Texas System Cancer Center and School of Medicine, Houston

Efforts to define policies on withholding or withdrawing life-sustaining procedures from hopelessly ill patients are a relatively recent development. In 1976, when two major hospitals publicly announced their protocols in treating the hopelessly ill, the *Journal* marked the event with an editorial titled "Terminating Life Support: Out of the Closet!"[1]

Since then, the subject of permitting patients to die has emerged into the open. The courts have issued several well-publicized decisions since the 1976 Quinlan case,[2-9] and legislatures in 15 states and the District of Columbia have enacted "natural death" acts (California, 1976; Idaho, 1977; Arkansas, 1977; New Mexico, 1977; Nevada, 1977; Oregon, 1977; North Carolina, 1977; Texas, 1977; Washington, 1979; Kansas, 1979; Alabama, 1981; District of Columbia, 1982; Vermont, 1982; Delaware, 1982; Virginia, 1983; and Illinois, 1983). Moreover, medical institutions have made public statements of "no code" policies.[10]

As medical technology has advanced, numerous articles in professional journals have dealt with various aspects of the subject, along with much discussion and debate of crucial ethical questions. However, the formulation of universally accepted guidelines for physicians treating the hopelessly ill has remained difficult. As Hilfiker states, "it is time we publicly examined our role in these situations, offered each other some guidelines, and came to some consensus about our responsibility."[11]

The present article, written by a group of experienced physicians from various disciplines and institutions, is an attempt to meet this need. We have not addressed the special questions surrounding treatment decisions for neonates and minors (a subject in itself) but have limited the scope of the paper to the irreversibly ill adult. Basic to our considerations are two important precepts: the patient's role in decision making is paramount, and a decrease in aggressive treat-

Reprinted, with permission, from *The New England Journal of Medicine* 1984 Apr. 12. 310(15):955–959.

Formulated at a meeting held at the Countway Library of Medicine, Boston, October 28–30, 1982, under the auspices of the Society for the Right to Die, New York.

Supported by a grant made in memory of Joseph S. Kornfeld.

ment of the hopelessly ill patient is advisable when such treatment would only prolong a difficult and uncomfortable process of dying.

The Patient's Role in Decision Making

The patient's right to make decisions about his or her medical treatment is clear. That right, grounded in both common law and the constitutional right of privacy, includes the right to refuse life-sustaining treatment—a fact affirmed in the courts and recently supported by a presidential commission.[10] Ideally, the right is exercised when the diagnosis and treatment are clear, the physician is skilled and sensitive, and the patient is competent and informed. Circumstances, however, are often less than ideal. In writing about "specific clinical and psychologic problems that may complicate the concept of patient autonomy and the right to die with dignity," Jackson and Youngner[12] have illustrated a number of factors that can interfere with appropriate decision making even if the patient's competency is not in question. Disease, pain, drugs, and a variety of conditions altering mental states may severely reduce the patient's capacity for judgment. Since these circumstances can fluctuate, competency can be lost and regained, requiring reevaluation at intervals.

The principal obstacle to a patient's effective participation in decision making is lack of competence, and only when competence is lacking can others substitute their judgment for that of the patient. Therefore, the assessment of competence is a critical issue. Although legal determination of incompetence may at times be a matter for court review, this step can be safely bypassed when there is unanimity on the part of the physician and others consulted—family and close friends, and psychiatrists, if indicated. In arriving at the determination of incompetence, the physician must coordinate the various evaluations and opinions and document them clearly in the medical records. We believe that a hopelessly ill patient's refusal of life-sustaining treatment is not in itself a reason to question the patient's competency, no matter what the personal values of the physician or family may be.

If the terminally ill patient's ability to make decisions becomes progressively reduced, the physician must rely increasingly on the presumed or prestated wishes of the patient. It helps if there is a longstanding relationship between patient and physician, but in fact many adults have no personal physician. Terminally ill patients are often cared for by specialists or members of house staff who do not know what the patient would have wished or may not have the time or experience to handle difficult problems of this kind. Under these circumstances. it becomes important to have other means of determining the patient's desires. A written statement, prepared in advance of the patient's illness and diminished decision-making capacity, can be helpful in indicating to the physician the patient's preference with respect to terminal treatment.[13] Such advance directions, or "living wills," are recognized by law in 15 states and the District of Columbia, and even in states where they have not been legally authorized, they provide important though not binding evidence of a patient's wishes.

Another aid to decision making in which the patient cannot participate effectively is a proxy, designated in advance by the patient to speak on his or her behalf.[14] This option has only recently been provided by law in a few states—either as part of the state's "living will" legislation (Delaware's Death with Dignity Act of 1982 and Virginia's Natural Death Act of 1983) or (in California) as an amendment to the durable-power-of-attorney statute, extending the authorization to health-care decisions.[15] Since the clinical circumstances of a future illness and available treatment options are unpredictable, a proxy chosen by the patient offers the advantage of decision making based on both an intimate knowledge of the patient's wishes and the physician's recommendations.

Neither the living will nor the proxy appointment is a perfect mechanism for projecting a patient's wishes into a period of future incompetency. The living will cannot predict all the various alternatives that become possible as acute illnesses arise, and in many cases, the document is not updated with any regularity. A proxy may not be available at the time of need, or he or she may have a conflict of interest, either emotionally or legally. Nevertheless, in spite of imperfections, the living will and the proxy can be of real assistance to the physician trying to decide the best course of treatment for the dying patient. In their absence, the physician must ascertain from family and friends the attitudes and wishes the patient would have expressed had competence been maintained.

The Physician's Role in Decision Making

The patient's right to accept or refuse treatment notwithstanding, the physician has a major role in the decision-making process. He or she has the knowledge, skills, and judgment to provide diagnosis and prognosis, to offer treatment choices and explain their implications, and to assume responsibility for recommending a decision with respect to treatment.

The physician's schooling, residency training, and professional oath emphasize positive actions to sustain and prolong life; the educational system has only recently given attention to ethical questions surrounding the intentional reduction of medical intervention. Physicians do not easily accept the concept that it may be best to do less, not more, for a patient. The decision to pull back is much more difficult to make than the decision to push ahead with aggressive support, and today's sophisticated and complex medical technology invites physicians to make use of all the means at their disposal—a temptation that must be recognized when evaluating how much or how little to do for the patient.

Coupled with the traditional pressures for aggressive treatment is the uncertainty of diagnosis and prognosis, making it difficult to predict the length and quality of the patient's life with or without treatment. If the attending physician is not expert in the particular area of the patient's illness, he or she should consult with those who are. If there is disagreement concerning the diagnosis or prognosis or both, the life-sustaining approach should be continued until reasonable agreement is reached. However, insistence on certainty beyond a reasonable point can handicap the physician dealing with treatment options in apparently hopeless cases. The rare report of a patient with a similar condition who survived is not an overriding reason to continue aggressive treatment. Such negligible statistical possibilities do not outweigh the reasonable expectations of outcome that will guide treatment decisions.

Physicians are strongly influenced by their personal values and unconscious motivations. Although they should not be forced to act against their moral codes, they should guard against being excessively influenced by unexamined inner conflicts, a tendency to equate a patient's death with professional failure, or unrealistic expectations.

Fear of legal liability often interferes with the physician's ability to make the best choice for the patient. Assessment of legal risks is sometimes made by lawyers whose primary objective is to minimize liability, whether real or imagined. Unfortunately, this may be done at the expense of humane treatment and may go against the expressed wishes of the patient or family. A recent case in California involving murder charges against two physicians who withdrew all life support from a comatose patient created a climate of heightened apprehension in the medical community.[16] The action taken against the physicians was the first and only such criminal case in U.S. legal history.[17] Fortunately, the charges were dismissed by the California Court of Appeal. Treatment of the dying patient always takes place in the context of changing law and changing social policy, but in spite of legal uncertainties, appropriate and compassionate care should have priority over undue fears of criminal or civil liability.

Another possible influence on the physician's thinking is consideration of monetary costs to society and the use of scarce treatment resources in the care of the hopelessly ill. In the past, cost was rarely an important factor in decision making, but today, as society tries to contain the soaring cost of health care, the physician is subject to insistent demands for restraint, which cannot be ignored. Financial ruin of the patient's family, as well as the drain on resources for treatment of other patients who are not hopelessly ill, should be weighed in the decision-making process, although the patient's welfare obviously remains paramount.

Communication with the Patient

When a physician discusses life-threatening illness with a patient, a number of questions arise. Is the patient capable of accepting the information? How much information should the patient be given? When should the physician inform the patient of a fatal illness? Can information be imparted without destroying all hope? There are no absolute answers to these questions, but the following principles seem reasonable.

Although some physicians and families avoid frank discussions with patients, in our view, practically all patients, even disturbed ones, are better off knowing the truth. A decision not to tell the patient the truth because of fear of his or her emotional or psychological inability to handle such information is rarely if ever justified, and in such a case the burden of proof rests on the person who believes that the patient cannot cope with frank discussion. The anxiety of dealing with the unknown can be far more upsetting than the grief of dealing with a known, albeit tragic, truth. A failure to transmit to the patient knowledge of terminal illness can create barriers in communication, and the patient is effectively placed in isolation at a time when emotional sharing is most needed.

The dying patient should be given only as much information as he or she wishes to handle. Some patients want to know every detail, whereas others, who have a limited ability to understand or a limited desire to know, want only the most general information.

The discussion of critical illness and the patient's right to accept or refuse life-prolonging treatment should occur as early as possible in the course of disease; ideally, it will already have taken place at a time when the patient was healthy. However, regardless of any discussions that may or may not have taken place, when fatal illness occurs, the physician—if possible, one with whom the patient has already developed rapport, not a stranger—should tell the patient of an unfavorable diagnosis or prognosis as soon as the information is firm. Such discussions may have to be repeated, since patients often find it difficult to assimilate all they need to know at any one time, and as illness progresses, continued communication will be required to meet changing needs.

When the prognosis is bad, the physician must help the terminally ill patient understand and deal with the prognosis and alternatives for treatment without destroying all hope. This can be done by reassuring the patient that he or she will not be abandoned and by emphasizing the positive measures that can be used for support. The emotional distress that accompanies such discussions is usually more than offset by the security of a consensus about terminal care.

Another important consideration with respect to doctor-patient communication is the matter of informed consent. There are three basic prerequisites for informed consent: the patient must have the capacity to reason and make judgments, the decision must be made voluntarily and without coercion, and the patient must have a clear understanding of the risks and benefits of the proposed treatment alternatives or non-treatment, along with a full understanding of the nature of the disease and the prognosis. Fulfillment of the third condition requires that the physician take the time to discuss the issues fully with the patient and outline the differences among alternatives, which are sometimes very difficult to estimate. Nevertheless, it is the physician's responsibility to ensure, as much as possible, that all the conditions for informed consent are met. In addition to being thoroughly informed, the patient must also understand clearly his or her right to make choices about the type of care to be received—a right many patients are not aware of. This is the cornerstone of all decision making and is the basis on which informed consent rests.

The preeminence of the patient's choice does not preclude the physician's responsibility to make and to share with the patient a personal judgment about what the patient should do. Patients often ask a trusted physician, "What would you do?" A direct answer is in order. Some patients want every possible day of life, regardless of how limited the quality, whereas others apparently prefer early death to prolongation of a very limited life on a day-to-day basis. Given what the physician knows about the individual patient, some order of preference for available treatment choices can be offered. In any case, it is unfair simply to provide a mass of medical facts and options and leave the patient adrift without any further guidance on the alternative courses of action and inaction.

The physician's traditional role as a source of comfort to patients and their families becomes especially important when the decision has been made to withhold treatment that prolongs dying. Competent patients who have chosen to be allowed to die may experience a resultant feeling of abandonment. The family may share this feeling on behalf of the dying patient and have difficulty grappling with the consequences of a decision in which they may or may not have played a part. Assiduous attention to the patient's physical and emotional comfort at this point is essential. The physician's availability at such times can be a source of great psychological comfort to both patient and family.

The physician has a special obligation to listen to the doubts and fears expressed by patients who are hopelessly or terminally ill. Although a rare patient may contemplate suicide, the physician cannot participate by assisting in the act, for this is contrary to law. On the other hand, the physician in not obligated to assume that every such wish is irrational and requires coercive intervention.

The Provision of Appropriate Care

Although relief of pain and suffering is the primary consideration in the care of all hopelessly ill patients, differences in patients' disabilities dictate differences in the appropriate form and intensity of their care.

Levels of Care

It can be useful for the physician and other medical personnel to designate the level of care for the hopelessly ill patient that is appropriate at a given stage of the disease process. In this way the treatment goal can be addressed logically and openly. The physician should bring nurses and other health-care personnel into discussions concerning the level of therapy for an individual patient, since they are in close and frequent communication with the patient and his or her family. Decisions about care should be carefully documented in the record, and all appropriate personnel should be aware of them.

General levels of care can be described as follows: (1) emergency resuscitation; (2) intensive care and advanced life support; (3) general medical care, including antibiotics, drugs, surgery, cancer chemotherapy, and artificial hydration and nutrition; and (4) general nursing care and efforts to make the patient comfortable, including pain relief and hydration and nutrition as dictated by the patient's thirst and hunger. Although the program of care must be individualized, since every patient is unique, these four levels of treatment should be considered and discussed with the patient, the family, and other health-care personnel. Certainly, the competent patient has a right to know that such variations in approach exist.

Patients who require only the fourth level of care (comfort) are usually those clearly in the terminal phase of an irreversible illness. For such patients, routine monitoring procedures, including daily temperature, pulse, and blood-pressure readings, may be discontinued. Diagnostic measures, such as blood tests and x-ray films, may be omitted except when required to relieve an uncomfortable or painful condition. Antibiotics need not be administered for pneumonia or other infections. Certain mechanical interventions, such as urethral catheterization, may increase overall comfort and thus be justified, but any mechanical or surgical intervention should be discouraged if it does not accomplish the aim of making the patient comfortable.

Naturally or artificially administered hydration and nutrition may be given or withheld, depending on the patient's comfort. If these supports are to be withheld or withdrawn, however, the physician must be sensitive to the symbolic meaning of this step. The provision of food and water is so important symbolically that family, friends, and staff need to understand that many patients in a terminal situation are not aware of thirst or hunger. Everything done for the patient at the fourth level of care should meet only the test of whether it will make the patient more comfortable and whether it will honor his or her wishes. Any actions that withhold a form of treatment should be clearly discussed with interested parties and documented in the record.

Individualizing Treatment

The Competent Patient

In treating patients who are generally alert but are dying of a progressive illness, such as cancer, the physician must be especially sensitive to their need for relief from pain and suffering. Aggressive treatment in response to this need is often justified even if under other circumstances the risk of such treatment would be medically undesirable (e.g., it would result in respiratory depression). The level of care to be provided should reflect an understanding between patient and physician and should be reassessed from time to time. In many cases neither intensive care nor emergency resuscitation is desired by the patient and his or her family; there may be a wish only for comfort, with general medical treatment given solely to provide relief from distress.

When the facilities provided by an acute-care hospital are not essential to the comfort and dignity of the dying patient, he or she should be moved to a more appropriate setting, if possible. Care at home or in a less regimented environment, such as a hospice, should be encouraged and facilitated.

The Incompetent Patient

Patients with brain death.[18–20] Patients with irreversible cessation of all functions of the brain, determined in accordance with accepted medical standards, are considered medically and legally dead, and no further treatment is required.

Patients in a persistent vegetative state.[19,21] In this state the neocortex is largely and irreversibly destroyed, although some brain-stem functions persist. When this neurologic condition has been established with a high degree of medical certainty and has been carefully documented, it is morally justifiable to withhold antibiotics and artificial nutrition and hydration, as well as other forms of life-sustaining treatment, allowing the patient to die. This obviously requires careful efforts to obtain knowledge of the patient's prior wishes and the understanding and agreement of the family. Family attitudes will clearly influence the type of care given in these cases.

Severely and irreversibly demented patients. Patients in this category, most of them elderly, are at one end of the spectrum of decreasing mental capacity. They do not initiate purposeful activity but passively accept nourishment and bodily care.

When the severely demented patient has previously made his or her wishes known and when there is intercurrent illness, it is ethically permissible for the physician to withhold treatment that would serve mainly to prolong the dying process. When there is no prior expression or living will and when no family or advocate is available, the physician should be guided by the need to provide the most humane kind of treatment and the need to carry out the patient's wishes insofar as they are ascertainable.

Severely and irreversibly demented patients need only care given to make them comfortable. If such a patient rejects food and water by mouth, it is ethically permissible to withhold nutrition and hydration artificially administered by vein or gastric tube. Spoon feeding should be continued if needed for comfort. It is ethically appropriate not to treat intercurrent illness except with measures required for comfort (e.g., antibiotics for pneumonia can be withheld). For this category of patients, it is best if decisions about the handling of intercurrent illness are made prospectively, before the onset of an acute illness or threat to life. The physician must always bear in mind that senseless perpetuation of the status quo is decision by default.

Elderly patients with permanent mild impairment of competence. Many elderly patients are described as "pleasantly senile." Although somewhat limited in their ability to initiate activities and communicate, they often appear to be enjoying their moderately restricted lives. Freedom from discomfort should be an overriding objective in the care of such a patient. If emergency resuscitation and intensive care are required, the physician should provide these measures sparingly, guided by the patient's prior wishes, if known, by the wishes of the patient's family, and by an assessment of the patient's prospects for improvement.

Conclusions

Few topics in medicine are more complicated, more controversial, and more emotionally charged than treatment of the hopelessly ill. Technology competes with compassion, legal precedent lags, and controversy is inevitable. The problem is least troublesome when an informed patient and an empathetic physician together confront a clearly defined outlook. We have tried to outline a reasonable approach that is useful even when these ideal circumstances do not obtain. Our recommendations cannot resolve all conflicts, provide simple formulas, or comprehensively address the wide range of issues involved in caring for the hopelessly ill patient, but they are intended to offer some clarification and support for those who bear the social responsibility of deciding whether to forgo life-sustaining treatment for the hopelessly ill.

We are indebted to Edwin H. Cassem, M.D., for his review of the manuscript and to Peg Cameron, Marjorie Zucker, Ph.D., and Alice Mehling for editorial assistance.

References

1. Fried C. Terminating life support: out of the closet! N Engl J Med 1976; 295:390–1.

2. *In re Quinlan*, 70 N.J. 10, 355 A. 2d 647 (1976).

3. *Superintendent of Belchertown State School* vs. *Saikewicz*, 373 Mass. 728, 370 N.E. 2d 417 (Mass. 1977).

4. *In re Dinnerstein*, 380 N.E. 2d 134 (Mass. App. 1978).

5. *Staz v. Perlmutter*, Florida 362 So. 2d 160 (Fla. App. 1978); affirmed by Florida Supreme Court, 379 So. 2d 359 (1980).

6. *Severns v. Wilmington Medical Center, Inc.* et al, Del. Supr., 421 A, 2d 1334 (1980).

7. *In re Spring*, 405 N.E. 2d 115 (1980).

8. *In re Eichner* (Fox), Ct. of App., 52 N.Y.S. 2d 266 (1981).

9. *In re Storar*, Ct. of App., 52 N.Y. 2d 363, 420 N.E. 2d 64. 438 N.Y.S. 2d 255 (1981).

10. President's Commission for the Study of Ethical Problems in Medicine and Biomedical and Behavioral Research. Deciding to forego life-sustaining treatment. Washington, D.C.: Government Printing Office, 1983:236–9.

11. Hilfiker D. Allowing the debilitated to die: facing our ethical choices. N Engl J Med 1983; 308:716–9.

12. Jackson DL, Youngner S. Patient autonomy and "death with dignity": some clinical caveats. N Engl J Med 1979; 301:404–8.

13. Bok S. Personal directions for care at the end of life. N Engl J Med 1976; 295:367–9.

14. Relman AS. Michigan's sensible "living will." N Engl J Med 1979; 300:1270–2.

15. Durable power of attorney for health care [SB 762 (Keene) Ch. 1204 Stats 1983].

16. Nelson H. Life-support court edict leaves physicians cautious. Los Angeles Times. October 31, 1983.

17. Kirsch J. A death at Kaiser Hospital. California November 1982:79ff.

18. A definition of irreversible coma: report of the Ad Hoc Committee of the Harvard Medical School to Examine the Definition of Brain Death. JAMA 1968; 205:337–40.

19. Grenvik A, Powner DJ, Snyder JV, Jastremski MS, Babcock RA, Loughhead MG. Cessation of therapy in terminal illness and brain death. Crit Care Med 1978; 6:284–91.

20. Guidelines for the determination of death: report of the medical consultants on the diagnosis of death to the President's Commission for the Study of Ethical Problems in Medicine and Biomedical and Behavioral Research. JAMA 1981; 246:2184–6.

21. Optimum care for hopelessly ill patients: a report of the Clinical Care Committee of the Massachusetts General Hopsital. N Engl J Med 1976; 295:362–4.

Competence to Refuse Medical Treatment: Autonomy vs. Paternalism

George J. Annas, J.D., M.P.H., Boston University Schools of Medicine and Public Health, Boston

Joan E. Densberger, M.P.H., student, Boston College Law School, Boston

Introduction

Competent individuals are at liberty to make their own medical treatment decisions; incompetent individuals are not. Thus, competence and liberty are inextricably interwoven. Competence is broadly defined as the capacity to understand and appreciate the nature and consequence of one's actions. The vagueness of this definition, coupled with the dearth of legal literature on the subject, make competence determinations ripe for arbitrariness and pose a danger to individual liberty.[1] A determination of incompetence, or even a suspicion of it, can be used to justify paternalism by physicians and family members.[2]

Perhaps the most famous example of the paternalistic approach occurred in the treatment of Dr. Barney Clark, the recipient of the world's first artificial heart. Because he was so sick and so near death, and because his surgeon, Dr. William DeVries, believed that Clark really had no choice but to accept the artificial heart, the informed consent process was incomplete and paternalistic.

Instead of focusing on the unprecedented experimental nature of the implant, and planning for contingencies such as a "halfway success" with a live, but permanently hospitalized and incompetent patient, Dr. DeVries focused on the potential "therapeutic" aspects. This focus not only deprived Dr. Clark of the information needed to give an informed consent to the implant, but also deprived him of any opportunity to participate, either by prior decisions or naming a proxy, in decision making concerning the three major surgical procedures performed after the initial implant.[3] Dr. DeVries has justified his approach by arguing that, "He was too old for a transplant and there were no drugs that would help; the only thing that he could look forward to was dying."[4] The rhetoric was that only Barney Clark could make this decision. The reality was that by ignoring significant aspects of the procedure, and labelling it therapeutic experimentation, Clark was treated as incompetent and the choice was made for him.[5]

Although a discussion of rational suicide is

Reprinted with permission from the author and the *Toledo Law Review* 1984. 15:561.
Partial funding for the research for this article was furnished by Concern for Dying, 250 W. 57th St., New York, NY. The authors acknowledge the major contributions of the Legal Advisors of Concern for Dying to Part III of this article, and that of Professor Leonard Glantz to all parts of it.
When this article was written, Ms. Densberger was a student at Suffolk University Law School, Boston

beyond the scope of this article, the case of Elizabeth Bouvia illustrates some of the problems encountered in determining competence. Ms. Bouvia is a twenty-six year old cerebral palsy victim who has suffered from her disease since birth. She entered a hospital as a potential suicide, and later asked the staff to attend her while she refused all nutrition so that she might die of starvation.[6] In pursuit of this objective, she sought a restraining order to prevent the hospital staff from force feeding her. At the hearing, the testimony focused on her competence. While almost all of the physicians who testified found her competent, all agreed that recent events such as her inability to find employment, her financial problems, her separation from her husband, and her inability to have a child contributed to her decision to want to die.[7] Questions concerning the effects of stress, depression, physical impairments, and the "rationality" of a decision on a person's competence were argued. The trial judge found that Ms. Bouvia was mentally competent, but nonetheless refused to enjoin the physicians at Riverside Hospital from force feeding her because of the "profound effect" it would have on the doctors.[8] This extremely complicated and controversial case demonstrates the confusion surrounding the issues of when a determination of competence is appropriate and on what basis it should be made, and even what the consequences of a determination should be.

Most competence determinations, of course, are not front page news. They are made routinely in our nation's hospitals and nursing homes without fanfare or resort to the courts.[9] In all cases, however, what is at stake is that the right to make treatment decisions could be transferred from the patient to some other person.

The right to consent to or refuse treatment, even in the extreme case in which treatment might prolong life, tests the potency of our conviction to take autonomy seriously. The advent of effective medical technologies to sustain life has made competence more critical because the stakes in decision-making are higher. Cases involving refusals by patients and their surrogates of mechanical ventilators, cancer chemotherapy, kidney dialysis, surgery, and nasogastric feeding have all been litigated.[10]

In Section I of this article, we briefly review the legal pedigree of the right to consent to and refuse treatment. Section II deals with the problems of determining competence. In Section III, we suggest steps, including model legislation, to help promote and reaffirm the principle of self-determination in the medical care setting.

I. The Right to Consent to and Refuse Treatment

A. Overview

The presumption of Anglo-American law is that every competent adult is at liberty to consent to or refuse any proposed medical treatment.[11] When a physician's recommendation is refused, however, conflict becomes almost inevitable and its resolution is seldom easy.[12]

The legal right to refuse treatment is part of the common law right to self-determination.[13] In the last twenty years, the right to refuse treatment has gained additional judicial recognition as a right embodied in the constitutional right to privacy.[14] By enunciating a right to self-determination in matters of bodily integrity, in which the right to refuse treatment is implicit, the law "intends to enclose everyone in an invisible shield and to give each person the *right to decide* when to lower the shield and when to keep it in place."[15]

The President's Commission for the Study of Ethical Problems in Medicine and Biomedical and Behavioral Sciences (President's Commission) also has viewed self-determination as a shield "valued for the freedom from outside control it is intended to provide."[16] It is a manifestation of the desire to be an instrument of one's own and "not of other men's acts of will."[17] "[S]elf-determination overrides practitioner-determination even if providers [are] able to demonstrate that they [can] accurately assess the treatment an informed patient would choose."[18] Courts around the country have upheld the competent individual's freedom to make decisions regarding his own medical care even if the potential outcome (often death) is not viewed favorably by the courts.[19]

The right to refuse treatment also has been characterized as an aspect of the right to privacy implicit in the liberty provisions of the United States Constitution. In *Whalen v. Roe*, Justice Stevens suggested that the right encompassed something beyond the least common denominator of the Court's prior decisions with respect to marital choice, procreation, contraception, and child rearing, and embraced both a general "individual interest in avoiding disclosure of personal matters" and distinct "*interest in independence in making certain kinds of important decisions.*"[20]

The two leading right to refuse treatment cases from the state courts also have relied heavily on the constitutional right to privacy in upholding the right of a patient to refuse life-sustaining treatment. In the case of Karen Ann Quinlan, the New Jersey Supreme Court focused on the constitutional right of privacy in its analysis.[21] The *Quinlan* court concluded that "presumably this right is broad enough to encompass a patient's decision to decline medical treatment under certain circumstances, in much the same way as it is broad enough to encompass a women's decision to terminate pregnancy under certain circumstances."[22] In *Superintendent of Belchertown v. Saikewicz*,[23] the Massachusetts Supreme Judicial Court rejected the state's argument that permitting patients to refuse life saving treatment would undermine the state's legitimate interest in protecting the "value of life." The court stated that:

> The constitutional right to privacy, as we conceive it, is an expression of the sanctity of individual free choice and self-determination as fundamental constituents of life. *The value of life as so perceived is lessened* not by a decision to refuse treatment, but *by the failure to allow a competent human being the right of choice.*[24]

B. The Role of Competence

Although the right to refuse treatment is a legally and ethically recognized right, the ability to exercise it in the hospital remains problematic since only competent individuals have this right and the determination of competence is uncertain. Competence is *the* crucial issue since a lack of competence, or even the questioning of an individual's competence, deprives the individual of the liberty to make treatment decisions.[25]

The quality of consent is determined by examining four characteristics: voluntariness, competence, information, and understanding.[26] Although the courts have not explicitly required understanding as an element in making disclosures in the informed consent process, we believe that a proper definition of competence makes the understanding requirement implicit in informed consent. Competence is a capacity, but the most meaningful way to test for competence in a particular situation is to determine if the patient actually understood the information necessary to provide "informed" consent. If he did, he obviously had the capacity to understand it.

C. Informed Consent and Competence

The informed consent doctrine requires that a patient be given material information, information that might influence a patient's decision, including information about his condition, the proposed treatment, including its risks and benefits, and its alternatives. Implemented in good faith by the physician, informed consent enhances both self-determination and rational decision-making.[27] It is assumed that an informed patient has sufficient information on which to base a decision to accept or reject proposed treatment.[28] Thus, it is important to assess the patient's capability to understand and appreciate the information disclosed so that we can be confident it is *his* decision when he makes it.

Infants and comatose patients provide clear examples of patients who are incapable of making decisions regarding medical care. There are equally obvious cases where the patient is capable of making such decisions. Unfortunately, there are also many borderline or gray cases from the perspective of the physician, who wants both to honor the patient's wishes (respect autonomy) and deliver good medical care (promote the patients' well-being), when these two objectives seem to conflict.[29] These are often cases in which the capacity of the patient to participate in the medical decision-making process appears questionable or where the physician believes that the patient's refusal is not authentic but is instead a product of psychological, sociological, and perhaps, economic factors.[30] Such cases are dealt with in a variety of ways with varying degrees of arbitrariness, including sincere attempts to determine patient competence objectively.[31] At issue in all of these cases is the freedom of the individual to exercise the right to refuse treatment and accept the consequences of his own decision. To minimize arbitrariness and avoid imposing our values on those who may not share them, we must carefully consider when undertaking a determination of competence is warranted and how the determination shall be made.

II. Problems of Determining Competence

A. Approaches to Competence

A variety of approaches have been suggested to determine competence. The President's Commission identified three: outcome, status, and function. Under *the Outcome Approach*, decisions which do not reflect community values are used as evidence of incompetence. Under *the Status Approach,* an individual's competence is based on his physical or mental status (i.e., consciousness, age, mental or physical diagnosis). The *Functioning Approach* focuses on the individual's actual functioning in decision-making situations.[32]

Most commentators have assumed that the functioning approach is the correct approach, and have tried to better define the attributes needed to function competently. One philosopher has suggested, for example, that we can require any one of four increasingly strict standards: (1) *free action,* which involves a voluntary and intentional choice; (2) *authentic decision,* which is a decision that reflects the individual's values; (3) *effective deliberation,* which is an evaluation of the specific alternatives and their consequences; and (4) *moral reflection,* which is, in addition to effective deliberation, reflection on and acceptance of the moral values upon which the decision is based.[33] Two psychiatrists have used an analogous classification of increasingly difficult tests and suggested the following four possible tests: (1) evidencing a choice; (2) evidencing an understanding of relevant issues; (3) rationally manipulating the relevant information; and (4) in addition to (2) and (3), an appreciation of the nature of the situation.[34] In their words, "[a]ppreciation is distinct from factual understanding in that it requires the subject to consider the relevance to his immediate situation of those facts he has understood previously in the abstract."[35] The authors regard this as the "strictest" standard; we also believe it is the most reasonable one and, if fairly applied, the one that is most appropriate in hospital and nursing home settings. This type of "functioning" approach, as recommended by the President's Commission, avoids the pitfalls of second-guessing an individual's personality implicitly in the authentic decision and moral reflection test. The functioning approach also helps insure that the decision the patient makes is one he realizes will have consequences for himself. In addition, the test has a solid legal pedigree in the context of treatment refusals.[36]

The appreciation test of competence is, for example, used by the Massachusetts Court of Appeals in *Lane v. Candura.*[37] Mrs. Candura was a 77-year old widow and a diabetic who was suffering from gangrene in the right foot and lower leg. She had undergone two previous amputations (a toe and a portion of her right foot) and at the time of the second amputation, an arterial bypass had been performed in an attempt to decrease the probability of recurrences of gangrene. Her attending physicians recommended that the leg be amputated without delay. After some vacillation, she refused the operation and persisted in that refusal. The trial court held that Mrs. Candura was "incapable of making a rational and competent choice to undergo or reject the proposed surgery to her right leg. To this extent her behavior is irrational. She has closed her mind to the entire issue to the extent that the court cannot conclude that her decision to reject further treatment is rational and informed. . .."[38] The trial court concentrated on the fact that she had "closed her mind" and thus seemed to focus on "autonomy as effective deliberation." Ultimately, however, this appears to have been less important to the trial court than her actual decision which the court characterized as "irrational", thus falling into the "outcome approach" trap.[39] The Court of Appeals, on the other hand, concentrated on her ability to "appreciate" her situation and its alternatives. The court reversed the trial court's decision and stated that "Mrs. Candura's decision may be regarded by most as unfortunate but on the record in this case it is *not* the *uninformed decision* of a person incapable of appreciating the nature and consequences of her act."[40]

It is often difficult to separate objectivity in determining the relevant facts from subjectivity in the imposition of values in a competence determination. What should be considered a fact question, that is, whether a person is capable of understanding and appreciating the nature and consequences of his actions, can be transformed into a value question focusing on the reasonableness of the patient's decision. The criteria on which competence determinations are made in both law and medicine can be seen as a fact and value hybrid, the value aspects comprised of the competing values held by the patient, family, staff, and state. Of these, the patient's values must be determinative to protect liberty.

A more fundamental distinction between adjudication of competence in law and a competence determination in medicine is the presumption of competence. The legal rule is that competence is presumed. All proceedings to test the competence of a person to perform a certain act begin with a presumption of competence which continues unless the contrary is shown. The burden of proof is on the individual contesting competence.[52] Moreover, a person who is incompetent to function responsibly in one context may be competent in others.[53] In medicine, however, the prevailing supposition is often presumption of incompetence. Medical skepticism of patients' capacities for self-determination can be traced to the time of Hippocrates, who advised fellow practitioners to:

Perform [these duties] calmly and adroitly, concealing most things from the patient while you are attending to him. Give necessary orders with cheerfulness and sincerity, turning his attention away from what is being done to him; sometimes reprove sharply and emphatically, and sometimes comfort with solicitude and attention, revealing nothing of the patient's future or present condition,[54]

Jay Katz noted that "Hippocrates . . . recommeded this posture to physicians because he doubted patients' capacity for self-determination."[55] These attitudes were reflected in professional codes of ethics throughout the nineteenth and early twentieth centuries, and continue to be reflected in practice today.[56]

We must guard against physicians who presume patient incompetence. Education may be the long term solution. More immediately, however, it seems desirable to agree on a simple competence assessment test that can be administered at the bedside. Such a test, if based on "understanding and appreciation" and not on any technical medical or psychiatric judgment, should be usable by any reasonable person, including a family member or physician. Its existence will enhance patient autonomy to the degree that its use changes the physicians' attitudes in the direction of greater appreciation of patients' decision-making capacity.

The court of appeals noted that "[u]ntil she changed her original decision and withdrew her consent to the amputation, her competence was not questioned."[41] The doctors readily accepted her consent to the two initial amputations, and only questioned it when she disagreed with their judgment about her treatment. The court made it clear that competence is *not* to be judged by a standard of medical rationality, that is, what her physicians consider the only reasonable decision. Instead, the court pointed out that the relevant factors were her understanding of the "proposed operation" and the consequences of refusing it. According to the court, "[Mrs. Candura] has made it clear that she does not wish to have the op-

eration even though that decision will in all likelihood lead shortly to her death."[42]

This test of competence (the capacity to understand and appreciate the nature and consequences of one's acts) has been used by other courts in similar circumstances, and is probably the most precise concept of competence that we will be able to develop.[43] It can be restated in the medical care context by saying that if an individual understands and appreciates the information needed to give an informed consent, then that individual is competent to give both an informed consent and to refuse consent. We support use of this test because its content will vary with the actual treatment decision, and the risks and alternatives that face the patient, but not with the status of the patient or the decision made by the patient. This functional test is also the one used to determine if a minor is "mature" enough to consent to medical care.[44] This is appropriate since it avoids the use of a "status approach" and places primary emphasis on the minor's functional ability to make the specific treatment decision.

B. When Competence Is Questioned

Use of the "outcome approach" by physicians, as in the *Candura* case, is probably the rule rather than the exception: competence is typically questioned only when a patient refuses to consent to a recommended treatment.[45] Testimony before the President's Commission is consistent with this view: "coherent adults are seldom said to lack capacity (except, perhaps, in the mental health context) when they acquiesce in the course of treatment recommended by their physician."[46]

Without a specific, consistent basis for questioning and determining competence, the patient's reason for refusal, an easily identifiable target for criticism, can too easily become justification for paternalism. Thus, there may be a substitution of the physician's own judgment and values for those of the patient, including the physician's conception of a "good" or "bad" reason. The physician may also attempt to establish a cause-effect relationship between some kind of mental or physical factor (e.g., depression or blood loss) and the undesirable decision, thus enabling him to invalidate that decision on "medical" grounds and to proceed with his own decision.[47] Second-guessing a competent patient's decision by questioning the reasons for refusal is unjustified paternalism, as is labelling a person incompetent because of his stated reasons for refusing treatment.

C. Fact or Value Question?

Competence is viewed legally as a question of fact. In *Grannum v. Berard*, for example, the Washington Supreme Court stated that "[t]he mental capacity necessary to consent to a surgical operation is a question of fact to be determined from the circumstances of each individual case."[48] In *Candura*, "[t]he principal question [was] whether the facts established by the evidence [justified] a conclusion of legal incompetence."[49] Some physicians have erroneously concluded that "[t]he law has tended to address competency as a fixed attribute of an individual, a characteristic in itself with an inherent stability."[50] On the contrary, courts recognize that competence can change from day to day, and have done a remarkable job of considering all of the patient's characteristics in making what in law must be a yes or no decision at a particular point in time. Physicians are surely correct in asserting a continuum of competence. Yet, this does not answer the basic question of whether a particular patient is to lose the liberty to make his or her own decision about a particular treatment. Ultimately, the decision by both courts and physicians is likely to be based upon a value judgment. In the words of Justice Oliver Wendell Holmes: "General propositions do not decide concrete cases. The decision will depend on a judgment or intuition more subtle than any articulate major premise."[51]

D. Determining Competence

The President's Commission recommended that for the sake of "consistency and accuracy" and for the "protection of the right to self-determination" that health care professionals and institutions "develop clear policies to assess incompetence."[57] The Commission, however, did not offer much guidance as to how such policies should be developed or what they should be beyond advising that such determinations should generally be made at the bedside and that "routine recourse to the courts" should be avoided.[58] Although we do not wish to delineate precise policies, it is our hope that the following suggestions will be helpful in the development of methodologies for assessing competence.

A competence determination requires substantive criteria and procedural rules. Both aspects of the determination are important. The substantive criteria have special significance, however, because if they are unsound, the validity of the determination will be suspect regardless of the fairness of the procedures employed.

In determining whether or not the individual understands and appreciates the nature and consequences of the proposed consent or refusal, we believe physicians will find that asking the patient the following questions will be useful in making an objective determination provided that the patient has received the information needed to give an informed consent:

1. What is your present physical condition?

2. What is the treatment that is being recommended for you?

3. What do you and your doctor think might happen to you if you decide to accept the treatment? [This could be modified in appropriate circumstances to ask specifically about risks involved in the treatment, including those of most concern to the patient.]

4. What do you and your doctor think might happen to you if you decide not to accept the recommended treatment?

5. What are the alternative treatments available (including no treatment) and what are the probable consequences of accepting each?

Competence rests ultimately on an ability or capacity to understand and appreciate the nature and consequences of one's decision. It seems appropriate to test this ability in the medical care setting by using a basic informed consent interview. In this interview, one would carefully explain the nature of the proposed treatment, its likely risks and benefits, the alternatives (including no treatment) and their risks and benefits, and ideally before the patient is asked to consent, make a determination as to whether or not the patient actually understands this basic information. By making the competence determination *before* asking for consent, one avoids the "outcome approach" pitfall of labelling a patient incompetent on the basis of the patient's refusal.[59]

There are, of course, complicating factors. A patient who vacillates poses a problem to the physician attempting to discern what the patient wants. What is at stake in vacillation, however, is not incompetence, but indecisiveness. In cases where treatment is immediately necessary to sustain life or prevent serious harm, reasonable treatments can be performed to promote society's interest in health without significantly undercutting the patient's liberty interest, since the patient has made no decision.[60]

If a question persists in a nonemergent situation, treatment cannot be forced until a determination is made (either at the bedside or in court) that the patient is incompetent to make the decision regarding his care in the specific instance and a proxy named to act for the patient.[61]

Another potential complicating factor is mental illness. The existence of mental illness does not always constitute incompetence, although it may.[62] A case in which mental illness would cause incompetence is one in which the illness itself prevents the patient from understanding and appreciating the nature and consequences of his decision. For example, a delusional patient who is being treated for pulmonary abscess and refuses to have bronchoscopic drainage of his lesion because he believes he has no lung problems at all, but is convinced he has some foreign matter stuck in his nose, might properly be considered incompetent to refuse treatment.[63]

E. The Role of the Psychiatrist

Psychiatric evaluation of treatment refusals probably does not occur as frequently as it should. In the only study of treatment refusals in general hospitals, for example, it was found that out of 105 patients who refused treatment, only seven were seen by psychiatrists as a result. All of these were cases in which the patient had a past psychiatric history or was overtly depressed or psychotic.[64] On the other hand, when a psychiatrist is called, the purpose is almost always to have the patient declared incompetent so that treatment can be given over the patient's refusal. Accordingly, it is critical that the consulting psychiatrist have a good understanding of the limits of his or her role in this situation. The psychiatrist should concentrate on making a competence determination, not treating the patient. To avoid drawing inferences colored by his own values,[65] the psychiatrist should make a determination as to the presence or absence of mental disease. If a mental disease or illness is found, he should ask if it interferes with the patient's ability to make a decision. Approaches to the patient may vary, but the substantive test the psychiatrist applies should be one that first identifies (with the help of hospital counsel if necessary) the information needed for the patient to give an informed consent, and then determines the patient's understanding and appreciation of this information.

At the outset, the psychiatrist should determine, "What's going on here?" Who is challenging the patient's capacity for decision-making in a particular case? Is it the family? the physician? the nursing staff? In some cases it will be appro-

priate for the psychiatrist to interview the challenger to discover the motivation behind the action. This approach might exhume an underlying problem or tension which had previously been undisclosed or simply gone unnoticed by others. The psychiatrist must also decide for whom he or she is acting as an agent. Is it the hospital? the physician? the patient?[66] It seems likely that the approach and findings of a psychiatrist genuinely acting on behalf of the patient with only the patient's interests in mind would differ from the psychiatrist acting on behalf of a colleague when asked to examine a "troublesome" patient.

The limited amount of literature on treatment refusals has placed a heavy emphasis on the difficulties of dealing with a patient's "transient feelings of despair and hopelessness" and feeling of depression.[67] Physicians may improperly view a person's mood as a justification to treat without consent on the grounds that it will pass and the patient will change his mind.[68] Many have also argued that seriously injured persons, such as those suffering spinal cord injuries or serious burns, may experience shock, grief, pain, depression, and adverse psychological effects from powerful drugs.[69] Sometimes such feelings can be effectively treated with "supportive psychotherapy" or antidepressant drugs.[70] If these treatments are indicated and not refused by the patient, it is certainly appropriate to pursue them. On the other hand, if the competent patient refuses such treatment and persists in a refusal of treatment, that refusal should be honored. The relevant question is whether a mood such as depression has become so severe as to undermine one's ability to understand and appreciate the nature and consequences of his decisions. If it has not, it alone does not justify a determination of incompetence.

F. A Caveat

It has been noted that in some cases, such as troublesome or otherwise undesirable patients, physicians may be too quick to accept a refusal because they really do not want to treat the patient anyway.[71] In such cases, refusal may be taken at face value and used as an excuse to abandon the patient when abandonment may be neither justified morally nor consistent with the patient's legal rights. Although the patient has a right to refuse treatment, it remains the physician's legal responsibility to ensure that the patient understands the consequences of that refusal. In a recent Calfornia Supreme Court decision,[72] for example, a seemingly healthy young women refused her physician's recommendation that she be given a PAP smear on two different occasions over a ten-year period. She later developed cervical cancer and died. In a lawsuit brought by her surviving children against the physician, the court held that the "fiduciary qualities" implicit in the doctor-patient relationship obligated the physician to make sure that the refusal of an important, recommended procedure was "informed." Thus, the court determined that the doctor had an obligation to discuss these potential consequences of the patient's refusal of the tests with the patient.[73] In the coming era of Diagnostic Related Groups, managed health care, and cost containment, health care providers may have a financial incentive to terminate or not initiate expensive treatment.[74] It is vital that such incentives not lead to uncritical acceptance of a patient's treatment refusal: promoting autonomy requires us to ensure that decisions are based on *informed* consent.

G. Summary

Competence is primarily a fact question that can be answered without reference to medical expertise. Properly understood, a relative, a friend, a nurse, or any other person familiar with the individual and the standard of competence should be able to make a reasonable assessment. This objectivity is important. On the other hand, as a practical matter it will generally be the patient's attending physician who makes the initial assessment of competence. Thus, it is essential that the physician understand the relevant test so that it can be properly applied. Although there is probably no ideal way to make a decision as potentially complex as the one with which the physician is confronted, the physician must nonetheless become comfortable with the fact that a truly autonomous decision may not be synonymous with the medically-best decision, and that this is not inharmonious with moral or societal values. What matters most in making a decision about what will be done to the body of another is that the values and will of the patient are honored. As H. Tristram Englehardt has put it:

> When the patient decides that the future quality of life open to him is not worth the investment of pain and suffering to attain that future quality of life, that is a decision proper to the patient . . . one must be willing, as a price for recogniz-

ing the freedom of others, to live with the consequences of that freedom: some persons will make choices that they would regret were they to live longer.[75]

III. Reaffirming the Right to Refuse Treatment: A Proposed Model Act

Although the right of a competent adult to refuse treatment is firmly entrenched in both common and constitutional law,[76] cases continue to recur in which individuals are treated despite their competent objections or withdrawal of consent.[77] Because of this problem and the centrality of the right to refuse treatment to patient autonomy, we believe it is appropriate for society periodically to reaffirm its commitment to this principle. Indeed we believe that the clear articulation of an individual's right to refuse medical treatment is a proper subject for legislation. In addition, even though presently competent patients may be afforded the right of refusal, they may be treated after they become incompetent, even though they might not have wished treatment in such circumstances. To safeguard against treating previously competent individuals against their will, many individuals and groups have proposed "living wills"[78] in which an individual may set forth his treatment wishes in the event he later becomes incompetent and thus unable to speak for himself. More than a dozen states have passed living will or "death with dignity" legislation.[79] This movement underlines the seriousness of the public sentiment in this area. Nonetheless, we believe most of the recently passed and debated proposals are too narrow and limited, and that right to refuse legislation designed to enhance patient autonomy:

• Should not be restricted to the terminally ill, but should apply to all competent adults and mature minors;

• Should not limit the types of treatment an individual can refuse (e.g., to "extraordinary" treatment) but should apply to all medical interventions;

• Should permit individuals to designate another person to act on their behalf and set forth the criteria under which the designated person is to make decisions;

• Should require health care providers to follow the patient's wishes and provide punishment for those who do not; and

• Should require health care providers to continue to provide palliative care to patients who refuse other intervention.

The Model Legislation

The specific provisions of our proposal are set forth in the Appendix to this article. The model proposed was developed by the Legal Advisors of Concern for Dying.[80] The Model Act has already been introduced into the Florida legislature and has won the critical acclaim of the President's Commission. The Commission has stated: "In terms of its treatment of such central issues as the capacity to consent and the standard by which a proxy decision maker is to act, the Right to Refuse Treatment Act is carefully crafted and in conformity with the Commission's conclusions."[81] Many sections of the Act are self-explanatory, but some merit additional comment. No specific form or document is included because we believe the individual's wishes will be more likely to be set forth if his own words are used.

The right being reaffirmed is the right to refuse treatment implicit in any meaningful concept of individual liberty. Living will statutes, on the other hand, usually rely on a vaguely articulated "right to die" which we believe has no legal pedigree.[82] We include both adults and mature minors in the purview of the act because we believe minors who understand and appreciate the nature and consequences of their actions should be afforded self-determination and not forced to undergo medical treatment against their will.

The proposed Act is aimed at protecting the autonomy of not only the terminally-ill patients, but also those who are not terminally ill. All persons merit respect and autonomy. Moreover, if we do not raise our sensitivity regarding respect for the nonterminal patient's right to autonomy, it is extremely unlikely that the rights of terminal patients will be respected. The Act also applies to patients like Karen Ann Quinlan who, although in a hopeless, persistent vegetative state, do not suffer from an underlying, terminal illness.

The most critical definition in the Act is that of "competence" and a determination of competence should be made in a manner consistent with that discussed in Part II of this article. The

President's Commission noted that "by combining a proxy directive with specific instructions, an individual could control both the content and the process of decision-making about care in case of incapacity."[83] Our proposal incorporates this suggestion by permitting the declarant to both define what interventions are refused, and to name an authorized individual to make decisions consistent with his desires as expressed in the declaration.[84] The Act recognizes that some providers may have different belief systems than the people they care for as patients, and attempts to outline a realistic transfer procedure which respects the ethical views of both parties. The Act also recognizes, however, that the patient is most immediately affected by the treatment-refusal decision, since the patient's own future and quality of life are at stake. Consequently, when a patient's directive and a provider's views differ, the patient's directive must prevail over the physician's views in the rare occasions where transfer is impossible.[85]

Providers who follow the procedures outlined in this Act are relieved of liability under any civil, criminal, or administrative action. On the other hand, providers who abandon their patients or refuse to comply with valid declarations are subject to punishment. These offenders may face civil actions including charges of negligence and battery. Administrative sanctions may include license revocation, suspension or other disciplinary action by the state board of professional registration.

Other important sections of the Act make it clear that this method of refusing treatment is not exclusive, but in addition to any other methods recognized by law, that the refusal of treatment is not suicide, that a treatment refusal does not affect any insurance policy, and that regardless of refusals, palliative care must be given unless specifically refused by the patient himself.[86]

The Act is designed to promote the autonomy of competent adults and respect for their persons by enhancing the adults' right to accept or reject medical treatments recommended by their health care providers. It protects all patients who were once competent, both while they are competent and when they execute a declaration after they become incompetent. It provides that patients may execute a written, signed declaration setting forth their intentions on treatment and refusal decisions and permits patients to designate authorized individuals to make treatment decisions on their behalf should they become incompetent in the future. The Act upholds and clarifies consistent with the ethics of the medical profession and shields complying physicians, witnesses, and authorized persons acting in good faith, from liability. In addition, the Act provides sanctions for those who violate its provisions.

IV. Conclusion

The rights of privacy and self-determination in medical care hinge upon the doctrine of informed consent. This doctrine is based on the notion that an individual's consent must be competent, voluntary, and informed. Competence, the ability to understand and appreciate the nature and consequences of one's decision, is the *sine qua non* of autonomy in the medical setting. While "understanding" has never been explicitly required prior to consent to a medical procedure, when competence is questioned, the best way to test it is to determine whether or not the patient actually understands the material information required to make his decision "informed." This test of competence is objective and enhances the patient's central role in medical decision-making about his own body. If we take consent seriously, we must permit the competent, voluntary, informed and understanding refusal of consent to stand as well; otherwise the entire concept of liberty in health care becomes hollow.

Some of the most difficult problems are confronted when we are no longer able to communicate our wishes to our care givers. By proposing model legislation that permits individuals to express their wishes for treatment in a declaration that is binding upon their care givers after the patient becomes incompetent, we enhance liberty and make it more likely that individuals will be treated in ways consistent with their own values rather than according to the value of others. Had Dr. Barney Clark signed such a document prior to the implantation of his artificial heart, for example, we would all have been much more comfortable in knowing that his wishes regarding the additional surgeries he endured were being followed. Without such documentation, we are left with the uncomfortable feeling that at some point Dr. Clark lost his human identity, and instead of the artificial heart being a means to keep him alive, he became a means to keep the artificial heart alive.[87]

Unusual for its drama and expense, Dr. Clark's experience relates to all of our potential medical experiences. How can we help insure that we do not lose our human individuality, our "right to privacy", in the face of medical technology designed to "save" us? Without pretending to answer this difficult question, we suggest that individual liberty will stand a better chance of surviving in the hospital environment if competence determinations are better understood and competent treatment refusals are honored.

Notes

1. See Appelbaum & Roth, Patients Who Refuse Treatment in Medical Hospitals, 250 *J. A.M.A.* 1296 (1983); Meisel, The 'Exceptions' to the Informed Consent Doctrine: Striking a Balance Between Competing Values in Medical Decisionmaking, 1979 *Wisc. L. Rev.* 413, 440; Green, Judicial Tests of Mental Incompetency, 6 Mo. L. Rev. 141 (1941).

2. Strictly speaking, paternalism only applies to competent patients. Yet, the vagueness of its definition can lead to individuals being incorrectly labeled as incompetent, and thus improperly having their decisions made by others. Paternalism has been variously defined in legal and philosophical literature. Legal definitions tend to concentrate exclusively on interference with an individual's liberty for his own good, and that is how the term is used in this article. One commentator has written: "By paternalism I shall understand roughly the interference with a person's liberty of action justified by reasons referring exclusively to the welfare, good, happiness, needs, interests, or values of the person being coerced." Dworkin, Paternalism, in *Morality and The Law* 107, 108 (R. Wasserstrom ed. 1971). Medical ethicists tend to see the concept as somewhat broader. For example, Allen Buchanan defines paternalism as "interference with a person's freedom of action or freedom of information, or the deliberate dissemination of misinformation, where the alleged justification of interfering or misinforming is that it is for the good of the person who is interfered with or misinformed. Buchanan, Medical Paternalism, 7 *Phil. & Pub. Aff.* 370, 372 (1978). James Childress identifies two characteristics of a paternalistic act: the motivation and intention is to prevent harm, and it involves a refusal to accept or to acquiese in an individual's choices, wishes and actions. J. Childress, Paternalism and Health Care, in *Medical Responsibility* 15, 18–19 (W. Robinson & M. Pritchard eds. 1979). More broadly yet, Charles M. Culver and Bernard Gert list the following four characteristics as defining paternalistic behavior:
   A is acting paternalistically toward S if and only if (A's behavior correctly indicates that A believes that):
   1. his acting benefits S
   2. his action involves violating a moral rule with regard to S
   3. his action does not have S's past, present, or immediately forthcoming consent

4. S is competent to give consent (simple or valid).

C. CULVER & B. GERT, *Philosophy In Medicine* 130 (1982). In adopting Dworkin's more narrow view in this article we do not mean to suggest that Culver and Gert are not correct in widening liberty to include violation of any "moral rule," but only to conclude that in the treatment refusal situation, liberty is properly the exclusive focus relating to paternalistic behavior. See also Gruzalski, When to Keep Patients Alive Against Their Wishes, in *Value Conflicts In Health Care Decisions* 171, 172–79 (B. Gruzalski & C. Nelson eds. 1982).

3. *N.Y. Times,* Apr. 17, 1983, § 1, p 44. (One on December 4, 1982 to correct air leaks in lungs, one on December 14, 1982 to replace a cracked valve, and one on January 14, 1983, because of nosebleeds.) The consent form he did sign had promised him that only he would make the decisions to undergo such procedures; nevertheless, they were all made for him because he was deemed incompetent:

> 2.2. I further understand that additional chest surgeries may be required in the event the device needs to be replaced or repaired which *will be explained to me and will be done with a new consent form signed by me for each such procedure* and that in all likelihood, general anesthesia with its attendant risks would be necessary in connection with such procedures.
> 2.3. I also understand that the use of the artificial heart may necessitate additional instrumentation and studies in order that adequate information may be obtained concerning its functioning, and such instrumentation and studies are expected to consist of or be similar to those involved in cardiac catherization but may include other procedures, with attendant risks, discomfort and inconvenience. *Each of these new procedures will have a consent form which must be signed before they are performed* (emphasis added).

4. *Newsweek,* Dec. 13, 1982, 35–36.

5. Making the decision for experimental heart procedures on the basis that the "doctor knows best" has strong historical precedents. Dr. Christiaan Barnard, who performed the first human heart transplant in 1967, argued that his patient really had no choice: "He was at the end of the line . . . For a dying man it is not a difficult decision . . . If a lion chases you to the bank of a river filled with crocodiles, you will leap into the water convinced you have a chance to swim to the other side. But you would never accept such odds if there were no lion." Likewise, Dr. Denton Cooley argued about the first recipient of a temporary artificial heart, Haskell Karp, "He was a drowning man. A drowning man cannot be too particular what he's going to use as a life preserver." Annas, Consent to the Artificial Heart: The Lion and the Crocodiles, 13 *Hastings Center Rep.* 20 (April, 1983).

6. Bouvia v. County of Riverside, No. 159780 (Super. Ct. Cal. Dec. 16, 1983).

7. See Transcript of Bouvia case, see above. [hereinafter cited as Transcript].

8. Transcript p. 1242–43.

9. See, e.g., Brown & Thompson, Nontreatment of fever in Extended-Care Facilities, 300 *New Eng. J. Med.* 1246 (1979).

10. *In re* Earle Spring, 380 Mass. 629, 405 N.E.2d 115 (1980) (kidney dialysis); Custody of a Minor, 375 Mass. 733, 379 N.E.2d 1053 (1978) (chemotherapy); Lane v. Candura, 6 Mass. App. 377, 376 N.E.2d 1232 (1978) (surgery to remove gangrenous leg); *In re* Quinlan, 70 N.J. 10, 355 A.2d 647 (1976) (mechanical ventilator); *In re* Conroy, 188 N.J. Super. 523, 457 A.2d 1232 (1983), rev'd, 190 N.J. Super. 453, 464 A.2d 303 (1983) (nasogastric feeding); Matter of Application of Plaza Health and Rehabilitation Center, No. 84-1 Infancy (N.Y. Sup. Ct. Onodaga Cty Feb. 2, 1984) (Miller, J.) (force feeding).

11. See generally G. Grisez, *Life and Death With Liberty and Justice* 87–88 (1979).

12. See above, p. 88–89.

13. Schloendorff v. Society Hosp., 211 N.Y. 125, 105 N.E. 92 (1914). In 1914, a patient's right to self-determination was expressed in the Schloendorff case by Judge Cardozo in which he stated that "[e]very human being of adult years and sound mind has a right to determine what shall be done with his own body. . . ." Id. at 129, 105 N.E. at 93. Although Schloendorff has been hailed as a "celebrated case," (President's Commission for the Study of Ethical Problems in Medicine and Biomedical and Behavioral Sciences, 1 *Making Health Care Decisions* 20 (1982) [hereinafter cited as *Health Care Decisions*]) it is better seen as rhetoric. DICKENS, The Right to a Natural Death, 26 McGill L.J. 849 (1981). The right articulated by Judge Cardozo was a qualified right and its exercise was predicted on a condition (sound mind) which unfortunately left much room for ambiguity and varied interpretation. A better enunciation of the right to refuse treatment based on self-determination can be found in Natanson v. Kline, 186 Kan. 393, —, 350 P.2d 1093, 1104 (1960). In Natanson, the exercise of the right to refuse treatment was contingent upon the individual being of "sound mind." The Court said in dictum:

> Anglo-American law starts with the premise of thorough-going self-determination. It follows that each man is considered to be master of his own body and he may, if he be of sound mind, expressly prohibit the performance of life-saving surgery, or other medical treatment. A doctor might well believe that an operation or form of treatment is desirable or necessary but the law does not permit him to substitute his own judgment for that of the patient. . . .

14. In a series of decisions, the United States Supreme Court has tied the right of control over one's body to the fundamental right of privacy. Thus, a person has a right to use contraceptives free from state interference, Griswold v. Connecticut, 381 U.S. 479, 485 (1965); to obtain an abortion from a willing physician in the first trimester of pregnancy free from state interference, Roe v. Wade, 410 U.S. 113, 163, (1973); and to seek abortion services without permission of a parent or spouse, Planned Parenthood v. Danforth, 428 U.S. 52, 58 (1976).

15. G. GRISEZ, supra note 11, p. 88 (emphasis supplied).

16. *Health Care Decisions*, supra note 13, p. 45.

17. I. BERLIN, Two Concepts of Liberty, in *Four Essays on Liberty* 118, 138 (1969), quoted in *Health Care Decisions*, supra note 13, p. 45.

18. See *Health Care Decisions*, supra note 13, p. 45.

19. See Satz v. Perlmutter, 362 So. 2d 160 (Fla. Dist. Ct. App. 1978), aff'd 379 So. 2d 359 (Fla. 1980); *In re* Estate of Brooks, 32 Ill. 2d 361, 205 N.E.2d 435 (1965); *In re* Quakenbush, 156 N.J. Super. 282, 383 A.2d 785 (1978); Erickson v. Dilgard, 44 Misc. 2d 27, 252 N.Y.S.2d 705 (Sup. Ct. 1962). Cf. Judge Hews in Bouvia, "We all earnestly hope that this young woman will realize that there is hope in life and that now because of the action taken by her she can be a symbol of hope to others similarly situated if she changes her purpose." Bouvia v. County of Riverside, No. 159780 (Super. Ct. Cal. Dec. 16, 1983).

20. Whalen v. Roe, 429 U.S. 589, 596 (1977) (emphasis supplied).

21. *In re* Quinlan, 70 N.J. 10, 38, 355 A. 2d 647, 662 (1976), cert. denied sub nom., Garger v. N.J., 429 U.S. 922 (1976).

22. Quinlan, 70 N.J. at 40, 355 A.2d at 663.

23. Superintendent of Belchertown v. Saikewicz, ___ Mass. ___, 370 N.E.2d 417 (1977).

24. See above, p. ___, 370 NE.2d at 426 (emphasis supplied).

25. Legal Advisers, Concern for Dying, The Right to Refuse Treatment: A Model Act, 73 *Am. J. Pub. Health* 919 (1983).

26. G. ANNAS, L. GLANTZ & B. KATZ, *Informed Consent to Human Experimentation: The Subject's Dilemma* 53 (1977) [hereinafter cited as *Human Experimentation*].

27. See above, p. 33–38.

28. See above, p. 29–31.

29. Gruzalski, supra note 2, p. 171. And see examples in Jackson & Young, Patient Autonomy and Death With Dignity, 30 *New Eng. J. Med.* 404 (1979).

30. For a good discussion with illustrations of difficult cases see Rodin, et al., Stopping Life-Sustaining Medical Treatment: Psychiatric Considerations in the Termination of Renal Dialysis, 26 *Can. J. Psychiatry* 37 (1981).

31. Two psychiatrists have stated that:
    involuntary treatment of patients deemed by the staff to be incompetent was a common practice. It should be noted that the staff in several of the hospitals studied appeared to have a uniform *rule of thumb* to determine incompetency, namely that a patient be disoriented and incoherent. . . . Once a patient fell into this category, he or she was often restrained (using arm and leg restraints and "Posey" vests), treated with sedative and antipsychotic medication to control disruptive or annoying behavior (e.g., loud screaming), and given whatever treatment short of surgery or intrusive diagnostic procedures (generally classified as those that would require anesthesia) the physicians deemed necessary.
    Appelbaum & Roth, Treatment Refusal in Medical Hospitals, in 2 *Health Care Decisions*, supra note 13, p. 474, app. D (emphasis added).

32. HEALTH CARE DECISIONS, supra note 13, at 170.

33. Miller, Autonomy and the Refusal of Lifesaving Treatment, 11 *Hastings Center Rep.* 22, 27 (Aug. 1981).

34. APPELBAUM & ROTH, *Competency to Consent to Treatment* (1977).

35. See above, p. 954.

36. See supra notes 10 and 19.

37. Lane v. Candura, 6 Mass. App. Ct. 377, 376 NE.2d 1232 (1978).

38. See above, p. 379, 376 NE.2d at 1233.

39. At least two of the physicians who testified in the Bouvia case fell into the "outcome" trap. See Bouvia v. County of Riverside, No. 159780 (Super. Ct. Cal. Dec. 16, 1983). The chief of psychiatry at the hospital, Dr. Donald E. Fisher, testified that Ms. Bouvia's decision not to accept food was a "bad decision," "impaired," and one that he would not honor. Dr. Fisher was asked if Elizabeth Bouvia had changed her mind and decided to eat, would that decision be a "competent health care decision on her part." The doctor responded, "I think it would be." Transcript, supra note 7, at 590, More generally, Dr. Thomas M. Heric, called by the petitioner, testified: "Doctors like patients to agree with them. When a patient agrees with me, the patient is rational. When an 80 year old lady refuses to have a massive resection of her bowel for wide-spread cancer, then I send her to a psychiatrist, because she is not agreeing with me, so she is irrational." See above, p. 1021.

40. Lane v. Candura, 6 Mass. App. Ct. at ___, 376 N.E.2d at 1236 (emphasis added).

41. See above, p. at ___, 376 N.E.2d at 1235.

42. See above.

43. See, e.g., *In re* Osborne, 294 A.2d 372 (D.C. 1972); *In re* Quackenbush, 156 N.J. Super. 282, 383 A.2d 785 (Morris County Ct. 1978); *In re* Melideo, 88 Misc. 2d 974, 390 N.Y.S.2d 523 (Sup. Ct. 1976); *In re* Yetter, 62 Pa. D. & C.2d 619 (C.P. of Northampton County 1973). The requirements of "understanding and appreciating" cut across other areas of legal competence determinations. The two terms are also used together in determining the capacity necessary to enter into a contract. 2 *Black, Rescission and Cancellation*, p. 735 (2d ed. 1929). See also discussion in Green, supra note 1, pp. 147–52. While these terms can be criticized as vague, they are given meaning by the specific context in which they are used. In contracts, for example, by the nature of the particular transaction and its consequences; in wills, by the nature and extent of the property involved and the individual's relationships with others; and in the case of refusing treatment, with the elements necessary to give or withhold an informed consent. The degree of understanding and appreciation may vary from case to case, just as the degree of bodily invasion varies. In an analogous situation, the "reasonable degree of rational understanding" needed to be found competent to stand trial will "vary from the charge of petty theft to a charge of murder or kidnapping." Annas, Book Review, 54 *B.U.L. Rev.* 863, 866 (1974).

44. See discussion, *Human Experimentation*, supra note 26, pp. 70–73.

45. See supra note 39.

46. *Health Care Decisions*, supra note 13, p. 61. See also C. CULVER & B. GERT, supra note 2, p. 61; Meisel, supra note 1, p. 451.

47. See Starkman & Young, Evaluation and Management of the Patient Who Refuses Medical Care, *6 Primary Care* (1979); see also, e.g., Lane v. Candura, 6 Mass. App. Ct. 377, ___, 376 N.E.2d 1232, 1235 (1978); Meisel, supra note 1, pp. 446–47. We agree with those who argue that paternalism is never a justification for imposing treatment on a competent patient. On the other hand, we recognize that there may be extremely unusual circumstances which to many would justify paternalistic behavior for brief periods of time, and that focusing on the definition of "competence" rather than the elements justifying paternalism may simply be a smokescreen. For example, C. CULVER & B. GERT, supra note 2, specify three (and only three) factors that are relevant to justifying a paternalistic intervention:

1. The moral rule(s) which is (are) violated;
2. The probable amount of evil caused, avoided, or ameliorated by the moral rule violation (probable amount includes the kind and severity of the evil, the likelihood that the evil will occur, and the probable length of time it will be suffered);
3. The rational desires of the person(s) affected by the moral rule violation. See above, p. 148.

Culver & Gert argue further that to justify paternalistic behavior we must be prepared to publicly advocate that the violation be universal; "that it would be irrational for S not to choose having the rule violated with regard to himself." More specifically, to be strongly justified, all rational persons must be prepared to agree "that the evil prevented by universally allowing the violation would be greater than the evil caused by universally allowing [the evil caused by permitting liberty]." See above, p. 149. One example the authors use may be helpful. They cite the example of Dax Cowart (who they identify only as Mr. L), the 26-year-old Texan who was badly burned over more than 65% of his body and for more than 9 months had undergone a variety of procedures and operations. He was also subjected to very painful daily "tankings" that involved being placed in a tub of antibacterial solution to prevent skin infection. He has previously objected to these treatments, and now clearly states he no longer can stand the pain of the treatments, does not believe his outcome will be acceptable to him, and wants the tankings stopped. We agree with the authors that to continue treatment over Mr. Cowart's competent objections is unjustifiable paternalism. Using their own test they concluded that "[n]o rational person would publicly advocate this kind of violation because of the terrible consequences of living in a world where great pain could be inflicted on persons against their rational desires whenever some other person could do so by appealing to some different rational ranking of evils of his own." See above, pp. 152–53. On the other hand, what if Dax Cowart had only to undergo one week of painful tankings to be returned to an essentially normal life? Under these circumstances to prefer death might be labelled "irrational." The authors conclude that the physicians would be justified in acting paternalistically and treating the patient for a week over his objections, since "a rational person could publicly advocate this kind of violation" on a universal basis, see above, p. 154. This example, of course, raises the question of where and how one draws the line between a day, a week, a month, etc., of forced treatment and helps underline the subjectivity involved in making such a decision. Our own position is that one can continue treatment during a competence assessment, but if competence is established, no further treatment of the patient is permissible even though death would result, since we believe that the violation of liberty is far more serious an evil than apparently do Culver and Gert. The case of Dax Cowart is a well-known teaching case because of a videotape made of his treatment refusal in 1974 by the University of Texas Medical Branch in Galveston called "Please Let Me Die." Concern for Dying is currently producing an hour-long documentary of Mr. Cowart's medical treatment and subsequent recovery, which will be aired later in 1984.

48. Grannum v. Berard, 70 Wash.2d 304, ___, 422 P.2d 812, 814 (1967); see G. ANNAS, L. GLANTZ, & B.

Katz, *The Rights of Doctors, Nurses, and Allied Health Professionals*, pp. 80–82 (1981).

49. Lane v. Candura, 6 Mass. App. Ct. 377, ___, 376 N.E.3d 1232, 1235 (1978).

50. Roth & Appelbaum, Clinical Issues in the Assessment of Competency, 138 *Am. J. Psychiatry* 1462, 1466 (1981).

51. Lochner v. New York, 198 U.S. 45, 76 (1905) (dissent), quoted with approval in Green, Public Policies Underlying the Law of Mental Incompetency, 38 *Mich. L. Rev.* 1189, 1221 (1940) (competence determination context); see also supra notes 37–43 and accompanying text. See also Meisel, supra note 1, p. 452.

52. It has been suggested that it is therefore more appropriate to adopt the term "incompetence" determination, since this is what must be proven to deprive the patient of autonomy. Meisel, supra note 1, p. 442 n.104.

53. See also Green, supra note 1, pp. 158–59. Compare *In re* Holloway's Estate, 195 Cal. 711, 733, 235 P. 1012, 1021 (1925) with Faber v. Sweet Style Mfg. Co., 40 Misc. 2d 212, 216, 242 N.Y.S.2d 763, 768 (1963) (less mental capacity needed to make a will than a contract).

54. Hippocrates, Decorum, in 2 *Hippocrates* 297, 299 (W. Jones trans. 2d. ed. 1967).

55. Katz, Disclosure and Consent: In Search of Their Roots, in *Genetics and the Law* II 124 (A. Milunsky & G. Annas eds. 1980).

56. See above, pp. 123–24. Perhaps the most pervasive justification voiced for the "doctor knows best" attitude is the "thank you theory," i.e., the patient will later thank the doctor for ignoring his refusal. This justification has no basis, and, as Culver and Gert have stated, is neither a necessary nor sufficient condition to justify paternalism. As they note, the patient may either be a "grudging person" who never thanks anyone for anything, or one who is very obesiant toward physicians, and thus forgives and thanks them for everything. In the first instance thanks is not necessary to justify paternalism, and in the second it is insufficient. As the authors correctly note, "one must ask where the judgments about whether one will later be thanked come from." C. Culver & B. Gert, supra note 2, p. 161. The characteristics that lead one to adopt the "thank you theory" must be the same that justify paternalism generally.

57. *Health Care Decisions*, supra note 13, p. 173.

58. See above, p. 175.

59. Each case should, of course, be considered independently. However, as in law, although each competence determination should be pursued on a case-by-case basis, precedents should be established so that there are some principles to follow to assure greater equity and consistency in competence determinations. One author has suc-cinctly stated the importance of establishing principles in competence determinations which will serve to guide succeeding cases:

> Unless a decision about how to proceed in such a case is grounded on some relatively clear rationale, it may be only the product of that day's psychological outlook of the care provider, psychiatrist, hospital counsel, judge, or Institutional Review Board member whose opinion became decisive. . . . Because the case-by-case strategy [as thought of by the medical profession] is of itself empty of content, it may lull care providers, however well-intentioned they may be, into acting on the basis of values not shared by the patient.

Gruzalski, supra note 2, pp. 174–75. Cf. Rabkin, Gillerman & Rice, Orders Not To Resuscitate, 295 *New Eng. J. Med* 364 (1976) (recommending that the mental competence of patients to make decisions about their treatment be assessed on an ongoing basis). We believe respect for the individual's liberty demands that a competence determination be kept as narrow as possible and on point with the ability to perform the immediate task at hand; the ability to make a decision in a particular instance. We do, however, find reasonable the approach suggested by Roth and Appelbaum. They assert that

> [t]he magnitude of the intrusion on a patient's autonomy that is represented by the consequences of a finding of incompetency and the impact of allowing a competent patient to refuse potentially life-saving treatment both argue for a cautious approach to evaluation of competency, represented by at least two contacts with the patient on at least two different days.

Roth & Appelbaum, supra note 50, p. 1465.

60. E.g., Lane v. Candura, 6 Mass. App. Ct. 377, ___, 36 N.E.2d 1232, 1236 (1978) where the court stated "the fact that she has vacillated in her resolve not to submit to the operation does not justify a conclusion that her capacity to make the decision is impaired to the point of legal incompetence." See above.

In a case in the medical literature, a patient in a Medical Intensive Care Unit with a history of chronic obstructive lung disease was placed permanently on mechanical ventilation. The patient subsequently experienced "striking changes of mind almost daily" concerning his medical care and whether or not "he wanted maximal therapy." The staff evidenced great disagreement about which side of the patient's ambivalence to honor. Ultimately, when the patient developed a nosocomial pulmonary infection and experienced ventricular fibrillations, no efforts were made at cardiopulmonary resuscitation. In this case, the care givers never really knew what the patient wanted, since the patient had never made a clear decision. Continued treatment under these circumstances were certainly warranted, but the decision not to resuscitate seems problematic since there appears to have been no clear rationale for the decision. Jackson

& Younger, supra note 29, p. 405 (Case 1). When a patient is incompetent to make a decision, however, immediate steps should be taken to appoint a proxy decision-maker unless competence is likely to return before a treatment decision is required. Cf. Jackson v. Indiana, 406 U.S. 715 (1972):

> [A] person charged by a State with a criminal offense who is committed solely on account of his incapacity to proceed to trial cannot be held more than the *reasonable period of time necessary to determine whether there is a substantial probability that he will attain that capacity in the foreseeable future.* If it is determined that this is not the case, then the State must either institute the customary civil commitment proceeding that would be required to commit indefinitely any other citizen, *or release the defendant.*

See above, p. 738 (emphasis added).

61. The case of Elizabeth Bouvia illustrates what should not happen. The chief of psychiatry of Riverside General Hospital indicated that he would not honor her request not to be force fed unless she had "at least a six month history of virtual freedom from trouble." Bouvia v. County of Riverside, No. 159780 (Super. Ct. Cal. Dec. 16, 1983). See Transcript, supra note 7, pp. 596–97. In her case, such a requirement would have been virtually impossible to ever fulfill and would amount simply to a refusal to honor the patient's wishes. A useful comparison is the case of severely burned patients where survival with maximal treatment is unprecedented. A decision regarding "heroic" treatment can only be made with the patient's input if it is made very soon after the burn, and before massive doses of pain medication are required. Even under these extremely intense circumstances, 21 of 24 patients (or their families in cases where the patient was comatose or brain-injured) chose nonheroic care after being fully informed of their condition and options. Imbus & Zawacki, Autonomy for Burned Patients When Survival is Unprecedented, 297 *New Eng. J. Med.* 308, 309 (1977). We, of course, believe all burned patients should be given such an option. The study indicates, however, how well informed consent and informed refusals can work when the medical staff go out of their way to insure patient autonomy.

62. See, e.g., *In re* Yetter, 62 Pa. D. & C. 619 (C.P. of Northampton County 1973). Nor does temporary distortion of the patient's ability to choose because of pain, medication or a metabolic abnormality determine incompetency. Roth & Appelbaum, supra note 50, p. 1465. "Competency is not necessarily a fixed state that can be assessed with equivalent results at any one of a number of times. . . . Whenever the assessment of competency is being conducted in a nonemergency setting, more than one evaluation session should take place." See previous note; see also J. ROBERTSON, *The Rights of the Critically Ill* 42 (1983).

63. The case is described in Appelbaum & Roth, Treatment Refusal in Medical Hospitals, in 2 *Health*

Care Decisions, supra note 13, pp. 411, 432 app. D. The patient was not treated and died shortly thereafter. Apparently no attempt was made to determine his competence. This is what older legal cases referred to as the "insane delusion test." Specifically, to invalidate a contract or will it was insufficient that the maker was suffering from an insane delusion: the delusion had to be one that was "intimately related to the subject matter of the contract" or will. In contracts, for example, the question was whether the transaction was motivated by the delusion. If it was, the contract could be voided. Green, supra note 1, p. 151. Similarly, an insane delusion invalidates a will because it serves as improper motivation in its making. In one case, for example, the insane belief which arose before the testator's death that his wife had been unfaithful to him, and which led him to disinherit her, was sufficient to set aside the will. *In re* Honigman's Will, 8 N.Y.2d 244, 168 N.E.2d 676, 203 N.Y.S.2d 859 (1960). As applied to treatment refusals, delusions would only serve to make one incompetent to refuse treatment if they were the motivating factor behind the refusal, for example, if the patient thought he was immortal and thus would not die no matter what treatment he refused. Even if *some* of one's reasons for refusal are delusional, this still may not be sufficient to invalidate one's decision. For example, the fact that an elderly woman stated that one of her reasons for refusing an operation for breast cancer was that it would affect her ability to have babies and prohibit a movie career was insufficient to overcome her refusal because there was an independent and consistent reason voiced by her for the refusal: her fear that she would die if the surgery was performed. The court refused to overrule her decision simply because "some of her present reasons for refusal are delusional and the result of mental illness." *In re* Yetter, 62 Pa. D. & C. 619, 624 (C.P. of Northampton County 1973).

64. Appelbaum & Roth, supra note 1, p. 1300.

65. See, e.g., discussion of the court in Lane v. Candura, 6 Mass. App. Ct. 377, ___, 376 N.E.2d 1232, 1235 (1978).

> [The psychiatrist's opinion] appears to have been based upon (1) his inference from her unwillingness to discuss the problem with him that she was unable to face up to the problem or to understand that her refusal constituted a choice; (2) his characterization of "an unwillingness for whatever reason to consent to life saving treatment . . . as suicidal"; and (3) a possibility, not established by evidence as a reasonable probability, that her mind might be impaired by toxicity caused by the gangrenous condition.

See above, p. 376 N.E.2d p. 1235.

66. See generally T. Szaz, *Law, Liberty & Psychiatry* (1963).

67. See, e.g., Jackson & Younger, Patient Autonomy and "Death with Dignity." 301 *New Eng. J. Med.* 404 (1979); Rodin, et al., supra note 30, p. 542.

68. For example, in the case of Elizabeth Bouvia, her attending physician during the hearing, Psychiatrist Donald E. Fisher, argued that he believed that although Ms. Bouvia was legally competent, she would change her mood and her mind given time and resume eating. He accordingly felt justified in force feeding her with a nasogastric tube, and forcing psychotropic medication on her because he believed that these were life-saving procedures:

> Q. To what extent is giving her psychotropic medication a life-saving procedure?
>
> A. It may affect her mood, her attitude, her motivation to live.
>
> Q. Well, indeed, so might the surgical procedure/to improve her physical mobility/ . . . Why is the surgical procedure different in your mind than the psychototropic drugs . . . ?
>
> A. I think we are talking about two different periods of time. We are talking about tube feeding, psychotropic drugs, the movement, part of a procedure to keep a person alive. The orthopedic procedures, I think, are distant procedures and . . . could cover another time frame, another part of her life.

Questions from Attorney Richard Scott, Transcript 503–504. See generally, Annas, The Case of Elizabeth Bouvia: When Suicide Prevention Becomes Brutality, 14 *Hastings Center Rep.* 20 (April 1984).

69. E.g., Gruzalski, supra note 2, p. 172.

70. See examples in Appelbaum & Roth, supra note 31. In one case the authors reported that a woman who had previously had her left leg amputated because of vascular complications of diabetes refused to have her gangrenous right leg amputated as well. As in Candura, her physicians considered this decision "irrational." After a psychiatric consultation, she was placed on antidepressant medication (it was determined that she was depressed, but not incompetent) and changed her mind shortly thereafter, but before the medication was likely to have had any effect. Her "mood was clearly brighter . . . she no longer wanted to die . . . she also spoke hopefully of learning to walk with artificial limbs." See above, p. 433.

71. An example is provided by a 45-year-old man with a history of alcoholism who was admitted to the hospital the day after Christmas for gastrointestinal bleeding. He initially allowed the staff to use a nasogastric tube to lavage his stomach, but pulled it out several times and ultimately refused to have it reinserted. He also refused other procedures. The staff decided to transfer the patient, who resisted the idea and checked out against medical advice. See above, p. 446.

72. Truman v. Thomas, 27 Cal.3d 285, 611 P.2d 902, 165 Cal. Rptr. 308 (1980) (en banc).

73. See above, p. 294–95, 611 P.2d pp. 907–08, 165 Cal. Rptr. pp. 313–14.

74. See Brown, The Rationing of Hospital Care, in President's Commission for the Study of Ethical Problems in Medicine and Biomedical and Behavioral Research, 3 *Securing Access to Health Care* 253–84 (1983).

75. Quoted in Gruzalski, supra note 2, p. 174.

76. See supra notes 11–24 and accompanying text.

77. E.g., Satz v. Perlmutter, 362 So. 2d 160 (Fla. Dist. Ct. App. 1978), aff'd 379 So. 2d 359 (Fla. 1980); Foster v. Tourtellotte, Order CV 81-5046-RMT (Mx) (C.D. Cal. Nov. 16, 1981) (Takasugi, J.); *In re* Lydia E. Hall Hosp., 116 Misc. 2d 477, 455 N.Y.S. 2d 706 (Sup. Ct. 1982).

78. See, e.g., Concern for Dying, a New York-based educational organization which has distributed more than 5 million copies of the "living will" in the past 15 years. The rationale of the living will is that, with the advent of more effective medical technology, patients may have their lives prolonged painfully, expensively, fruitlessly and against their wills. By signing a prior statement, the patient hopes to avoid a technological imperative which commands that that which can be done must be done, and instead keep some control over medical treatment decisions. The organization's most recent version of the living will (Sept. 1983) is as follows:

> To My Family, My Physician, My Lawyer and All Others Whom It May Concern
>
> Death is as much a reality as birth, maturity and old age—it is the one certainty of life. If the time comes when I can no longer take part in decisions for my own future, let this statement stand as an expression of my wishes and directions, while I am still of sound mind.
>
> If at such a time the situation should arise in which there is no reasonable expectation of my recovery from extreme physical or mental disability, I direct that I be allowed to die and not be kept alive by medications, artificial means or "heroic measures." I do, however, ask that medication be mercifully administered to me to alleviate suffering even though this may shorten my remaining life.
>
> This statement is made after careful consideration and is in accordance with my strong convictions and beliefs. I want the wishes and directions here expressed carried out to the extent permitted by law. Insofar as they are not legally enforceable, I hope that those to whom this Will is addressed will regard themselves as morally bound by these provisions.
>
> Optional proxy statement: I hereby designate ___ to make treatment decisions for me in the event I am comotose or otherwise unable to make such decisions for myself.
>
> Possible additional provisions are:
>
> 1. Measures of artificial life-support in the face of impending death that I specifically refuse are:
>
> a) Electrical or mechanical resuscitation of my heart when it has stopped beating.
>
> b) Nasogastric tube feeding when I am paralyzed or unable to take nourishment by mouth.

c) Mechanical respiration when I am no longer able to sustain my own breathing.

2. I would like to live out my last days at home rather than in a hospital if it does not jeopardize the chance of my recovery to a meaningful and sentient life or does not impose an undue burden on my family.

3. If any of my tissues are sound and would be of value as transplants to other people, I freely give permission for such a donation.

79. Although specific provisions of these statutes vary, a typical statute allows patients to authorize the withholding or withdrawal of medical treatment in the event the patient becomes terminally ill. Most current "living will" statutes basically permit physicians to honor a terminally ill patient's directive not to be treated if the physician agrees that treatment is not indicated. This, of course, can be done in the absence of any statute; and the current statutes do not so much enhance patients' rights as they enhance provider rights (i.e., the physicians typically are granted immunity if they follow the provisions of the statute). See, e.g., ALA CODE §§ 22-8A-1 to 22-8A-10 (Supp. 1981); *Ark. Stat. Ann.* §§ 82-3081 to 82-3804 (Supp. 1981); *Cal. Health & Safety Code*] §§ 7185–7195 (*Deering Supp.* 1982); *D.C. Code Ann.* §§ 6-2421 to 2430 (Supp. 1982); *Del. Code Ann. tit.* 16, §§ 2501–2509 (1982); *Idaho Code* §§ 39-4501 to 39-4508 (Supp. 1982); *Kan. Stat. Ann.* §§ 65-28, 101 to 65-28, 109 (Supp. 1981); *Nev. Rev. Stat.* §§ 449.540–449.690 (1979); *N.M. Stat. Ann.* §§ 24-7-1 to 24-7-11 (1981); *N.C. Gen. Stat.* §§ 90-320 to 90-322 (1981); *Or. Rev. Stat.* §§ 97.050–97.090 (1981); *Tex. Rev. Civ. Stat. Ann.* art. 4590h §§ 1-11 (Vernon 1982); *Vt. Stat. Ann. tit.* §§ 5251–5262 (1982); *Wash. Rev. Code Ann.* §§ 70.122.010–70.122.905 (West 1982). See generally G. J. ANNAS, L. H. GLANTZ, B. F. KATZ, *The Rights of Doctors, Nurses, and Allied Health Professionals* 220–23 (1981); G. Grisez, J. M. Boyle, *Life and Death With Liberty and Justice* 223–43 (1980); KEYSERLINGK, *Sanctity of Life or Quality of Life* (1981); R. VEATCH, *Death, Dying and the Biological Revolution* 199–201 (1976); Beraldo, Give Me Liberty and Give Me Death: The Right to Die and the California Natural Death Act, 20 *Santa Clara L. Rev.* 971 (1980); Dickens, The Right to Natural Death, 26 *McGill L.J.* 847 (1981); Hand, Death with Dignity and the Terminally Ill: The Need for Legislative Action, 4 *Nova L.J.* 257 (1980); Havens, *In re* Living Will, 5 *Nova L.J.* 466 (1981); Kaplan, Euthanasia Legislation: A Survery and a Model Act, 2 *A. J. Law & Med.* 41 (1976); Kite, The Right to Die a Natural Death and the Living Will, 13 *Tex. Tech. L. Rev.* 99 (1982); Kutner, The Living Will: Coping with the Historical Event of Death, 27 *Baylor L. Rev.* 39 (1975); Kutner, Due Process of Euthanasia: The Living Will, a Proposal, 44 *Ind. L.J.* 539–54 (1969); Stephenson, The Right to Die: A Proposal for Natural Death Legislation, 49 *U. Cin. L. Rev.* 228 (1980); Walters, The Kansas Natural Death Act, 19 *Washburn L.J.* 519 (1980); Law Reform Comm of Canada, Euthanasia, Aiding Suicide and Cessation of Treatment (Working Paper 28) (1982); Yale Law School Model Bill, in *Society for the Right to Die Legislative Handbook* 23–26 (1981).

80. The Legal Advisers Committee of Concern for Dying was formed in 1980 and took on the development of a model bill as one of its first projects. In addition to the authors of this article, who are chairman & research assistant respectively, the committee consists of lawyers from across the United States and others involved in the drafting of the model bill. Members included Leonard H. Glantz (Boston U. School of Public Health); Barbara F. Katz (U. Massachusetts Medical Center); Margaret Somerville (McGill Law School); J. Dinsmore Adams (New York); C. Dickerman Williams (New York); Richard Scott (Los Angeles); Jane Greenlaw (U. of Rochester, NY); Kenneth Wing (U. No. Carolina Law School); Joseph Healey (U. Connecticut Medical School) and John Robertson (U. Texs Law School). The Committee met approximately every six months over a three year period, and their model bill was adopted by the Board of Directors of Concern for Dying in January, 1983 and published in 73 *Am. J. Pub. Health* 918 (1983).

81. President's Commission For The Study Of Ethical Problems In Medicine And Biomedical And Behavioral Reasearch, *Deciding to Forego Life-Sustaining Treatment* 148 (1983). The Commission did add, however, that they believed "[g]reater opportunity for review of determinations of incompetency and of proxy's decisions may be needed . . . to protect patients' self-determination and welfare." See above. It is our hope that this article will serve to address this concern of the Commission's.

82. The "right to die" was essentially the right Ms. Bouvia asserted in seeking a court injunction to forbid the medical staff from force feeding her while she starved herself to death in the hospital. See supra notes 6, 39, 61, and 68.

83. 1 *Making Health Care Decisions*, supra note 13, p. 159.

84. Existing durable power of attorney statutes are collected in 1 *Making Health Care Decisions*, supra note 13, pp. 155–60. Their problems are discussed in Legal Problems of the Aged and Infirm—the Durable Power of Attorney-Planned Protective Services and the Living Will, 13 *Real Property, Probate & Trust* 1 (1978). To clarify the application of the durable power of attorney to medical treatment decisions, California has recently amended its durable power of attorney statute, and it is likely that other states will follow California's lead. One would also be obligated to respect the patient's prior directive regarding the withholding of IV or nasogastric feeding under the Act. The law on withholding nutrition from an incompetent patient is currently ambiguous. See Annas, Nonfeeding: Lawful Killing in California, Homicide in New Jersey, 13 *Hastings Center Rpt.* 19 (Dec. 1983) for a discussion of the cases of *In re* Conroy, supra note 10, currently on appeal to New Jersey Supreme Court and Barber & Nejdl

v. Superior Ct., 2 Civil No. 69350, 69351 (Ct. of App. 2d Dist., Div. 2, Oct. 12, 1983) (among the issues are whether feeding, by whatever means, is properly considered a medical "treatment"). Even under the Act, prisoners would not be permitted to starve themselves to death for political or personal motives not related to their medical conditions. See Annas, Prison Hunger Strikes: Why Motive Matters, 12 *Hastings Center Rep.* 21 (Dec. 1982) for a discussion of the four cases that exist on this issue: Zant v. Prevatte, 248 Ga. 832, 286 S.E.2d 715 (1982) (right to privacy includes right of a competent prisoner to starve himself to death); Von Holden v. Chapman, 87 A.D.2d 66, 450 N.Y.S. 2d 623 (App. Div. 1982) (state has a compelling interest to prevent suicide); White v. Narick, 292 S.E. 2d 54 (W. Va. 1982) (state has a compelling interest in preserving life); and Commissioner v. Meyers, 399 N.E. 2d 452 (Mass. 1979) (state can force prisoner to obtain kidney dialysis where motivation is to manipulate his placement in the prison system because of its compelling interest in upholding orderly prison administration).

85. This may at first seem harsh, but we believe that the balance between the physician's personal ethics or the ethics of the medical profession, and the liberty interest of the patient will always be tipped by the patient's interest in being free from nonconsensual medical interventions. See, for example, the discussion of medical ethics as a "compelling state interest" by the Massachusetts Supreme Court in Belchertown State School v. Saikewicz, 373 Mass. 728, 370 N.E.2d 417 (1977), where the court concludes that honoring a patient's refusal is consistent with prevailing medical ethics, but even if it weren't: "if the doctrines of informed consent and right of privacy have as their foundations the right to bodily integrity . . . and control of one's own fate, then those rights are superior to the institutional considerations [maintenance of the ethical integrity of the medical profession]." See above, p. ___, 370 N.E.2d p. 417. Under this Act, for example, if the physicians at Riverside General Hospital could not transfer Ms. Bouvia or find a physician there who would continue caring for her without forcing feeding by I.V.'s or a nasogastric tube, they would be obligated to respect her refusals of these interventions. See supra notes 6–8 and accompanying text.

86. There is no time limit to the validity of declarations, just as there is no time limit on ordinary wills or on donations made under Uniform Anatomical Gift Acts. The primary protection regarding the wishes of a person is the requirement for two witnesses to certify that they believe the person understood what he was signing and did it voluntarily. We have not restricted the individuals who can be either witnesses or authorized persons (e.g., to exclude the attending physician or relative who might benefit under a will) because we think this unnecessarily implies bad faith on the part of categories of individuals and unnecessarily restricts the autonomy of a person to pick his own proxy

and witnesses. A second protection for the declarant is that revocation is made easy. But the intent to revoke must be specific. Merely signing a blanket hospital admissions form that "consents" to whatever treatment physicians at the hospital wish to render is insufficient indication of revocation of a declaration. While a relative may sabotage a patient's wishes, the Act relies on good faith and criminal penalties to discourage this.

87. Dr. Clark acknowledged this in a videotaped interview with his surgeon, Dr. DeVries. Dr. DeVries asked: "It's been hard for you, hasn't it Barney?" Dr. Clark replied: "Yes, its been hard, but the heart itself has pumped right along, *I think its doing well*," *N.Y. Times*, March 3, 1983, at 1, col. 8 (emphasis supplied).

Appendix
Right to Refuse Treatment Act

Section 1. Definitions
"Competent person" shall mean an individual who is able to understand and appreciate the nature and consequences of a decision to accept or refuse treatment.

"Declaration" shall mean a written statement executed according to the provisions of this Act which sets forth the declarant's intentions with respect to medical procedures, treatment or nontreatment, and may include the declarant's intentions concerning palliative care.

"Declarant" shall mean an individual who executes a declaration under the provisions of this Act.

"Health care provider" shall mean a person, facility or institution licensed or authorized to provide health care.

"Incompetent person" shall mean a person who is unable to understand and appreciate the nature and consequences of a decision to accept or refuse treatment.

"Medical procedure or treatment" shall mean any action taken by a physician or health care provider designed to diagnose, assess, or treat a disease, illness, or injury. These include, but are not limited to, surgery, drugs, transfusions, mechanical ventilation, dialysis, resuscitation, artificial feeding, and any other medical act designed for diagnosis, assessment or treatment.

"Palliative care" shall mean any measure taken by a physician or health care provider designed primarily to maintain the patient's comfort. These include, but are not limited to, sedatives and pain-killing drugs; non-artificial, oral feeding; suction; hydration; and hygienic care.

"Physician" shall mean any physician responsible for the declarant's care.

Section 2

A competent person has the right to refuse any medical procedure or treatment, and any palliative care measure.

Section 3

A competent person may execute a declaration directing the withholding or withdrawal of any medical procedure or treatment or any palliative care measure, which is in use or may be used in the future in the person's medical care or treatment, even if continuance of the medical procedure or treatment could prevent or postpone the person's death from being caused by the person's disease, illness or injury. The declaration shall be in writing, dated and signed by the declarant in the presence of two adult witnesses. The two witnesses must sign the declaration, and by their signatures indicate they believe the declarant's execution of the declaration was understanding and voluntary.

Section 4

If a person is unable to sign a declaration due to a physical impairment, the person may execute a declaration by communicating agreement after the declaration has been read to the person in the presence of the two adult witnesses. The two witnesses must sign the declaration and by their signatures indicate the person is physically impaired so as to be unable to sign the declaration, that the person understands the declaration's terms and that the person voluntarily agrees to the terms of the declaration.

Section 5

A declarant shall have the right to appoint in the declaration a person authorized to order the administration, withholding, or withdrawal of medical procedures and treatment in the event that the declarant becomes incompetent. A person so authorized shall have the power to enforce the provisions of the declaration and shall be bound to exercise this authority consistent with the declaration and the authorized person's best judgement as to the actual desires and preferences of the declarant. No palliative care measure may be withheld by an authorized person unless explicitly provided for in the declaration. Physicians and health care providers caring for incompetent declarants shall provide such authorized persons all medical information which would be available to the declarant if the declarant were competent.

Section 6

Any declarant may revoke a declaration by destroying or defacing it, executing a written revocation, making an oral revocation, or by any other act evidencing the declarant's specific intent to revoke the declaration.

Section 7

A competent person who orders the withholding or withdrawal of treatment shall receive appropriate palliative care unless it is expressly stated by the person orally or through a declaration that the person refuses palliative care.

Section 8

This act shall not impair or supersede a person's legal right to direct the withholding or withdrawal of medical treatment or procedures in any other manner recognized by law.

Section 9

No person shall require anyone to execute a declaration as a condition of enrollment, continuation, or receipt of benefits for disability, life, health or any other type of insurance. The withdrawal or withholding of medical procedures or treatment pursuant to the provisions of this Act shall not affect the validity of any insurance policy, and shall not constitute suicide.

Section 10

This Act shall create no presumption concerning the intention of a person who has failed to execute a declaration. The fact that a person has failed to execute a declaration shall not constitute evidence of that person's intent concerning treatment or nontreatment.

Section 11

A declaration made pursuant to this Act, an oral refusal by a person, or a refusal of medical procedures or treatment through an authorized person, shall be binding on all physicians and health care providers caring for the declarant.

Section 12

A physician who fails to comply with a written or oral declaration and to make necessary arrangements to transfer the declarant to another physician who will effectuate the declaration shall be subject to civil liability and professional disciplinary action, including license revocation or suspension. When acting in good faith to effectuate the terms of a declaration or when following the direction of an authorized person appointed in a declaration under Section 5, no physician or health care provider shall be liable in any civil, criminal, or administrative action for withholding or withdrawing any medical procedure, treatment, or palliative care measure. When acting in good faith, no witness to a declaration, or person authorized to make treatment decisions under Section 5, shall be liable in any civil, criminal, or administrative action.

A person found guilty of willfully concealing a declaration, or falsifying or forging a revocation of a declaration, shall be subject to criminal prosecution for a misdemeanor [the class or type of misdemeanor is left to the determination of individual state legislatures].

Any person who falsifies or forges a declaration, or who willfully conceals or withholds information concerning the revocation of a declaration, with the intent to cause a withholding or withdrawal of life-sustaining procedures from a person, and who thereby causes life-sustaining procedures to be withheld or withdrawn and death to be hastened, shall be subject to criminal prosecution for a felony [the class or type of felony is left to the determination of individual state legislatures].

If any provision or application of this Act is held invalid, this invalidity shall not affect other provisions or applications of the Act which can be given effect without the invalid provision or application, and to this end the provisions of this Act are severable.

A Summary of *Values in Conflict: Resolving Ethical Issues in Hospital Care*

Paul B. Hofmann, Emory University Hospital, Atlanta

Recognizing the importance of helping hospitals address the growing number and complexity of ethical dilemmas associated with caring for patients, the American Hospital Association's (AHA) General council established the Special Committee on Biomedical Ethics in June 1983. Among its 15 members were trustees, physicians, administrators, nurses, clergy, and a health care journalist. Legal counsel was provided by AHA staff as well as an adjunct legal task force.

The Committee was given two years to complete its charge: to identify the major biomedical ethical issues facing hospitals and to formulate guidelines to assist hospitals in developing institutional policies and processes for decision making on these issues.

Responding to a sense of urgency, the committee prepared and the Association approved and distributed two documents prior to publication of its report. Hospitals throughout the country received guidelines on the organization, composition, and function of ethics committees in March 1984 and a policy on the patient's choice of treatment options in March 1985.

Values in Conflict: Resolving Ethical Issues in Hospital Care, the committee's complete report, was published in July 1985. This chapter will focus on the major findings and recommendations of the report.

Overview

Given the diversity of the nation's hospitals (their size, location, mission, and ownership), the committee concluded that it would be unwise and presumptuous to create a set of bioethical recipes. Instead, it attempted to develop basic principles and guidelines to serve as a foundation for institutional policies and procedures reflecting the unique characteristics of each institution. The report stresses three major objectives of these policies.

First, these policies should be the basis for educational programs to assist health care professionals in resolving value conflicts. Second, hospital policies and practices should clearly acknowledge the patient's responsibility for decision making and, in addition to supporting the patients' fundamental right of self-determination, should support appropriate roles for their families and hospital staff. Third, and perhaps most important, policies should facilitate the resolution of dilemmas at the level closest to the pa-

Mr. Hofmann is the chairman, American Hospital Association Special Committee on Biomedical Ethics.

tient, at the lowest cost, and ordinarily without resort to the courts. Although particularly difficult cases might require judicial intervention, the committee recommended that policies identify the types of issues that may require legal counsel.

Making Patient Care Decisions

The rights of patients to influence decisions affecting their care was the central theme dominating committee discussion of informed consent, patient decision-making capacity, treatment selection, and do-not-resuscitate decisions. The report stressed the importance of collaborative decision making between the patient and the physician. In addition, because a hospital setting can intimidate patients and illness or injury frequently compromises decision-making capacity, the report urges hospitals to develop policies and practices to compensate for these factors.

Informed Consent

The committee was concerned that informed consent often is viewed simplistically as a signature on a standard form. Proper informed consent should represent the patient's voluntary decision based on an understanding of the proposed action and its benefits, risks, and alternatives; therefore, hospital policy should encourage discussion about the purposes and consequences of both routine and special procedures. Hospital staff should realize that many procedures that they view as "routine" are not recognized as such by the patient.

Hospitals share three specific responsibilities with their medical staffs in regard to informed consent. First, they are accountable for ensuring that proper informed consent has been obtained for diagnostic and therapeutic procedures. Second, they should facilitate educational programs to reinforce the necessity of obtaining valid consents. Third, they must ensure that patients are aware of their right to request additional information and/or to reject proposed procedures.

Patient Decision-Making Capacity

In most cases, there is little doubt about the patient's capacity to make a valid decision. In others, it is not always clear when a patient's physical condition, emotional status, intelligence, or legal standing may affect decision-making capacity.

The committee concentrated on the definition and assessment of capacity, barriers to capacity, and steps to be considered in cases of in-capacity. Decision-making capacity was defined as the patient's ability to make choices that reflect an understanding and appreciation of the nature and consequences of one's actions and of alternative actions, and to evaluate them in relation to personal preferences and priorities. A critical distinction was made between *decision-making* capacity and the legal term *competency*. The committee observed that a minor, who is legally not competent, may have considerable decision-making capacity, and a temporarily impaired adult who has not been declared incompetent may lack the ability to make an informed decision. The committee also distinguished between a patient's capacity to make some decisions versus all decisions. Even patients with limited capacity should be permitted and encouraged to make decisions regarding menu selection and other relatively routine issues. Allowing the patient to make as many of these decisions as possible demonstrates respect for the patient and increases the patient's sense of autonomy.

Although recognizing that the attending physician is principally responsible for assessing decision-making capacity, the committee believed that other members of the health care team as well as the patient's family and friends may provide information and observations useful in evaluating the patient's ability to make appropriate decisions. In case of strong disagreement or doubt about a patient's capacity, a psychiatric consultation may be helpful or necessary. Such consultation may also be required to obtain a formal judgment of incompetence. The committee, concerned about the possibility of both premature and extended assumptions of incapacity, recommended that decisions be reviewed as the patient's condition changes.

The committee urged that hospitals be aware of common barriers to patient decision-making capacity, such as various language and hearing difficulties. Hospitals have a responsibility to assist in making interpreters available, and physicians should remain sensitive to the temporary effects of medications and the different stages of a patient's illness. The use of chemical restraints, described later in the report, also can influence the patient's ability to make an informed decision.

In cases of incapacity, the committee urged that every effort be made to protect the patient's interests through surrogate decision making. Usually the choice of an appropriate surrogate is obvious, but the primary qualifications are that the person knows the patient best, has been a close confidant, and can represent the patient's best interests. Information from living wills, durable powers of attorney, previous communications, and lifestyle preferences may provide information regarding what the patient would have decided before becoming incapacitated. With reference to assessment of competency and/or appointment of a legal guardian, the most common circumstances that suggest the need for such action are: "(1)the incapacity is [of the patient] great and likely to be prolonged, and there is no obvious surrogate; (2)the capacity of the patient is questionable, and the decision to be made is significant; (3)the views of the surrogate are strongly at variance with medical judgment or the patient's known views; or (4)the choice of the individual to serve as surrogate is controversial and all efforts to resolve the matter at the hospital level have failed; and (5)family members radically disagree about the course of action in the case of a patient who lacks adequate decision-making capacity."

The Decision to Refuse Treatment

The right of the patient to refuse specific treatment or all treatment is generally recognized and upheld by both state legislation and the courts. The committee believed that hospitals should permit patients with decision-making capacity to exercise this right within the context of the institution's mission and society's role in preserving the ethical integrity of the health care system and health care professionals.

A refusal certain to cause the patient's death raises obvious ethical issues. The hospital must consider not only the patient's views, but also legal requirements and ramifications, the perspectives of those involved in caring for the patient, and the hospital's mission. When these factors cannot be reconciled, patients who have asked that life-sustaining treatment be withheld or discontinued may be placed in an adversarial role with the hospital and the physician. The committee recommended that recourse to judicial intervention should be reserved for when the patient, or surrogate if the patient is comatose or otherwise mentally incapacitated, prefers court procedures or the issues resist resolution at a less formal level.

Do-Not-Resuscitate Decisions

Do-not-resuscitate (DNR) decisions are usually made when a resuscitation effort appears inap-

propriate in terms of the patient's overall condition and personal values. In the absence of a specific directive not to resuscitate, normal resuscitation procedures should be initiated. Committee members unanimously agreed that all hospitals should have policies addressing when, how, and by whom DNR decisions should be made and documented.

If the patient is capable of making a decision, a DNR order should result only from collaborative and consensual decision making. Furthermore, if a patient does not agree to a proposed DNR order, it should not be written, even if a previous preference for no resuscitation efforts was expressed.

If the patient is incapacitated, advance directives such as living wills and previous communications with physicians, family members, or friends can serve as a proxy for the patient's preference. In case of disagreement between an appropriate surrogate and the physician, the committee suggested that mechanisms for institutional review, such as an ethics committee, should be available.

DNR decisions should be recorded as formal orders by attending physicians. In addition, the medical record should document discussions with the patient (or surrogate), family members, and health care professionals caring for the patient, as well as the relevant data contributing to the DNR decision. Hospitals should have procedures to ensure that DNR orders are regularly reviewed. The institution should also determine whether housestaff or nursing personnel may refuse to cooperate with such orders and, if so, how they can exercise this option in an acceptable manner.

Caring For Patients

The committee agreed that interactions on virtually every level among and between hospital employees, physicians, patients, and their families have ethical dimensions. The report's second major section highlighted a number of representative ethical issues associated with caring for patients. These included maintaining confidentiality, using restraints, providing continuity of care, disclosing errors and negative outcomes, identifying problems of professional competence, establishing ethics committees, and protecting the moral prerogatives of the health care institution and health care professionals.

Confidentiality

Patients have the right to expect that all communications and records pertaining to their care will be treated as confidential. Despite this widely accepted principle, changes in the hospital environment, including new laws and regulations and activities of third-party payers, are affecting the range and type of information considered confidential. The committee concluded that hospitals should maintain policies that protect and support a climate conducive to confidentiality. For example, the use of patient information in education and research should be addressed, and hospital policy should emphasize that subsidization of the patient's care by public funds must not be allowed to reduce either an individual or organizational commitment to preserving confidentiality.

Hospital policy should also reflect the institution's position on other key elements of this issue, including the right of patients to have access to their records, except as restricted by state law. In addition, it is essential that conditions be noted when the right of confidentiality may be overridden, for example, when the patient's life or safety is endangered, when substantial and foreseeable harm to a third party can be prevented, when the interests or rights of the public are jeopardized, or when there is a legal obligation to report certain communicable diseases, injuries or other conditions.

Restraints on Patients

The use of physical or chemical restraints requires a judgment that weighs the risks to the patient or others against the obligation to respect the patient's right of autonomy and self-determination. Although the committee was aware that this topic was prominently covered in discussions of psychiatric services, several members expressed concern that restraints may often be applied prematurely or inappropriately in general hospitals.

Because the potential for abuse of restraints is great, the report urges hospitals to develop policies that describe the proper use of safety vests, wrist, and other physical restraints, and chemical restraints such as tranquilizers. The committee also recommended that a hospital's policy should indicate who is entitled to authorize restraints.

The policy should also provide guidance on: documentation of the types of patient behavior requiring restraints; appropriate communication with the patient and the patient's family about the need for restraints; documentation of this discussion in the medical record; proper fitting of a physical restraint or titration of a chemical restraint to minimize the risk of harm to the patient; and the frequency with which physical restraints should be checked and chemical restraints reassessed to ensure maximum patient safety, comfort, and freedom.

Continuity of Care

The hospital is seldom in a position, either in terms of mission or finances, to meet the community's entire spectrum of health care needs. However, the committee believed that the institution has a moral obligation to facilitate continuity of care for patients upon discharge. If a hospital cannot provide a needed service because of resource limitations, it should work with community agencies and other organizations to help facilitate its provision.

With the continued deemphasis of expensive inpatient services, there should be greater incentives to coordinate ambulatory services, home health care, hospice programs, and a wide range of similar activities. In many communities, citizens will expect the hospital to exercise a leadership role. A failure to take the initiative or to respond to the challenge could compromise the hospital's reputation for being sensitive to the health needs of its service area population.

Medical Errors and Negative Outcomes

Health care professionals realize that some medical errors and negative outcomes are inevitable, but a hospital's response in such situations has significant ethical ramifications. Diagnostic and treatment errors, nosocomial infections, unanticipated complications, and adverse results must certainly be minimized. When they do occur, however, full and timely disclosure should be the standard response. The committee concluded that partial or nondisclosure, allegedly to serve the patient's or the family's best interest, is rarely defensible. Delays or attempts to hide the truth are neither morally nor legally acceptable alternatives.

Provider Competence

The committee drew an important distinction between unfortunate mistakes and patterns of care that suggest incompetent, illegal, or unethical behavior. Every hospital has a moral and legal responsibility to ensure that its employees and physicians provide care that meets acceptable standards. Therefore, each institution should have clearly defined, publicized, and convenient mechanisms for receiving, investigating, and acting on allegations of impropriety. These mechanisms (for example, patient representatives, ombudsmen, social workers, chaplains, and administrators) should be accessible to patients, their families, and friends, as well as to physicians, employees, and volunteers. Creating an atmosphere conducive to proper disclosure can be achieved if the hospital's efforts are thorough, confidential, and provide for timely investigation and corrective action.

Ethics Committees

Although hospital ethics committees are not new, the report of the President's Commission for the Study of Ethical Problems in Medicine and Biomedical and Behavioral Research and the "Baby Doe" regulations have stimulated legitimate interest in their role and potential value. Consequently, the committee developed *Guidlines on Hospital Committees on Biomedical Ethics*, which were distributed to all AHA institutional members in March 1984, following approval by the AHA General Council. The document notes that ethics committees can serve a variety of useful functions, but they should not assume decision-making authority. By serving in an advisory capacity, facilitating educational programs on biomedical ethical issues, and accepting similar duties, an ethics committee can make a significant contribution to enhancing a hospital's sensitivity to the ethical dilemmas confronting its many constituencies. Size, composition, access to the committee, its place in the hospital's organizational structure, and frequency of meetings will vary from one institution to another. Ethics committees have limitations, and they should not be viewed as a panacea. If carefully planned, however, an ethics committee can become an invaluable resource to both sectarian and nonsectarian hospitals.

Moral Prerogatives in Deciding on Services

Every hospital must make decisions on the range of services it will provide. These decisions are usually based upon the community's perceived need for a service, its compatibility with the hospital's mission, the service's availability elsewhere, the hospital's ability to provide the service, and the hospital's financial viability. The hospital's moral prerogative to remain solvent makes economics a legitimate consideration. In exercising this prerogative, the committee recommended that hospitals develop mechanisms to subsidize unprofitable but necessary services.

The personal values of a health care professional may conflict occasionally with those of colleagues or patients. To the extent possible, a hospital should accommodate employees who object to participating in certain procedures by arranging for other personnel to substitute. However, depending upon staff resources, such an arrangement may not always be practical. In this situation, the patient's needs must receive the highest priority. Hospitals should encourage employees to inform their supervisors of moral convictions that may affect their performance. The committee also recommended that support be provided to staff to help them cope with the emotional stress of dealing with difficult ethical issues.

Service Mix

Rising consumer expectations and the rapid development of new medical knowledge are colliding with pressures to contain health care costs. In the absence of a national health policy, hospitals are left with an implicit responsibility to establish guidelines on service mix, use of new technology, and organ transplantation. Therefore, informal rationing can and does occur. The committee believed that all of these issues have complex ethical implications for hospitals.

Determination of service mix has become a more vital undertaking as the result of an increasingly competitive marketplace for health care in general and hospitals in particular. Compromises and trade-offs will be necessary. Some decisions may create confusion, anxiety, or anger if they are not communicated effectively to employees, physicians, and the community. The committee noted that to continue services without regard for their impact on revenue and expenses would be fiscally irresponsible; to pursue business practices without regard for service access and outcomes would be morally reprehensible. Trustees, medical staffs, and administrators should be held accountable for reconciling such dilemmas.

New Technology

Decisions regarding the acquisition of new technology should not be made exclusively on economic merits. Because many technological advances in medical care increase rather than decrease costs, other factors should be considered. The committee believed that technology's influence on existing services, other facilities in the community, the number of potential beneficiaries, personnel and space requirements, and competing capital requirements are among the issues that should be evaluated systematically.

Objective analysis can be difficult when funds are contributed and strong opinions are expressed by influential individuals. In addition, operating costs as well as other consequences frequently are disregarded or underestimated when technology is acquired primarily for the prestige that it allegedly brings to the institution. The committee cautioned hospitals to approach decisions about new technology with a full appreciation of their impact on the institution, its staff, and the community in relation to noneconomic issues, including ethical issues.

Organ Transplantation

Although most hospitals are not involved in organ transplantation activity, the number of transplant programs is increasing as a result of the introduction of new surgical techniques, better tissue matching, and the availability of new immunosuppressive drugs. The committee suggested that hospitals should rely essentially on the same principles as for acquisition of other innovative technology, with some significant additional considerations. Often, resource consumption associated with transplant procedures exceeds initial assumptions. Similarly, acquisition of organs is usually much more difficult than is anticipated. The most obvious ethical challenge is posed by a pool of transplant candidates that is almost always greater that the number of acceptable donor organs.

Rationing of Services

As mentioned previously, inconsistent rationing of services is a current reality. However, as most rationing is informal and implicit, ethical ramifications are largely ignored. Limiting the number of medically indigent patients served, allocating intensive care beds, and restricting specific services for various reasons are usually the rule, not the exception. The committee realized that rationing was likely to become more prevalent.

To the extent possible, hospital leadership should acknowledge the existence of rationing so that its ethical dimensions can be better understood and addressed by the hospital.

Conclusion

The last chapter of the committee's report briefly describes several challenges that confront hospitals now and will intensify in the future. Some primarily institutional challenges include the reevaluation of hospital missions, cooperating with competitors, ethically sound advertising, the provision of cost-efficient services, assuring appropriate services for the elderly, and the reallocation of resources for research, teaching, and patient care. Other challenges raise fundamental health policy questions. How should access to health care be assured and who should pay for it? How can society be assured that advances in medical science and research will be applied wisely? When does prolongation of life become prolongation of dying? What are the implications of a shift from publicly funded to privately funded scientific research? What responsibility should individuals have for the consequences of their harmful lifestyle decisions? How much of funding should be allocated for health care as opposed to other essential needs? What amount of total health care dollars should be expended on research and prevention as opposed to direct patient care?

Noting that none of these questions could be easily answered, the committee emphasized that differing values inherent in treatment and other health care decisions demand continuing attention. A glossary, bibliography, case studies, and other resource material were included in the report's appendixes to assist hospitals in pursuing topics of special interest.

Not all bioethical dilemmas can be predicted with confidence, and most will be characterized by uncertainty, ambiguity, tension, and conflict. Through judicious use of the committee's report, it is hoped that hospitals will become more effective in creating an environment in which ethical issues in patient care can be met in a compassionate and morally responsible manner that is sensitive to the needs of patients, their families, and health professionals.

Legal Perspectives on Institutional Ethics Committees

Alexander M. Capron, LL.B., Department of Law, University of Southern California, Los Angeles

There are several ways to gain a legal perspective on the subject of hospital or, more generally, institutional ethics committees. I intend to pursue two of them: first by looking at the law *and* ethics committees, and then by turning to the law *of* ethics committees.

I. The Law *and* Ethics Committees

To understand something about the relationship of the law to ethics committees, one might well begin by examining the context in which attention to ethics committees arises. After exploring this context—or, one might say, the legal need for committees—I will examine the specific legal impetus for the current interest in ethics committees.

A. The Legal Context of Ethics Committees

Plainly, ethical questions are not new to medical practice or to health care institutions. Moreover, for some years already, institutions have turned to special committees for aid in setting ethical standards and in resolving problems as they arise. In fact, while the President's Commission, as part of its study on *Deciding to Forego Life-Sustaining Care,* found that only 1 percent of all hospitals in the United States—and only 4.3 percent of those with 200 or more beds—reported having ethics committees,[1] a much larger percent of Catholic hospitals have long had committees charged with considering ethical matters.[2] These groups have usually concerned themselves with questions that are of particular interest to these religious institutions, such as whether it is permissible for non-Catholic physicians practicing in the hospital to perform sterilizations, and so forth.

When the term "hospital ethics committee" is used today, however, it has a different meaning. The present concern arises from a realization that an increasing number of hard choices are occurring in the care of very sick and dying patients, from the newborn nursery to the geriatric nursing home. The hope is that we will find some means of making those choices that better protects all the interests at stake, particularly those of vulnerable patients.

Reprinted with permission from the author and the *Journal of College and University Law* Spring. 11(4):417–431.
Adapted from a presentation made by Professor Capron to a Statewide Conference on Hospital Ethics Committees, sponsored by West Virginia Hospitals, Inc., on September 15, 1984.

The interests involved in these choices might seem a more appropriate topic for philosophers and physicians, but I do not believe that a discussion of law would be fruitful without also attending to the value questions involved. The reason that this area of medical care has become so complex is that there is no simple way to resolve the tension between several ethical precepts—respect for personal autonomy and protection of human life—which are fundamental in our society and important for lawmakers and interpreters.[3] Moreover, given the many different people whose interests are implicated in any particular decision about life-sustaining treatment, it often requires a three-dimensional matrix, and not a mere two-dimensional grid, just to describe the interrelationship of even the autonomy and life-protection values, to say nothing of the other values implicated, which involve familial solidarity, professional goals, and institutional integrity and solvency. Thus, the legal context of ethics committees today must include a recognition that no simple formula can be substituted for the process of choice, and that any individual or group participating in that process has to be able to respond appropriately to ambiguity and conflict.

A decade ago, the intensive care unit—with its ability to prolong functioning in comatose patients who were dependent on the respirator—surfaced in public consciousness as the locus of some very difficult ethical questions. Some of those issues were resolved as society came to accept the conclusion at which medicine had already arrived, namely that certain patients—those lacking all functions of the entire brain, including the brain stem—were dead and could therefore be removed from respirator support.[4]

Yet the adoption of statutes incorporating a modern "definition" of death resolved only the easiest cases—those of bodies that could be maintained on a respirator for just a brief period even with the most intensive support. This left the more difficult cases, in which medical intervention could keep a patient just short of death for an indefinite period—with no real prospect of ever recovering. Such cases raised a host of issues. The law has done a fairly adequate job of addressing a few of these issues, principally those that call for a procedural response. For example, cases and statutes have made it possible for people to determine who will act as their surrogates if they become incapable of deciding about their own medical care;[5] the law has also clarified what should happen when an incompetent patient has not appointed someone to act on his or her behalf.[6]

On substantive issues, however, the law has been—and in my view is likely to go on being—less helpful. Of course, some of the most important issues remaining are capable of being addressed in procedural terms. Thus, in response to the question "what objectives should a surrogate seek in making decisions about an incompetent patient's medical care?", the courts have replied that when a formerly competent patient's wishes are known, the surrogate should apply a "substitute judgment" standard, under which the surrogate would be guided generally by the patient's values and preferences and specifically by any explicit instructions from the patient about the types of care he or she wanted or rejected, in the context of various possible treatment outcomes; when the patient's preferences are unknown or unknowable (as with a child or some retarded adults), the surrogate should use the more objective "best interests" standard.[7]

Nonetheless, certain more basic questions about what care is required, and which interventions may be foregone, have not been resolved. The *Quinlan* case confronted that issue, but in the end did not fully resolve it.[8] Joseph Quinlan had petitioned to be appointed his comatose daughter's guardian for the purpose of consenting to the withdrawal of *all* treatment. By the time the New Jersey Supreme Court granted permission, the focus had shifted to removal of the respirator, on the assumption (not shared by some of the consulting neurologists) that this would lead to Karen's death. Now, however, when asked whether he would tell the physicians to remove the tubes that have supplied Karen with food for the past nine years, Mr. Quinlan replies with a simple, almost shocked reaction that that is her nourishment.

It is precisely this issue of artificial feeding that illustrates both the moral and human perplexity of the choices involved and the need for new processes and devices to aid in the making of these choices. Recently, in reviewing treatment decisions about seriously ill patients, appellate courts in California and Massachusetts and the New Jersey Supreme Court ruled that artificial feeding may be classified as a medical procedure (rather than always as ordinary care that should be provided to patients) and as such may be withdrawn when the burdens it imposes (especially for incurable, unconscious patients) outweigh its benefits.

The first two intermediate state appellate courts that addressed this issue had initially reached opposite results. In quashing the murder indictment of Drs. Neil Barber and Robert Nejdl for having ordered the withdrawal of the lines that supplied food and water to a patient who had been comatose for five days after surgery, a California Court of Appeals held that the artificial provision of nutrition should be treated like any other form of medical treatment.[9] Hence, the court held, when the benefits it provides for the patient are not proportionate to the burdens imposed, artificial feeding may be withdrawn on the instructions of the patient's surrogate decisionmakers (in this case, the wife and children of Clarence Herbert).

The second opinion in 1983 was issued by the Appellate Division of the New Jersey Supreme Court. It reversed an order permitting the removal of a nasogastric tube from an 84-year-old patient, Claire Conroy.[10] Suffering from severe organic brain syndrome, gangrene, arteriosclerotic heart disease, hypertension, diabetes mellitus, necrotic decubitus ulcers, and urinary tract infection, she lay in a fetal position, moaning but unable to speak, and weighing less than 50 pounds. The appellate court's conclusion that feeding remains obligatory for patients who are short of permanent unconsciousness was reversed in January 1985. The state's highest court held that there is no valid distinction between stopping treatment and not starting it and that when an existing treatment, including artificial feeding is declined by a patient or, in the case of an incompetent patient, is too burdensome and not curative, it may be withdrawn.[11]

In the meantime, in June 1984, the Massachusetts Appeals Court issued an opinion in the third case,[12] on which the Supreme Judicial Court had declined to take further action, that goes even further than the *Barber* case in California in authorizing the removal of artificial nutrition. Like the New Jersey decision in *Conroy,* the case arose in the context of a petition for advance determination of the right course of a guardian to follow, rather than after-the-fact in a criminal prosecution, and the patient was severely confused but not comatose. The Massachusetts physicians (like those caring for the patient in the California case) took the position that further artificial feeding was inappropriate; this serves as a reminder that court proceedings—which rest on the expectation of true adversariness—may not function well in the context of some institution decisions about death-and-dying. Moreover, another factor in the legal background of ethics committees emerged in the Massachusetts case: it involved the appointment of a stranger-guardian rather than a familiar-guardian (such as Mr. Herbert's family or Miss Conroy's nephew, Thomas Whittemore). Thus, the guardian and the court were faced with the task of discerning what was best for the 92-year-old patient with severe mental illness, without the benefit of long acquaintance or a reliable expression of her personal views while still competent.

At the time of the Massachusetts litigation, the patient, Mary Hier, had had a gastrostomy tube surgically implanted in her abdomen for ten years because she was unable to ingest food orally. Over that time she had repeatedly pulled out the tube. Sometimes it could be reinserted through the old entrance hole (or stoma); other times, open abdominal surgery was needed to insert it anew. Her current admission to the hospital arose when the physician at her nursing home was unable to reinsert the tube through the stoma after she pulled it out several times in the prior week. She was sustained through intravenous feeding, which is useful only for a limited time and "mainly for hydration rather than as a source of an adequate and balanced diet."[13]

The physicians (and, in turn, the guardian and the judge) considered six ways of feeding Mrs. Hier, but concluded that only surgery to reinsert the gastrostomy tube was feasible. Although such an operation is routinely successful, with less than 5% mortality, in Mrs. Hier's case the court found the complications "considerable," the chances of success "somewhat questionable," and the risk of mortality "somewhat higher" (perhaps 20 percent or more),[14] so that most of her physicians were against it.

The trial court had found that Mrs. Hier would forego the surgery if she were competent to choose. The basis for this conclusion seems highly problematic because it was based on the "substituted judgment" standard, although most courts and commentators would limit the standard to situations when a patient's competent wishes can be ascertained. Plainly, in this case, such a determination was not possible because Mrs. Hier had been a highly confused mental patient for many years. The people trying to decide for Mary Hier were at least in a better position than those who had earlier been faced with the question whether to put Joseph Saikewicz, a sixty-seven-year-old mentally retarded resident of a state institution through a course of cancer che-motherapy.[15] In Mrs. Heir's case, her reaction to the feeding tubes was known, while for Joseph Saikewicz, it was hypothetical.

These three cases, on the cutting edge of life-and-death decision making in health care insti-tutions, are important in the present context as reminders of three things. The cases illustrate just how difficult the decisions that have to be made are, especially when they concern the care of el-derly and demented patients without immediate relatives or other surrogate decision makers who are certain about their views on life-prolonging treatment. Second, as stated by all the courts, these are decisions that should not—and cannot fea-sibly—become matters for routine judicial in-volvement; indeed, the delays and vagaries in these decisions shows how problematic it would be to rely primarily on the courts to decide about treatment terminations. And thus, third, the cases show the need for means closer to the actual lo-cus of decision making within the institution if the quality and appropriateness of the decisions are to be improved.

B. The Legal Impetus for Ethics Committees

Treatment situations (and their legal fall-out) of the type just described provide the legal *context* of institutional ethics committees. I turn now to the second aspect of the law *and* ethics commit-tees—namely, the legal *impetus* for these com-mittees.

The first explicit legal push toward the adop-tion of ethics committees came eight years ago in the *Quinlan* decision. Drawing on a very sketchy idea in a law review article by a physician,[16] the New Jersey Supreme Court stated that treatment could be withdrawn from Karen Quinlan, and other patients in comparable condition, if that was the wish of the guardian, acting on the advice of the treating physician that there was "no reason-able possibility of [the patient] ever emerging . . . to a cognitive, sapient state,"[17] provided that a "hospital ethics committee" concurred with this conclusion. Although it prescribed that the com-mittee should be multidisciplinary, the court ac-tually assigned it only the medical function of confirming Karen Quinlan's prognosis. Most commentators have concluded that the court was confused in creating a "prognosis committee" with nonmedical members.[18] It may be that, having itself performed the extra-medical task of weigh-ing the propriety of Mr. Quinlan's request, the

court found that the only remaining task *in the particular case before it* was to confirm Miss Quin-lan's current prognosis, while firmly intending in future cases for multidisciplinary ethics commit-tees to take on "multidisciplinary" sorts of tasks, not limited to prognosis.[19] At the least, one can say that having given dramatic legal impetus to the notion of ethics committees, the New Jersey Supreme Court also created a good deal of con-fusion about the appropriate scope of activities for such committees.

Although seminal, the *Quinlan* decision ac-tually did not start a bandwagon rolling for eth-ics committees; there was no rush to start the committees between 1976 and 1983. Indeed, sev-eral courts, such as those in Massachusetts[20] and Washington,[21] explicitly disapproved of multidis-ciplinary ethics committees as part of the deci-sion making process. A much more explicit im-petus for hospitals to adopt ethics committees came in the wake of the famous 1982 Indiana case of *Infant Doe*. In that case, the Indiana Su-preme Court let stand a trial court decision per-mitting parents of a child with Down Syndrome to withhold the surgery the baby needed to cor-rect an intestinal blockage. The criticism of that outcome led the federal government to issue a series of directives and regulations, under Sec-tion 504 of the 1973 Rehabilitation Act, that pro-vided for means of investigating allegations of wrongful withholding of life-sustaining treat-ment to children born with handicaps.[22] A hos-pital found to have acquiesced in such a decision by a guardian could have all its federal fund-ing—including reimbursement for patients cov-ered by Medicare—cut off.

When the White House decided that the no-tices sent to hospitals in the wake of the Indiana decision were not sufficient to accomplish its ob-jectives, it ordered the Office of Civil Rights in the Department of Health and Human Services to issue explicit regulations in March 1983, which not only set forth the requirements about treat-ment but also established a 24-hour toll-free "hot line" on which complaints could be made, which would result in the dispatch of what came to be known as "Baby Doe squads" to review on-going treatment decisions in individual cases.[23] Shortly after these "interim final regulations" were is-sued, the American Academy of Pediatrics and other plaintiffs succeeded in having the United States District Court for the District of Columbia enjoin their enforcement, basically on the ground that the regulations had been issued without adequate notice and opportunity for comment, as specified by the Administrative Procedure Act.[24]

Rather than trying to reverse this decision, the Department reissued the regulations and asked for comments, specifically drawing commentators' attention to the recommendations of the President's Commission in its report on *Deciding to Forego Life-Sustaining Treatment.*[25] Among the recommendations in that report that drew particular attention was the Commission's suggestion that institutional ethics committees would provide better protection for patients' interests than federal intervention or even routine judicial review, especially when a decision is made not to provide life-sustaining care to a seriously ill newborn. In its comments, the American Academy of Pediatrics recommended that the Baby Doe hotline and squads be replaced by a requirement that the governing body of each hospital that provides care to children appoint an "infant bioethical review committee," or join with other hospitals in establishing joint committees.

In issuing its second, revised set of regulations at the beginning of 1984,[26] HHS retained the Baby Doe apparatus (despite the fact that an objective observer could easily conclude that the hot-line and squads have done more harm than good). But it also recommended that hospitals appoint what is called "Infant Care Review Committees." To encourage this step, HHS offered some carrots—and an apparent threatened stick for those who did not comply. The rules allowed hospitals with such a committee to list it on the notices posted in hospitals (before the phone numbers for the governmental agencies) as the first contact for complaints, and they also suggested that government investigators would pay greater deference to decisions that had been approved by such committees than those that had not.

As a result of litigation that swirled around the care of another handicapped baby born in October 1983 on Long Island—known in court papers as "Baby Jane Doe"—the continuing validity of the second set of Baby Doe regulations is also not in doubt. The United States Court of Appeals has ruled that the federal government's request to see Baby Jane's medical records is invalid because the regulations go beyond the scope of the 1973 Rehabilitation Act,[27] and the AMA has launched a suit—successful thus far at the trial court level—to enjoin the enforcement of the regulations.[28] Further controversy now attends the Child Abuse Act amendments and the regulations proposed thereunder, which are discussed elsewhere in this.

Nevertheless, the whole process has brought ethics committees to the forefront of discussion of these difficult issues of life-and-death. Most notably, the idea of ethics committees is now endorsed by many leaders in the medical community, in sharp contrast to the situation only a few years ago when the sentiment was strongly against such bodies.[29]

II. The Law *Of* Ethics Committees

As I said at the outset, I want to explore a second legal perspective as well—namely, the law *of* ethics committees. As should already be apparent, there are no detailed legal regulations or court decisions that control the operation of such bodies. The roles and functions of such committees have been described elsewhere, and are usually said to include education, guideline-writing, and case review.[30] Depending upon one's view of the current functions for institutional ethics committees, one will reach varying conclusions about several points with legal overtones:

1. Membership
2. Appointment and removal
3. Powers of the committee
4. Timing of committee action
5. Responsibility and liability
6. Record-keeping

A. Categories and Role of Members

The first issue is "Who's on the committee?" HHS regulations suggest a specific makeup for an ICRC. The next step may well follow the path of Institutional Review Boards [IRBs], which also grew out of federal guidelines in the mid-1960s for recipients of federal funds.[31] Now those have been transformed into detailed regulations that specify IRB membership, though the relationale behind the requirement of a diverse membership of eight or more people is not well articulated.[32] Anyone who knows anything about small group behavior knows that a committee made up of seven or eight people, only one of whom is in any sense an "outsider," is in effect an "inside" committee, except in rare cases when the one member from outside the institution is by chance such a dominant personality that all seven will yield whatever their views are.

Likewise, in terms of the professional makeup of an ICRC the dominance of health care professionals is still very pronounced. Is that a problem in any way? We would know the answer to that question only if we knew the philosophy that lies behind a multidisciplinary or multiconstituency committee. Is it, indeed, a committee that is intended to be "representative?" And if so, of whom? A particular community may sense that its views on treatment diverge from those of physicians and other decision makers at the hospital. That may be an illusion or it may be a view held by only a small number of people in the community; it appears, however, to have been an impetus to put noninstitutional people on ethics committees. It then becomes very important to ask: on what basis are those people to be chosen? Indeed, as to *all* members on the committee, one needs to know whether they should represent certain views or attempt to work as a committee and come up with an amalgam view, some new consensus. I do not think that the question has been answered by the Baby Doe II regulations or by the proposed child abuse regulations. Yet this is a question that every institution must answer for itself if it is not simply going to respond in a reflexive fashion that a multidisciplinary committee is, for self-evident reasons, the preferable format.

B. Appointment and Removal

Second, who should have what authority to appoint and remove ethics committee members? And, indeed, does the appointment involve only the members or does it include designating a chairman? Plainly, the latter question takes on considerable importance if, as is likely to be the case, the chairman is given specific powers (such as screening cases and negotiating with administrators) beyond those held by all the members.

Additionally, institutions must decide whether appointment to the committee will be for a particular term of service, and what will be the grounds for removal? This is also an issue that IRBs faced in particular cases, often with very little advance preparation. For IRBs, lack of explicit foresight to this question has resulted in certain disgruntled parties suggesting that abuses occurred in the committee process, giving at least the appearance of manipulation when the committee did not cooperate in the way the institution wanted.

Authority and independence are issues about which one must be very sensitive in writing the charter of an ethics committee. Some institutions have what they call an ethics committee which in reality is merely a panel of consultants—often the "wise heads" of the institution who have long demonstrated an interest in ethical dilemmas and who are willing to consult with others about them. Do such people have any real authority? What if their views are distasteful to the powers-that-be in the institution? It may also be important for legal and administrative reasons to know whether a particular committee is one appointed by the board or by the medical staff. To whom does the committee report? For a variety of reasons—including indicating the seriousness of the subject for the institution—there are good reasons for having the committee be a creature of the board, though there are some pragmatic reasons (as described below) for lodging the committee with the medical staff.

C. Committee's Powers

Third, what powers does the committee have? People frequently assert that an ethics committee should be "advisory." But if so, advice given to whom and with what effect? Does the advice go to the medical staff as a whole, to the particular attending physician who is caring for the patient, or to the patient and family?

When a committee is not facing difficult cases that cause a great deal of controversy, it may be that committee powers will not be a major issue; they will give advice to whomever seeks their advice and leave it at that. What happens, however, if members of the committee disagree with each other? Would there be a vote to determine the committee's collective judgment? Some people doubt that it is appropriate for the committee to search for general consensus rather than simply being a forum for ideas to be discussed and all options to be laid on the table. Yet without some sense that an entire ethics committee is going to come to a conclusion as a group on the case it is involved in, it seems strained even to use the word "committee" to describe it, rather than a "panel of independent consultants" or perhaps a "seminar of ethical educators." To call it a committee suggests that the group will come to some kind of closure on the issues that it addresses.

Yet along with closure on a decision comes responsibility, which raises another issue about disagreements. Suppose the committee (or even certain members of the committee) disagrees with others in the decision making process, particularly the family and physicians? In many contexts the law will be looking over the shoulder of the committee, not only the federal law with the threat of intervention by a Baby Doe squad from Washington, but also state laws on homicide and child abuse and neglect. Those laws are backed up by reporting provisions, particularly the child abuse and neglect laws, which require reporting suspected cases of neglect that endanger a child to a protective agency, prosecutor, or court, depending on the jurisdiction. If a failure to provide (or parents' refusal to consent to) a particular medical or surgical treatment could be characterized as abuse or neglect, and committee members (or some of them) disagree with the decision not to treat, what is their responsibility? Do they at that point remain merely "advisory?" If their duty includes "blowing the whistle," everyone would then know that if a case if brought to the committee and the decision leaves some committee members uncomfortable, the result will be intervention by a state or federal official.

D. Timing of Committee Action

When should committee action occur? Though the assumption seems to be that review will be prospective, the President's Commission also noted that there may be a need for retrospective review to avoid cases falling through the cracks. If one had only prospective review, a convenient way of avoiding conflicts would be not to raise an issue for ethics committee review until the decision was so far along that the committee would have no effect and the case would become moot (e.g., by the patient's death). Furthermore, prospective review is going to be a difficult task because it must often be done on short notice. So some after-the-fact review seems inevitable. Such review is likely to appear less "advisory" and more "investigatory."

And what precisely should trigger review? One of the arguments over ethics committees has focused on whether they should be optional, on the one hand, or mandatory, on the other.[33] In favor of an optional committee, it is said committees ought to be available for those cases in which people want to use them—for example, at the request of the family where there has been internal disagreement or disagreement between family and physicians, or at the request of physicians or nurses, again because of professional divisions or failure to agree with the family decision makers.

But such optional review is not the whole picture in light of those federally required no-

tices in the nurses' station that invite anonymous phone calls. The notices list the committee (in those institutions that have one) as the first resource for the telephone caller. What is going to happen when such calls come in? Is that enough to trigger an investigation or a committee meeting? These questions illustrate the importance of being clear about the powers of the chairperson. When one of those calls comes in, will the chairperson automatically convene the whole meeting, or should the committee have a protocol that says, perhaps, that the chairperson performs initial investigations? What happens if the chairperson's investigation (as has been true of the overwhelming number of the calls that have come to HHS) shows no basis for going further? Or that there is a minor problem of miscommunication, or that the person who made the phone call was simply misinformed about the treatment that was or was not being given to the patient? Can such cases be disposed of without committee review? It took about 12 years in the area of IRBs to get to the point where the federal regulations distinguish between those cases in which review can be waived, those in which it can be expedited, and those cases for which full review by the committee is required. If we are going to start developing ethics committees, we might well learn from the experience with IRBs and be a little more procedurally sophisticated about how cases are going to be handled.

Alternatively, on the mandatory side, are there any cases that must be reviewed? The President's Commission suggested that a non-treatment decision of a neonate that is likely to lead to death would be an appropriate category for mandatory review, particularly when the neonate is burdened by an unremediable handicap that might lead some people not to be fully protective of its life.[34] What about the withdrawal of treatment that is not life-supporting—for example, the decision not to treat spina bifida which is not imminently life-threatening but which is projected to have a major effect on the child's longevity and functioning? These are many such questions that an institution ought to resolve, under the heading "What Triggers What Kind of Review?"

E. Responsibility and Liability

Many people want committees created to protect patients (and especially to preserve lives). Yet some people also favor ethics committees in the belief that they will protect physicians or hospitals. Such an objective is not necessarily improper; for example, suppose it were phrased as desiring to free physicians to treat according to their best clinical judgment, without the distortion introduced by variations in the degree to which they are "risk averse" to litigation.

Yet there is danger here as well. A committee that helps physicians, nurses, and patients and their relatives think through the ethical and social implications of their decisions is one thing. A committee that appears to lift the burdens of complex decisions off their shoulders entirely may end up dispersing responsibility to the extent that no one bears it. The seeds of this problem were sown as early as the *Quinlan* decision, in which it was explicitly suggested, as a strength of an ethics committee, that it would diffuse responsibility and remove the sense of legal liability. A certain amount of concern for legal risk serves as a healthy reminder of the weighty nature of the decisions one is making.

In addressing questions about liability one must turn for analogies, in the absence of direct judicial or legislative guidance, to the law on such bodies as hospital tissue (pathology) committees and credentials committees. For example, in *Larson v. Mithallal*,[35] the plaintiff sued the hospital for negligently awarding staff privileges to his physicians. The Appellate Division of the New York Supreme Court denied the plaintiff's motion to discover the records of the hospital's credentials committee on the ground that New York law protects proceedings and records "relating to the performance of a medical review function." Many states have similar laws. Indeed, even when a physician sues, the results may be the same. In *Straube v. Larson*,[36] a physician sued the hospital's chief administrator for damages based on the actions of the hospital's disciplinary committee. The Oregon Supreme Court disallowed transcripts of the committee's proceedings as evidence.

The question then becomes whether an ethics committee is a medical review committee. The answer may depend in part on the terms of the general state statute or perhaps of any new, specialized statute that those who favor such committees may be able to persuade their state legislature to adopt. The current federal regulations (with their quasi-requirement of ethics committees) would not determine the issue or provide any cloak of confidentiality not given by state law. Furthermore, the precise manner in which the committee is chartered (by the trustees? administrators? medical staff?) and appointed (only physicians or others, including laypeople? only

people connected with the hospital or outsiders as well?) could affect the outcome, as well as whether the committee's members are encompassed under the umbrella of the institution's liability insurance policy. These are important issues for every institution to study and resolve before establishing a committee.

Generally, the law looks with disfavor on privileges that make unavailable material that might be helpful to fact-finders in resolving an issue. The rationale for confidentiality of "peer review" records—that it is necessary for candid evaluation of professionals' performance, which in turn leads to better internal discipline and correction of problems—is coming increasingly under challenge.[37] It is far from self-evident that a court, in interpreting a confidentiality statute, would regard contemporaneous "review" of an unfolding life-and-death drama by an ethics committee as comparable (on grounds of the public policy rationale for the statutory privilege) to after-the-fact review of cases by a pathology committee or review of a physician's staff privileges by a credential committee which, although prospective, does not relate to the welfare of a particular patient-at-risk.

F. Records

Finally, there is the question of record keeping. Suppose a physician is sued in a case that the committee had reviewed, but the committee members are not joined as defendants. The committee's records in the case might still be of great interest to the plaintiff—how did the physician view the issues at the time decisions had to be made? Did the committee agree? And so forth. Under state law, even if the committee's records are generally protected, the statement of a party (such as a physician) to the committee (as recorded by in whatever fashion) may be discoverable.[38]

Of course, this could mean that if the committee members *were* all made parties-defendant in a suit, the committee's whole record of the case could be discovered.

Outside the context of litigation, questions about the accessibility of a committee's records could also arise under a Freedom of Information Act (FOIA) request,[39] if such committees are viewed as creatures of the federal government because of the history of their creation because of the Medicare/Medicaid funding received by the institutions establishing them. An analogous area of law concerns the status of Professional

Standards Review Organization (PSRO) records. The PSRO system was created by Congress to allow control of Medicare/Medicaid costs through self-regulation by the medical profession, and the statute specifically provides for the confidentiality of PSRO records. In *St. Mary's Hospital v. Philadelphia PSRO, Inc.*[40] Judge Green held that PSRO records are not discoverable. The decision rests in part on *Forsham v. Harris,*[41] in which the Supreme Court ruled that the receipt of federal research funds by the University Group Diabetes Program did not make their records those of a "federal agency" (and hence discoverable under FOIA through the Department of Health, Education and Welfare) even though the Group's activities were subject to "extensive, detailed, and virtually day-to-day supervision" by federal officials. On this basis, one would conclude that the law of ethics committees probably does *not* include public access to records under the Federal FOIA—but that is neither certain nor persuasive of the outcome under a state FOIA, particularly for a state-run hospital.

In sum, one would have to conclude that there are a host of legal issues regarding institutional ethics committees, of which the list just presented is merely illustrative not exhaustive.[42] It seems likely that even when a conscientious committee attempts to address these issues, many will remain unresolvable in the current state of the law. Accordingly, one might despair of this undertaking. That is not the intended message of this essay, and I would find that a regrettable outcome. Compared with the alternatives, ethics committees seem attractive, despite the unfavorable and very uncomfortable atmosphere created by the federal government's unnecessarily interventionist and punitive posture on the issue of familial decision making about very sick newborns. Each institution will have to develop a means of improving the quality of life-and-death decisions that is appropriate to institutional circumstances. For many, perhaps most, some form of "ethics committee" should probably be part of that response.

Notes

1. President's Commission for the Study of Ethical Problems in Medicine and Biomedical and Behavioral Research. *Deciding to Forego Life-Sustaining Treatment: A Report on the Ethical, Medical, and Legal Issues in Treatment Decisions* 161 (1983) [hereinafter *Deciding to Forego Treatment*].

2. Kalchbrenner, Kelly & McCarthy, Ethics Committees and Ethicists in Catholic Hospitals, 64 *Hospital Progress* 47 (Sept. 1983).

3. See generally Cantor, A Patient's Decision to Decline Life-Saving Medical Treatment: Bodily Integrity Versus the Preservation of Life, 26 *Rutgers L. Rev.* 228 (1973).

4. See President's Commission for the Study of Ethical Problems of Medicine and Biomedical and Behavioral Research, Defining Death: A Report on the Medical, Legal and Ethical Issues in the Determination of Death (1981).

5. See, e.g., *Deciding to Forego Treatment,* supra note 1, at 389–437 (setting forth state statutes and proposals on "durable power of attorney" and other means of appointing proxy-decision makers).

6. See, e.g., *In re* Quinlan, 70 N.J. 10, 355 A.2d 647, cert. denied, 429 U.S. 922 (1976); *In re* Storar, 52 N.Y.2d 363, 438 N.Y.S.2d 266, 420 N.E.2d 64 (1981); cert. denied, 454 U.S. 858 (1981).

7. *In re* Conroy, No. A-108, Sept. Term 1983, Slip. op. at 47–50 (N.J., Jan. 17, 1985) (establishing two best interests tests: "limited-objective," when there is trustworthy evidence of a patient's wishes, albeit not enough to meet the standards for "substitute judgment," and "pure-objective," which requires greater evidence of burdens to the patient because there is not trustworthy evidence of the patient's wishes).

8. *In re* Quinlan, 70 N.J. p. 55, 355 A.2d at 671.

9. Barber v. Superior Court, 147 Cal. App. 3d 1006, 1016, 195 Cal. Rptr. 484, 490 (1983).

10. *In re* Conroy, 190 N.J. Super. 453, 464 A.2d 303 (App. Div.), cert. granted, 95 N.J. 195, 470 A.2d 418 (1983).

11. *In re* Conroy, No. A-108, Sept. Term 1983, Slip op. (N.J., Jan. 17, 1985).

12. *In re* Hier, 18 Mass. App. Ct. 200, 464 N.E.2d 959 (1984).

13. See above, p. 203, 464 N.E.2d at 961.

14. See above, p. 204, 464 N.E.2d at 962.

15. Superintendent of Belchertown v. Saikewicz, 373 Mass. 728, 370 N.E.2d 417 (1977).

16. Tell, The Physician's Dilemma—A Doctor's View: What the Law Should Be, 27 *Baylor L. Rev.* 6 (1975).

17. *In re* Quinlan, 70 N.J. 10, 55, 355 A.2d 647, 671–72 (1976).

18. See, e.g., Annas, Reconciling Quinlan and Saikewicz: Decision Making for the Terminally Ill Incompetent, 4 *Am. J.L. & Med.* 367, 378–79 (1979).

19. I am indebted to Professor Alan J. Weisbard for this suggestion.

20. Superintendent of Belchertown v. Saikewicz, 373 Mass. 728, 370 N.E.2d 417 (1977).

21. *In re* Coyler, 99 Wash. 2d 114, 660 P.2d 738 (1983).

22. 47 *Fed. Reg.* 26027 (1982).

23. 48 *Fed. Reg.* 9630 (1983).

24. American Academy of Pediatrics v. Heckler, 561 F. Supp. 395 (D.D.C. 1983).

25. 48 *Fed. Reg.* 30846 (1983).

26. 49 *Fed. Reg.* 1622 (1984).

27. United States v. University Hosp., 729 F.2d 144 (2d Cir. 1984).

28. American Hosp. Ass'n v. Heckler, 585 F. Supp. 541 (S.D.N.Y. 1984), aff'd, Nos. 84-6211 and 84-6213 (2d Cir. Dec. 27, 1984).

29. Strain, The American Academy of Pediatrics Comments on the "Baby Doe II" Regulation, 309 *New Eng. J. Med.* 443 (1983).

30. See, e.g., *Institutional Ethics Committees and Health Care Decisionmaking* 22–30, 149–200 (R. Cranford & A. Doudera, eds. 1984); *Deciding to Forego Treatment,* supra note 1, pp. 160–165.

31. See generally President's Commission for the Study of Ethical Problems in Medicine and Biomedical and Behavioral Research, *Protecting Human Sub-jects:* A Report on the Adequacy and Uniformity of Federal Rules and Their Implementation (1981).

32. See 45 C.F.R. Part 46 (1983).

33. Robertson, Committees as Decision Makers: Alternative Structures and Responsibilities, in *Institutional Ethics Committees and Health Care Decision Making,* supra note 29, p. 85.

34. *Deciding to Forego Treatment,* supra note 1, p. 227.

35. 72 A.D.2d 806, 421 N.Y.S.2d 922 (1979).

36. 287 Or. 357, 600 P.2d 371 (Or. 1979).

37. Goldberg, The Peer Review Privilege: A Law in Search of A Valid Policy, 10 *Am. J.L. & Med.* 151 (1984).

38. See Lenard v. New York Univ. Medical Center, 83 A.D.2d 860, 442 N.Y.S.2d 30 (1981).

39. 5 U.S.C. § 552 (1976).

40. No. 78-2943, Slip. op. (E.D. Pa. 1980).

41. 445 U.S. 169 (1980).

42. See Levine, Questions and (Some Very Tentative) Answers About Hospital Ethics Committees, *Hastings Center Rep.* 9 (June 1984).

Ethics Committees: Promise or Peril?

Richard A. McCormick, S.J., S.T.D., Rose F. Kennedy Institute of Ethics, Georgetown University, Washington, DC

The recent attention focused on ethics committees can be traced to three sources. First, in 1976, there was the New Jersey Supreme Court's ruling in the Karen Quinlan case. The court held that a physician who wishes to withdraw life-sustaining medical treatment from a patient and be free from civil or criminal liability, must receive an ethics committee's reinforcement of the prognosis that the patient will never return to "a cognitive, sapient life,"[1] Second, in its report, *Deciding to Forego Treatment,* the President's Commission for the Study of Ethical Problems in Medicine and Biomedical and Behavioral Research discussed the potential for, and advocated further research into, hospital ethics committees.[2] Finally, in response to the then-proposed "Baby Doe" regulations issued by the United States Department of Health and Human Services (HHS), the American Academy of Pediatrics proposed as an alternative the formation of infant bioethical review committees; the HHS final rule acknowledged this concept and endorsed the use of "infant care review committees."[3]

Overall, our experience of the effectiveness of such committees is too recent to be of much help. The significant literature is at most only seven years old, and much of it does not draw upon experience; rather, it attempts to structure future committees. Estimates of the frequency of ethics committees range from 41 percent of Catholic hospitals,[4] to only one percent of United States hospitals,[5] although this difference may be due in part to the varying definitions used by the surveys. In other words, we have a flock of questions and doubts. Building on such an incomplete and embryonic experience is hazardous, tentative, and likely to be a bit speculative. In the following overview, I propose to give a sense of the conditions leading to the use of these committees and a brief summary of the functions and problems. It is offered in the spirit of stimulating thought and provoking discussion; at this stage, that is what I judge we need.

Reprinted, with permission, from *Law, Medicine & Health Care* 1984 Sept. 12:4):150–155. Copyright 1984, American Society of Law and Medicine, 765 Commonwealth Ave., Boston.
Based on a keynote address delivered at the conference, Institutional Ethics Committees and Healthcare Decisionmaking, held in Detroit, April 1984, co-sponsored by the Mercy Health Corporation and the American Society of Law and Medicine.

Cultural Variables and Background Conditions

By examining the background conditions or cultural variables that led to the idea of ethics committees, we may be foreshadowing to some extent the purpose these committees have and the role they should come to play. I will mention eight variables.

The Complexity of Problems

With the growing sophistication of medical technology and the expansion of treatment options, the ethical and medical dimensions of many decisions have become indistinct and complex. Since both health care personnel and health care institutions presumably wish to engage in "ethically acceptable" practices, they begin to look for help in gray areas. An example of a situation in which individuals turned to a court for help is that of the Houle infant, who died following court-ordered emergency surgery at Maine Medical Center in 1974.[6] Born 15 days earlier, the child was horribly deformed. His entire left side was malformed; he had no left eye, was practically without a left ear, had a deformed left hand, and some of his vertebrae were not fused. He could not be fed by mouth for he was afflicted with a tracheo-esophageal fistula, through which air leaked into his stomach, and fluid from the stomach pushed up into the lungs. As Dr. André Hellegers noted at the time: "It takes little imagination to think there were further internal deformities."[7]

As the days passed, the condition of the child deteriorated. Although the tracheo-esophageal fistula, the immediate threat to his survival, could have been corrected with relative ease by surgery, the parents refused to consent to the surgery on their baby because of the complications and deformities. Several doctors in the Maine Medical Center disagreed with that decision, and took the case to court. The Maine Superior Court ordered the surgery, and ruled: "At the moment of live birth there does exist a human being entitled to the fullest protection of the law. The most basic right enjoyed by every human being is the right to life itself."[8]

It is, of course, still unsettled whether a decision to withhold life-saving surgery is always a denial of the right to life. In the case of the Houle baby, the parents and their advisors obviously thought not, while several physicians thought that it did. These complex issues continue to lead to similar disagreements in other situations.

The Range of Options

This is very closely connected with the point just made but is distinct from it. In discussing how treatment decisions should be made for incompetents whose wishes about treatment cannot be determined, Robert Veatch and I proposed a double principle: the patient's best interest and the family's self-determination. In other words, the basic criterion was the patient's best interest. The initial determination of this should reside with the family or family surrogates. In an article discussing this idea, we cautioned:

> Of course, the principle of familial self-determination cannot ride unchecked. Society's responsibility to assure that the interests of its incompetent members are served will place some limits on familial autonomy. In cases, however, where a family is willing to make such decisions . . . the state should intervene only when the familial judgment so exceeds the limits of reason that the compromise with what is objectively in the incompetent one's best interests cannot be tolerated.[9]

This implies that the notion of "best interest" could include a range of acceptable behaviors. What are the outside limits of that range? How is that range determined? It has become increasingly clear that such a determination exceeds the perspective of an individual and that a group might be expected to approximate more nearly (even if not always achieve) the "reasonable person standard."

Protection

In today's litigious atmosphere, health care decisions are repeatedly exposed to legal redress. The problem is only intensified by highly questionable judicial utterances. One thinks of Judge Robert Muir's assertion that those who removed Karen Quinlan's respirator would be subjected to New Jersey's homicide laws.[10] One thinks of Judge Robert Wenke's sweeping dicta in the Nejdl-Barber case: "Murder is the shortening of life;"[11] and "the morality of the defendants' conduct, the purity of their motives, common practice in this type of situation, and the wishes of the decedent's family are all of no weight in the resolution of this motion. The answer lies in the law of the state."[12] One thinks of the threat of financial sanctions by the federal government in Baby Doe-like cases.[13]

Such developments have understandably

surrounded many treatment decisions with fear of liability. Yet, ethics committees do not exist to dispel fear. Robert Veatch astutely noted that an ethics committee should not be expected "to offer legal protection if it concurs with a treatment refusal decision that is eventually contested."[14] However, I believe that decisions are much less likely to be contested if they have the backing of an ethics committee, for the decision will be seen to surpass individual (possibly idiosyncratic and "interested") perspectives and very likely to conform to public standards of the acceptable.

Nature of Judgments in Clinical Decisions

The term "medically indicated" is very frequently used to support and eventually justify treatment decisions of all types, including withholding or withdrawal of life-support systems. If treatment decisions were simply a matter of medical indications, then these decisions would be exclusively within the competence of medical personnel.

Such is not the case, however, as has become especially clear in the past decade. Edmund Pellegrino has usefully distinguished four components of the notion of the patient's best interest.[15] The first is "medical good," which refers to the effects of medical intervention on the natural history of the disease being treated, or to what can be achieved by the application of medical knowledge. It could be cure, containment, prevention, amelioration, or prolongation of life. Thus, a respirator can be used to achieve complete recovery, to tide a patient over a crisis, to discover the underlying cause of the problem, or to discover whether the illness is terminal. The tendency of physicians is to equate medical good with the patient's overall good. Such an equation involves two fallacies. First, if any procedure can be done, it ought to be done. All dimensions of patients' good are deflated into medical good. The second fallacy is the expansion of medical good to include quality-of-life criteria. Thus, if treatment of defective newborns would result in a life without meaningful relationships, it is said to be not medically indicated. This intermingling of types of "the good" exceeds medical competence. Whether a life is worth living is not measurable by medical means. The second component of the patient's best interest is the patient's preference, that is, what the patient thinks is worthwhile. The scientifically correct decision, to be good in this sense, must be placed within the context of the patient's particular life situation, value system, and religious beliefs. The third component is the "good of the human as human." Unique to humans is the very capacity to set life-plans, to make choices. This capacity is frustrated if the patient's choices are not free. Therefore, other things being equal, that treatment is preferable or good that preserves the very capacity to choose. The final component of the patient's best interests is the "good of the last resort." This refers to the good which gathers all others and is their base and explanation. The good of last resort grounds, and provides intelligibility to, other choices. For instance, for many persons, this good refers to God, and God's plans for them in their lives. The good of last resort will or should inform the patient's preferences.

In the ideal decision, these components are congruent. Whatever the case, the clinical decision must attend to all of the components. It is thus clear that "best interests" is a broad human judgment, not a narrowly scientific one. And once that is understood, it becomes clear that competences other than medical competence can shed light on the clinical decision. We have become newly aware of this in recent years,[16] and that awareness is the backdrop for the emergence of interdisciplinary ethics committees.

The Emergence of Patient Autonomy

The understanding of the complexity of the concept of a patient's best interests accompanies the emergence of patient autonomy as a key value in decision making as a component of patient dignity. The shift from a beneficence-oriented ethic with its correlative paternalism of practice has moved rapidly in the past 15–20 years. This shift can lead to conflicts between a patient's judgment and physician-institution judgment or policy. Conflicts suggest mediation and arbitration.

The Emergence of Economic Considerations

Paul Starr has shown that beginning in the late 1960s, the economic structure of the health care system began to change dramatically.[17] Corporations set up by investors to make profits entered the business of health care and competed with voluntary nonprofit hospitals for federal and private insurance money. Such corporations built or acquired such facilities as general hospitals, nursing homes, health maintenance organizations, ambulatory surgical centers, renal dialysis centers, diagnostic laboratories, and home care services. A huge new industry has arisen.

Private, not-for-profit hospitals began to mimic their profit-making competitors with aggressive marketing strategies. They have reorganized their corporate structure to allow for the acquisition of satellite and affiliated institutions, charitable foundations that own businesses.[18]

In the midst of all this, health care, once regarded as a social good, a moral right of the citizen even if poor, is now being marketed and sold for a profit.[19] Investor-owned corporations with their business philosophy are increasingly taking over the patient population. Professional autonomy is being diminished. As Relman summarizes:

> Hospital and clinic managers, reporting to corporate executives rather than to members of the medical staff, will have more responsibility—and physicians less— for the critical decisions that determine where the money and medical technology will go. More physicians will be salaried employees and fewer will be independent fee-for-service practitioners.[20]

Obviously, ethical questions abound in this economic shift, and they are, by and large, questions of policy. For instance, how can physicians continue to serve their patients' interests first and foremost when their professional judgments are so easily exposed to the economic interests of their employers? The use of diagnosis related groups in hospitals can operate as a contemporary symbol of this problem. Where protective and distributive policies are concerned, neither the for-profit employer nor the for-profit employee (physician) are alone the most disinterested guarantors of a patient's best interest.

Religious Convictions of Some Groups

I refer here above all, but not exclusively, to such problems as sterilization in Catholic hospitals. The moral teaching of the Catholic Church on this matter is absolute and adamant: "Thou shalt not directly sterilize." Yet, two factors complicate this posture. First, there is widespread theological dissent on the point. Second, hospitals have always had to deal pastorally with conflicting situations in applying these strictures. In some places, committees have been seen as appropriate vehicles to achieve a livable policy—to permit yet to control. What typically happens is that sterilizations in Catholic hospitals are forbidden unless a hospital committee decides that, in a

particular case, the patient meets the criteria established by the institution for an exception. Some institutions (e.g., those in Canada) spell out the criteria quite specifically in medical terms. Others leave the matter quite general ("overall good of the patient"). Still others leave the criteria unstated and proceed on a case-by-case basis.

Individual Decisions, as Affected by the Plurality of Publics

By this last culturable variable, I refer to a characteristic of our atmosphere. Decisionmaking is no longer simply a one-on-one affair. Increasingly, health care personnel must be responsive to a variety of publics, Medicare and Medicaid agencies, group practice sensitivities, religious policies, state or federal legislation, and, as suggested above, the "corporate third party." Some of the values for which these publics stand compete with each other. Resolution of such conflicts may not be achieved through medical or scientific judgments; rather, such resolutions call for policy decisions that range far beyond medical expertise.

These are just a few of the considerations or "cultural variables" that have led the way to the concept of ethics committees. I now refer to a dimension of these variables that further complicates health care decisions and underlies the need for a broadly representative mechanism in health care facilities. That dimension is uncertainty: nearly all of the variables mentioned are clouded by present division and future uncertainty.

A few examples show the problems that occur because of this uncertainty. For example, emphasis on patient autonomy is certainty a healthy reaction to an excessive paternalism. But is it possible that such an emphasis can become an overemphasis? For instance, is there not a point where information flow and physicians' prescriptions are covered by the doctor-patient relationship of mutual trust? The patient comes to the physician with a single purpose: cure or relief. Should we not assume that the overarching purpose within a trusting relationship means that the patient may not want to know about every minute detail, about even the most unlikely of outcomes? Childress and Beauchamp illustrate the dilemma well:

> A woman had a fatal reaction during urography. The radiologist indicated that he did not warn this patient (or any other

patients) of a possible fatal reaction to urography because it would not do any good. "I could have told her," he said, "that there was a chance she might have a reaction and even die. After calming her down I would then have told her that she had seen two urologists in the past week and both of them had told her she needed urography. I have done 6,000 to 8,000 urograms in the past 13 years and no one has ever had a fatal reaction. We have been doing urograms at this hospital for at least 25 years and no one has ever had a fatal reaction. Because the indications for urography were great and the chances for a reaction were remote I am sure I would have convinced Mrs. E. . . . to have the procedures. She would have then had the reaction and died and the fact that I warned her would have done Mrs. E. . . . absolutely no good." According to the American College of Radiology, "Our responsibility is to our patients and to do what is best for our patients medically. Informing patients of risks and possible death from urography may not be in the best interest of the patient and . . . it may be dangerous."[21]

Where do we draw the line between what reasonable people would want to know, and what they consider trivial and would not want to know? There is *present* conflict and *future* uncertainty here.

Another example would be the delicate question of withholding nutrition or hydration. Several recent articles have argued that where the patient is dying and comatose, intravenous fluids are not required.[22] Lynn and Childress apply this reasoning to one like Karen Quinlan in a persistent vegetative state.

> Thus, if the parents of an anencephalic infant or a patient like Karen Quinlan in a persistent vegetative state felt strongly that no medical procedures should be applied to provide nutrition and hydration, and the care givers agree, there should be no barrier in law or public policy to thwart that plan.[23]

Judge Lynn Compton in the Nejdl-Barber case would agree,[24] as do I. But many likely will not, from ethical and legal points of view. Daniel Callahan has manifested his profound uneasiness with these conclusions. He refers to a deepseated revulsion at stopping feeding, and argues that feeding is "a tolerable price to pay to preserve—with ample margin to spare—one of the few moral emotions that could just as easily be called a necessary social instinct."[25] Once again, present ethical division and future uncertainty form the climate for the ethics committee.

Similar analyses could be made of legal uncertainties, government involvement, ecclesiastical or political tensions and divisions, and financial uncertainties (e.g., the effect of diagnosis related groups on patient management). The liberal-conservative tension is likely to be present in all facets of health care.

The Problems of Ethics Committees

This analysis leads directly to the second part of my article: the problems of, and objections to, ethics committees. Because these committees are here to stay and are worthwhile, we should face their problems and objections unflinchingly and in their strongest form.

One of the largest problems is physician resistance. It is well known that many physicians are indifferent to, and frequently hostile to, what they regard as the "intrusion" of ethics on their turf. In my twenty-five years of experience with physicians, I have concluded that there are only two times when they will appear at ethics conferences: at grand rounds at 7:00 a.m., or on Friday or Saturday nights with cocktails and dinner, spouses included.

What is responsible for physicians' resistance? It may be due to the perseverance of the beneficence ethos, the "physician knows best" attitude rooted in the long, specialized training of the modern physician. This can translate into a one-sided emphasis on the privacy or the individualism of the physician-patient relationship, to the point where the ethical and legal dimensions are unwelcome.

The formulations of this problem vary, but only in minor ways. Recently, Morris B. Abram, former chairman of the President's Commission, and Susan M. Wolf, wrote: "We generally avoid empowering our Government to dictate private morality. The prospect of creating an institutional priesthood to dictate rules on medical ethics is abhorrent."[26] I agree with this principle, but I criticize the language. Note the phrase, "dictate private morality"—as though ethical deliberation means dictating rules, as if medical practice were a private matter. This is a common attitude of physicians toward ethics committees; they are worried that the committees will dictate rules on what is a private matter.

The problem is intensified when we recall that physicians are not simply practitioners. They are "feeders" in an increasingly competitive health care system; that is, they feed the patients to the hospitals, thereby providing hospitals with their profits. Hospitals do not want to alienate their feeders. To avoid doing so, hospital administrators could easiliy treat the committees as window-dressing.

Another problem that can arise in at least some cases where an ethics committee is concerned is confidentiality. It is a problem because relying on such a committee is not the same as seeking a professional consultation. The committee may include non-medical members of the hospital staff, or even members of the general public. Hospital staff cannot presume that patients have consented to a display of their cases before such a group, especially if the disclosure involves details of their private lives that most of us would want protected. I am sure that there are ways around this problem. But it must be recognized as a problem; too often it is not. I raised this issue with the Bioethics Committee of the American Hospital Association and was surprised to learn that several hospital administrators did not see it as a problem. There is still a lingering attitude that the professional secret is the secret whispered amongst professionals.

Committee members' lack of clinical knowledge is an objection that I have heard repeatedly. How can nonclinical people understand sufficiently the medical details upon which medical judgment is based? Clearly, there is substance to this objection, but it should function as a challenge rather than as an obstacle. Health care personnel must learn the art of translation, and nonclinical people must familiarize themselves with clinical attitudes and language. Unless such lines of communication are established, physicians will convert medical paternalism into ethical paternalism and will continue to view ethics committees as intruders. This will only delay the day when the patient's best interest is viewed as it should be—as involving a broad human (ethical) judgment, not simply a scientific or medical one.

Another problem is that of inhouse protectionism. Depending on the attitudes and disciplinary make-up of an ethics committee, it could begin to operate protectively for the institution and its practitioners. This is all the more possible where a legally threatening and highly competitive administrative atmosphere combines with an exaggerated notion of physician autonomy. Obviously, an attitude of inhouse protectionism can affect the quality of ethical deliberation and the ultimate credibility of an ethics committee. I do not see this as a major objection, but only as a potential problem against which we should guard.

We must also deal with the issue of pragmatic situationism. I have used a "dirty word" here because I want the objection to bite as deeply and as painfully as possible. Health care personnel are often deeply stamped with two attitudes: they are trained to get results; and they view each case as unique. In combination, these traits can lead to—although they need not—a rootlessness which is corrosive of morality. For example, after discussing the problem of defective newborns, Anthony Shaw writes:

> If an underlying philosophy can be gleaned from the vignettes presented above, I hope it is one that tries to find a solution, humane and loving, based on the circumstances of each case rather than by means of a dogmatic formula approach. (Fletcher has best expressed this philosophy in his book *Situation Ethics.* . . .)[27]

There are many ethicists who do not believe that the only alternative are Fletcherism and dogmatism. To state the problem in this way can easily result in a hopelessly muddled "geographical morality." This brings up the interesting question of what are the ethics of the ethics committee.

Another concern is that of legal accommodationism. There is the legitimate fear that ethics committees will be too narrowly focused on the law and that ethics may be diluted in the process. The law is, of course, very important, and it is clearly related to ethics. But the two are distinct. For example, a procedure may not be legally regulated and still be regarded as unethical.

Since ethics committees can easily be oversensitive to the felt need of consensus, many people distrust them. Such a felt need, it is asserted, can flatten the sharp differences that make for the ethically prophetic, the religiously distinctive element in ethics. Thus Margaret Steinfels, in her critique of the Ethics Advisory Board's conclusions on *in vitro* fertilization, wrote: "Proceeding in the manner of a body that hopes to reach a consensus, the Board both acknowledged and finessed the issues on which it could not agree by careful attention to the wording of its conclusions."[28] She argues that this is especially a danger when the composition of the committee favors the medical establishment and their "ethical imperatives."

Some argue that the process of review is too cumbersome. I have heard physicians express the fear that the very cases that are most problematic are those that lead themselves least to committee deliberation. Emergency cases and code decisions are examples of situations that require quick medical action.

Another concern has roots in the fear of exposure. Some health care personnel do not want things in writing when dealing with such uncertain areas. Some personnel especially want to avoid the exposure associated with "whistle-blowing."

Ethics committees also run the risk of offending the value pluralism so important to society. Health care personnel and patients represent a broad spectrum of values and religious orientations. A committee, it is argued, will almost necesssarily offend individual sensitivities as it attempts to arrive at the one, correct ethical conclusion or posture. Neonatal intensive care cases may be particularly vulnerable to this problem. Some parents feel that their emotional and financial resources should play a key ethical role in treatment-nontreatment decisions. Committees are likely to disagree or be insensitive to these concerns.

The lack of ethical expertise among committee members poses another problem. This relates closely to my fifth point concerning pragmatic situationism. For a committee to function in a disciplined way, a good deal of ethical education will be required of its members. There are practical problems associated with this education, however. Who will give it? Will committee members be open to it? Will they have the time?

Another contention is that diffusion of responsibility will be a natural result of committee deliberations. If advice is sought in difficult cases from an ethics committee, it is possible that a sense of responsibility for individual decisions will be dispersed to the point where no individual feels responsible. That this could be detrimental to patient care needs little elaboration.

These, then, are some of the problems and arguments that committees are likely to face. To all of them, there are persuasive answers. Nevertheless, the institutions that establish ethics committees would do well to weigh them in advance,

to circumvent unnecessary opposition and possibly obstacular tactics.

Functions

It is important to spell out clearly the mandate of an ethics committee, if for no other reason than to dispel the fear and antagonism of staff members, especially physicians—the fear of "intrusion" and antagonism toward "dictation." Briefly, there are four functions. First, there is the function of guidance, via consultation or review. This is *not* decision making. Rather, it is an attempt to spell out those values that constitute the context in which individual prudence must operate. Occasionally, the guidance may be judgmental, but I think that this will occur rarely. Under the title of guidance, the committee will also be the mechanism of court referral when there is patient (family)-physician disagreement. Second, an ethics committee can and should function frequently as a support mechanism for individual decisionmakers. This proved true, by and large, with the three federal bioethics commissions, and I see no reason why it should not be true of local ethics committees.

Third, there is the function of developing policies. This is perhaps a committee's most difficult function since it may touch on virtually everything: do-not-resuscitate policies, staffing, acquisition, and hospital organization (e.g., unionization policy). Indeed, these many and different areas strongly suggest the need for different committees with different personnel. The final function is education. A well-functioning committee should be a major educational tool within the hospital. Again, this task is enormous precisely because of the broad sweep of the policies to which the committee might address itself.

Recommendations

I have four basic, non-threatening recommendations. First, we should make use of the experience of institutional review boards. Clearly, these are different in composition and purpose from ethics committees, but they have dealt with ethical questions. Concretely, they have protected patients without unduly curtailing research and harassing physicians. Whatever we can carry over from them to ethics committees is likely to be supportive.

Second, those involved in ethics committees should move slowly. This caution refers to every aspect of the ethics committee: its composition, mandate, and workload. We are, after all, in relatively uncharted waters and haste or impatience can magnify problems.

Third, the make-up and functioning of the ethics committee should be reevaluated on a regular basis. Its work is too important to be abandoned to its own dynamic. Fourth, the committee should emphasize education. In the initial stages, it would be wise to spend what may seem to be an inordinate amount of time in the long run, but this establishes a common working framework and language for the committee.

Finally, attention should be paid to the necessity of personal compatibility. From my own— and others'—experience, I would say that a committed doubles its efficiency and halves its efforts if the individual members are personally compatible. Such compatibility dissipates obstinacy and creates openness to the views of others.

Are ethics committees a promise or a peril? They are a little bit of both, but they will be more of the former if we proceed with the care and foresight that their importance deserves.

References

1. *In re* Quinlan, 355 A.2d 647, 672 (N.J. 1976). It is clear that this is not properly the function of an ethics committee but, rather, of a "prognosis committee."

2. President's Commission for the Study of Ethical Problems in Medicine and Biomedical and Behavioral Research, Deciding to Forego Life-Sustaining Treatment: Ethical, Medical, and Legal Issues in Treatment Decisions (U.S. Gov't. Printing Office, Washington, D.C.) (1983) at 168–70 [hereinafter referred to as Deciding to Forego Treatment].

3. Nondiscrimination on the Basis of Handicap; Procedures and Guidelines Relating to Health Care for Handicapped Infants; Final Rule, 49 Fed. Reg. 1621, 1623 (January 16, 1984) (to be codified at 45 C.F.R. §84.55).

4. Kalchbrenner, J., Kelly, M. J., McCarthy, D. G., *Ethics Committees and Ethicists in Catholic Hospitals*, Hospital Progress 64(9): 47, 47 (September 1983).

5. Youngner, S. J., *et al.*, *A National Survey of Ethics Committees*, in Deciding to Forego Treatment, *supra* note 2, p. 448.

6. McCormick, R. A., *To Save or Let Die: The Dilemma of Modern Medicine*, Journal of the American Medical Association 229(2):172, 172 (July 8, 1974).

7. *Id., quoting* Obstetrical and Gynecological News (April 1974).

8. McCormick, *supra* note 6, p. 172, *quoting* Maine

Medical Ctr. v. Houle, No. 74-145 (Cumberland County Me. Super. February 14, 1974).

9. McCormick, R. A., Veatch, R.M., *The Preservation of Life and Self-Determination*, Theological Studies 41(2):390, 395–96 (June 1980).

10. *In re* Quinlan, 137 N.J. Super. 227, 261–63 (N.J. Super. Ct. Ch. Div. 1975).

11. People v. Barber, No. A 025586, slip op. p. 2 (Cal. Super. Ct. May 5, 1983).

12. *Id.* p. 4.

13. 49 Fed. Reg. 1640–42 (January 16, 1984) (to be codified at 45 C.F.R. §84, app. C.).

14. Veatch, R. M., *Ethics Committees: Are They Legitimate?* Ethics Committee Newsletter 1(2): 1, 2 (November 1983).

15. Pellegrino, E., *Moral Choice: The Good of the Patient and the Patient's Good*, in Moral Choice and the Medical Crisis (L. Kopelman, J. C. Moskop, eds.) (D. Reidel, Holland) (forthcoming 1984).

16. *See* Deciding to Forego Treatment, *supra* note 2, pp. 119–36.

17. P. Starr, The Social Transformation of American Medicine (Basic Books, Inc., New York, N.Y.) (1982) at 420–44.

18. *Id.* pp. 439–44.

19. *Cf.* Relman, A. S., *The Power of the Doctors*, New York Review of Books 31(5):29, 29 (March 29, 1984).

20. *Id.* p. 32.

21. T. L. Beauchamp, J. F. Childress, Principles of Biomedical Ethics (Oxford University Press, New York, N.Y.) (1979) at 255, *citing* Allen, R. W., *Informed Consent: A Medical Decision*, Radiology 119:233–34 (April 1976).

22. Lynn, J., Childress, J. F., *Must Patients Always Be Given Food and Water*, Hastings Center Report 13(5): 17 (October 1983); Micetich, K., Steinecker, P., Thomasma, D., *Are Intravenous Fluids Morally Required?* Archives of Internal Medicine 143: 975–78 (1983).

23. Lynn, Childress, *supra* note 22, p. 18.

24. Barber v. Superior Court, 195 Cal. Rptr. 484, 492–93 (Cal. App. 1983).

25. Callahan, D., *On Feeding the Dying*, Hastings Center Report 13(5):22, 22 (October 1983).

26. Abram, M. B., Wolf, S. M., *Public Involvement in Medical Ethics: A Model for Governmental Action*, New England Journal of Medicine 310(10): 627, 627 (March 8, 1984).

27. Shaw, A., *Dilemmas of Informed Consent in Children*, New England Journal of Medicine 289(17): 885, 889 (October 25, 1973).

28. Steinfels, M. O., *In Vitro Fertilization: "Ethically Acceptable" Research*, Hastings Center Report 9(3): 5, 5 (June 1979).

Ethics Committees: What We Have Learned

Sister Corrine Bayley, M.A., St. Joseph Health System, Orange, CA
Ronald E. Cranford, M.D., Neurological Intensive Care Unit, Hennepin County Medical Center, Minneapolis

In 1982, when the two of us were involved with the American Society of Law and Medicine in planning the first nationwide conference on ethics committees, we could not have predicted with any certainty how these committees would develop. We were then, and still are, optimistic that ethics committees can fill a significant void in the clinical setting. As ethical dilemmas become more complex and occur more frequently, a resource is needed that can provide education, recommend policies and guidelines, and be available for case review. Having said all that in the early 1980s, it is time now to take a look at what we have learned and to ask the question "Are ethics committees alive and well?"

They are clearly alive, having proliferated even faster than we thought they might. Several things account for this, not least among them the endorsement of several major professional associations[1] and the flurry of activity in the "Baby Doe" area. Surveys[2] show that the number of hospitals with ethics committees is in the range of 26 to 40 percent, most of them in not-for-profit hospitals. Our prediction is that within the next five years, the majority of hospitals will have ethics committees or infant ethics committees, or both.

To the question "Are the committees well?," we answer a qualified yes. Some are not only well but thriving. Others are stable, and a few others need a transfer to intensive care or, at the very least, a blood transfusion. Because practical experiences and creative suggestions for success have been documented elsewhere,[3] we will focus in this paper primarily on areas of difficulty and uncertainty, as well as make some predictions about future directions of ethics committees.

Committees are different from one another and have major mood swings within themselves. Talk to a committee one month and nothing has happened. Talk to it the next month—after a case review or a good educational session—and the positive energy is tangible. We find ourselves repeating one of the things we said at early ethics committee conferences: the ethics committee is not task-oriented like most other hospital committees. Therefore, the process will often be frustrating, and self-doubt will make several appearances. However, satisfaction results when, over time, committee members realize that they have become much more sophisticated in their understanding of ethical issues and in their ability to work through an ethical dilemma.

Committee Functions

The three primary functions of ethics committees, education, policy and guideline development, and consultation,[4] have been exercised with varying degrees of success. In our opinion, two of these functions, education and consultation, have been fraught with the most difficulties.

Many ethics committees are formed because several people in the hospital (primarily nurses, social workers, chaplains, physicians, and administrators) are uneasy about the lack of discussion and direction regarding ethical issues. For example, do-not-resuscitate (DNR) orders are being written by the physician without discussion with patients or families or, conversely, patients or families want a DNR order or limitation of other therapy, and physicians refuse to issue it. Concerns about informed consent, determination of competency, the role of families in decision making, and the validity of "living wills" overlap legal with ethical issues. People are unclear how to sort them out. Despite intense concern, many professionals, not to mention patients and families, feel isolated and powerless, as if they are the only ones who are uncertain or hesitant about these and other issues.

When committees first began to be formed, there was an almost audible sigh of relief. At last there would be a way to deal with all these issues and concerns! What committee members quickly recognized (if they were honest) was that no one on the committee had a much better idea than anyone else about how to think about the issues. Forming a committee was just the first step to better decisions. The second step was self-education.

Education

Self-education relies on a lot of factors that are not readily available to ethics committees. Resource people for one thing. In the past few years, a body of knowledge has developed regarding the nature of ethical decision making in clinical setting. Committee members need to be exposed to definitions, distinctions, ethical principles, and methodologies for approaching an ethical dilemma. Many committees have taken on this task with determination. Others have not fared so well. Since there is usually no one on the committee able to provide needed expertise, members may neither recognize that they need it nor know where to get it.

For some people, merely being a member of the committee convinces them that they have achieved some kind of legitimate expertise. That can be a dangerous assumption, particularly if the committee begins to do hospitalwide education, policy development, and case review before spending adequate time on self-education. Fortunately, most committees have one or two members who have a natural capacity for thoughtful reflection, and these members have usually become much more articulate over time.

A second problem with self-education is time. Most committees meet monthly for approximately 1-1/2 to 2 hours. Unless members read considerably and attend seminars in between, it will take years for even the the most dedicated of committees to progress very rapidly. In the past, committees often have had the luxury of time for study, but new committees will not be so fortunate. They are likely to be expected to produce educational programs for others, to develop policies and guidelines, and even be available for case reviews very quickly.

Finally, most committees have not been self-critical about how well they have accomplished their task of education, either for themselves or for the hospital community. Committees need to find a way to measure their efforts more accurately so that they will not become discouraged. Committees with the greatest success in hospitalwide education, for example, are those that have devised simple ways to measure their efforts. A committee that keeps careful track of attendance at its monthly ethics rounds can move quickly to expand publicity, improve the quality of speakers, or conduct small surveys about topics of interest if attendance begins to decline. This gives the committee an important sense of control. A committee that does not bother to find some way to measure its effectiveness is less likely to be aware of when responses to its efforts are changing. When no one shows up at a scheduled event, the committee is understandably discouraged and unsure of what to do to change the response. Committees do not have the time or resources to do complex evaluations, but a failure to perform any evaluation at all is an invitation to discouragement. Most committees are just beginning to get into hospitalwide education and should not find it too difficult to devise some way of measuring their effectiveness.

Despite problems, it is through education that committees can have their strongest effect, not least because good education can get people thinking more clearly and constructively about issues. We have observed that, after a year or two, committees have much more facility in distinguishing between ethical issues, medical issues, legal issues and administrative issues. For example, there is a big difference in the ethical implications of removing a ventilator from a patient who is brain dead and one who is irreversibly comatose. Similarly, once it is known that a patient is likely to recover consciousness, there should no longer by any ethical dilemma about whether to follow the family's wishes to discontinue all treatment. The decision should be postponed until it can be ascertained what the patient wants.

Developing Policies and Guidelines

The development of policies and guidelines is a task enthusiastically entered into by many committees, and for good reason. These documents are badly needed in most hospitals,[5] and developing them gives committee members a sense of accomplishment. This function overlaps nicely with that of education, since the presentation of a draft policy provides the occasion to gather a multidisciplinary group of professionals who will help implement it. The interaction and clarification that take place in these sessions prompt committees to remark that the process of developing and presenting the document can be as helpful as finally completing it.

Committees cannot accurately speak of "finally completing" policies or guidelines, because they need to be evaluated, reality-tested, and revised as new information becomes available. Many committees report having revised their DNR guidelines two or three times. In addition to DNR guidelines, documents most likely to be developed by ethics committees at this point include a description of committee functions, guidelines for making treatment decisions for seriously ill newborns, guidelines for foregoing life prolonging treatment, and guidelines for the determination of death and dealing with families of brain-dead patients.

Most of these documents have been called guidelines rather than policies primarily because committees were on uncertain ground in a new effort. Guidelines are advisory statements; policies reflect expected practice.

A recent trend is for some committees to recommend DNR policies rather than DNR guidelines. This is a logical evolution, as a standard of practice is beginning to emerge in this area, and hospitals will want some assurance that they are in step with it. It should be more than a guideline, for example, to insist that DNR orders be documented in the patient's chart.

In general, committees are more careful than they have been in the past about defining terms; being clear about whether something is mandatory or permissive and making distinctions between policies, principles, procedures, and guidelines (even if they are in the same document). Clarity in this area has not reached its peak; in the next few years committees will pay more attention to the way policies and/or guidelines are written. It is also likely that committees within their own geographic areas will do more networking and sharing of policies among themselves and with the public in community education sessions.

Consultation

Even though most committees follow the "party line" and mention education as their first function, success is almost always measured in terms of the consultation function. Increasingly, the two of us are asked how committees are handling consultations, how many are being done, whether a vote is taken, how (and whether) the whole committee is assembled for consultations, who can ask for a consultation, who is present, and so on. This is understandable because case reviews, unlike education conferences, are much more in tune with the usual nature of education in the medical setting. They are smaller in scale, case specific, active, rapid, and have definite resolutions. There is a concrete accomplishment and thus the committee members feel a sense of achievement.

Although understandable, the emphasis on consultation is distressing for several reasons. First, committee members need to develop expertise before they consult, not so much in knowing the right answers as in knowing the right questions. Second, a preoccupation with consultation can distract from the important business of education and policy and guideline development. Third, consultations will come soon enough, and when they do, the committee will naturally evolve the structure, or various structures, for dealing with them.

Some have noted difficulties with the use of the word consultation to describe what the committees are or should be doing.[6] Others have suggested substituting case conference or concurrent or prospective case review. Whatever it is called, this function of the ethics committee requires being available when the health care team, patients, and/or families want assistance in sorting through a difficult ethical decision.

Until now, consultations have been most often initiated by physicians, although as other staff members become more familiar with the functions of the committee (usually through individual committee members and/or through hospitalwide education) they are beginning to raise issues with individual members or with the committee as a whole. We believe that in the next few years patients and families will become more aware of the existence of ethics committees and will be more likely to contact them.

Initiation of consultation by someone other than the attending physician raises some sensitive issues, of course, particularly if the physician is perceived to be contributing to the problem. Experienced committees will recognize that difficulties are not resolved unless all the primary participants are involved. Thus, ethics committees will find ways to facilitate communication between and among the various parties, excluding no one.

Gathering the facts, naming the dilemma, setting priorities among ethical principles, and considering options are all part of a good consultation process. This can be done by one or more members of the committee or by the committee as a whole. It should be clear that committees or individual members do not make decisions; their role is to provide a forum for communication and to facilitate the process of decision making. Many times a formal recommendation is not needed, because a consensus will emerge. At other times, a formal recommendation may be appropriate. A practice is slowly emerging of making a brief note of the discussion and the recommendation of the committee on the patient's medical record. This is ordinarily done by the chairman of the ethics committee.

Prospective and Retrospective Reviews

Prospective review, which usually looks at the available options in a single case, and retrospective review, which looks at a group of cases as a class, has become, or will likely become, a regular function of ethics committees.

Prospective Review

Routine prospective review by ethics committees is not currently done in many places, but we anticipate that it will become routine, particularly in instances likely to be troublesome. Examples include foregoing treatment for certain categories of seriously ill newborns and treating or foregoing treatment of incompetent patients with no family or guardian. These reviews can provide due process and can obviate the need for routine court review, particularly in determining what is in the best interest of an incompetent adult with no surrogate decision maker.

Retrospective Review

Retrospective case review is a function of ethics committees that was not much discussed in the early 1980s. It has emerged in a few places recently as an activity that has potential for improving the quality of decision making in the hospital and in evaluating how clearly the committee policies and/or guidelines are being followed. Typical categories of cases include DNR, treatment of seriously ill newborns, and cases in which life-sustaining treatment was foregone.

Retrospective review has the potential for creating hostility, since it may appear that the committee is looking over physicians' shoulders and second guessing their decisions and actions. Because of this potential, education about retrospective review should stress that the purpose is not to fault actions in particular cases, but only to see whether there are problems that could be handled more effectively if there were better policies or guidelines in place. In this way, retrospective review differs considerably from prospective review.

It is worth noting that when ethics committees began to be discussed rather widely in the early 1980s, concern was voiced, mostly by physicians, that such committees would be an unwelcome intrusion into their territory. "I have made these decisions for years; why do we need a committee all of a sudden?" Explanation that the committees do not make decisions has not stilled all of these voices; however, many physicians have become staunch supporters of ethics committees, appreciating them as a resource rather than fearing them as a potential source of criticism.[7]

Committee Membership

Although there is agreement that ethics committees should be multidisciplinary, their composition varies. Size varies greatly, with the average number being 15 and the range from 6 to 30 members.

The most successful committees are not dominated by any one profession, but include relatively equal numbers of physicians and nurses (making up about two thirds), with the remainder composed of one or more social workers, clergy, administrators, board members, ethicists, attorneys, and lay persons.

The last three categories, ethicists, attorneys, and lay persons, deserve special mention because their role is evolving and often unclear.

Ethicists (or bioethicists) are those who have studied and written about the moral implications and ethical nature of health care decisions, either at the policy level or in the clinical setting. Usually they have degrees in philosophy or moral theology, although lawyers, physicians, nurses, and others who have studied bioethics are often considered practicing bioethicists. They bring a sensitivity to the committees' need for clarity, consistency, and principled reasoning. Although all committee members will need to learn how to think consciously within an ethical frame of reference, an ethicist can help to get that process started and can monitor the process.

The person who fills the ethicist role is not intended to provide "expert" moral judgments for the committee; moral judgments and ethical arguments should not be confused with each other. It cannot be emphasized too strongly that the ethicist's obligation is to help the committee maintain standards of ethical analysis, not to provide moral judgments.

Committees are frequently advised to include among their members a lawyer who is not a hospital employee. This works well if it is clear that the attorney is present to serve the same kind of professional function on the committee as do others: to bring expert knowledge that the committee members need. Nonhospital lawyers are preferred, not because they are better lawyers or know more about ethics, but because lawyers employed to protect the hospital's interest could be in a position of conflict. This is so particularly in areas in which the law is not clear and in which a hospital lawyer would be more likely to take a conservative legal position rather than to enter into a careful ethical analysis of the issue. The lawyer chosen should understand that the committee's focus is on ethics, not law. Legal knowledge is an important component but not the committee's primary focus.

Ethics committees are increasingly adding one or more lay members to their number. Primary reasons for this include the desire for credibility and accountability in the local community, the advantage of having a nonhospital perspective, and the significance of representing a primary group served by the institution. We think that more lay members will be added to committees as committee members themselves become more comfortable in their role and as a more educated public shows interest in serving on ethics committees.

As with the selection of all members, the committee should be less concerned with a lay person's background or function and more concerned with the quality of his or her thinking, attitudes, and temperament. Even the most representative committee will not do anyone any good if its members are not thoughtful, reflective, critical thinkers who are willing and able to move slowly, to tolerate substantial ambiguity, and to accept and respect one another.

Infant Ethics Committees

Because the U.S. Department of Health and Human Services (DHSS) has developed guidelines for infant care review committees, some people believe such committees are required by law. They are not. However, hospitals that treat newborns should be familiar with the 1984 Amendments to the Child Abuse and Neglect Prevention and Treatment Act, with its accompanying regulations.[8] The section on Infant Care Review Committees shows that the DHHS does not consider these to be ethics committees, but prognosis committees.

The treatment of newborns with serious disabilities is an area in which ethical dilemmas are rife. Hospitals should have policies or guidelines addressing these issues and a mechanism for review when there is disagreement about whether limiting treatment is appropriate.

When the American Academy of Pediatrics developed their "Guidelines for Infant Bioethics Committees"[9] some hospitals considered establishing a separate ethics committee for newborns. Usually these were hospitals who did not already have an ethics committee into which the function could be incorporated. Thus some facilities are in the rather unusual situation of having a committee that deals only with ethical issues in the care of infants. We believe that there may be good reason, particularly in hospitals with tertiary care status for the care of newborns, to have two separate committees. If there is only one committee, it should be broadly representative enough to consider a wider range of ethical issues than only for newborns.

Legal Concerns

Many questions have been raised about the legal situation of ethics committees, among them: Are records discoverable? Could committees or individual members be named in a lawsuit? Will liability insurance cover such eventuality? Could the committee increase the risk of liability in any way? Should the committee be a committee of the medical staff? Should patients be notified when they are discussed by the committee? What kinds of records should be kept? There are no definitive answers to most of these questions, although probable responses have been suggested, based on experience with other types of committees.[10]

We expect that courts will increasingly rely on recommendations from ethics committees and conversely, that fewer cases will be brought to court as individual practitioners rely on advice from ethics committees. Overall liability will decrease rather than increase, as ethics committees assist with good decision-making practices.

State statutes differ on the types of committees whose records are protected from discoverability and whose members are granted immunity. Generally, we think the question of whether to ensure non-discoverability for committee proceedings is much less important than ensuring that good records are kept. Minutes and other records[11] should demonstrate that choices were made after a thorough review of the facts and consideration of the ethical issues involved. Committees that are concerned about discoverability are organized as medical staff committees (at the present time, about half of them). Committees that are concerned about a more representative mix of members and more flexibility are organized as administrative or board committees.

It is likely that in the coming years there will be legislation requiring and/or protecting ethics committees. Although it may be too soon to consider such legislation, we expect it is ultimately inevitable. It will be important for ethics committees to stay on top of such proposals and develop written comments on them, preferably by networking with other committees. The cumulative experience of different ethics committees is of value in assessing the strengths and weaknesses of these committees. In addition, sharing experiences and insights will be helpful to the committees, and suggestions coming from a network should carry considerable weight with policymakers.

One of the issues, more ethical than legal in nature, that is increasingly debated is whether patients and/or families should be informed that their situation will be discussed with the ethics committee. At present, this is usually not done. We believe that, in order to honor patients' claims to confidentiality and to demonsntrate respect for patients, the presumption should be that notice will be given to patients whenever their case is reviewed by the committee. Should there be a decision not to notify the patient or family, committee members should be clear about why this choice was made.

The Future

Although the issues dealt with by ethics committees will continue to evolve primarily around individual treatment decisions, it is likely that members will become more interested in questions of social policy. Included are such concerns as providing health care to the medically indigent, trade-offs between preventive and high-technology care, and the allocation of resources.

Ethics committees may be looked to for guidance as allocation issues become more acute. This may happen either by their being drawn into choices about individual patients having access to treatment (for example, ICU beds or organ transplants) or by committees being asked to recommend policy to assist boards of directors in allocating resources. Involvement in patient selection is likely to be very controversial and may require a separate committee.

Ethics committee members have regularly indicated a great interest in learning about resource allocation issues but they are unsure of how they can apply this learning. Diagnosis-related groups (DRGs) may create ethical problems, but it is not obvious that ethics committees will have a major role in addressing those problems. Here again, providing education in the hospital about how financial issues create ethical problems may become the committees' most important role. If so, they will need to become more committed to education rather than consultation as their primary function.

It is also probable that, as the public becomes more aware of how it is affected by hospital policies, there will be greater lay representation on committees. Conversely, as more outsiders come to the committees, the committees will begin to move outside the hospital. We are already seeing networking and the sharing of expertise and resources among ethics committees within metropolitan areas and even within states. This is bound to increase. In addition, ethics committees will be sought after to provide greater public education and to create a bridge between hospitals and nursing homes with respect to the burgeoning ethical problems involved in geriatric care.

It appears to us that although there are many areas for improvement, the work of ethics committees has resulted in a positive difference in the institutions in which they function. Policies or guidelines now exist where before there was very little guidance; regular formal efforts to bring ethical issues to the attention of the hospital community are conducted; and the treatment of some patients has been improved as a result of committee discussions that clarified the ethical dimensions of clinical care. The committees are widely seen as a promising new undertaking, and enthusiasm about their potential value continues to be very strong. In fact, there is probably less criticism of ethics committees now than there was in the early 1980s.

Ethics committees have begun to alter the moral climate of institutions and break down some hierarchical barriers to acknowledge the values of patient, physician, nurse, others on the health care team, and society at large. More of this will happen in the long run. In the short run, committees continue to perform a critical function by virtue of their very existence: they are tangible evidence of an institution's concern with ethical issues in health care. Those who stay with this work will continue to grow in their own confidence and to teach others, both formally and informally. They may even surprise themselves as they realize how far down the path they have come, unclear though the way may have been at the beginning.

Notes

1. Among the professional associations that have endorsed institutional ethics committees are the American Medical Association, the American Hospital Association, the Catholic Hospital Association, the American Academy of Pediatrics, and several state hospital associations and medical societies.

2. Hospital ethics committees surveyed. *Hospitals* (1984 May 16.) 58(10): 52; Kalchbrenner, J., Kelly, M. J., and McCarthy, D. G. Ethics committees and ethicists in Catholic hospitals. *Hospital Progress* 1983 Sept. 64(9): 47–51.

3. See, for example, Cranford, R. E., and Doudera, A. E., editors. *Institutional Ethics Committees and Health Care Decision Making.* Ann Arbor, MI: Health Administration Press, 1984.

4. In the early 1980s, three functions of ethics committees were generally described. Recently, a fourth function is being suggested: retrospective case review.

5. See, especially, President's Commission for the Study of Ethical Problems in Medicine and Biomedical and Behavioral Research. *Deciding to Forego Life-Sustaining Treatment.* Washington, DC: U.S. Government Printing Office, 1983.

6. Purtillo, R. Ethics consultations in the hospital. *New England Journal of Medicine* 1984 Oct. 11. 311(15): 983–986.

7. A potential problem is that some physicians are more interested in ethics committees as a protection against liability than as a source of ethical insight.

8. The amendments were signed into law on October 9, 1984, as Public Law 98-457. The DHHS' final rule and model guidelines for infant care review committees are published in the *Federal Register.* April 15, 1985, pp. 14878–901.

9. Infant Bioethics Task Force and Consultants. Guidelines for infant bioethics committees. *Pediatrics.* 1984 Aug. 74(2): 306–310.

10. Cranford, R. E., Hester, F. A., and Ashley, B. Z. Institutional ethics committees: Issues of confidentiality and immunity. *Law, Medicine and Health Care.* 1985 Apr. 13(2): 52–60.

11. In addition to minutes, committees often prepare a separate record of patient care consultations and make notes on the chart.

Part 4

The Patient within the Hospital: Practice

In the end, the best ethical guide is experience. When waters are as thoroughly uncharted as those through which the hospital and patient must navigate these days—with each side being vulnerable to misjudgment, bad timing, knee-jerk thinking, and fear—perhaps the best we can hope for is to apply the lessons of the past within the context of societal, practical, legal, and clinical guidelines. Hospital and patient alike have wrestled with many of these issues before, no matter how much we would like to think that those who confront them today are pioneers.

Today, to be sure, the landscape is dotted with more mines. The law, once a stranger to such hospital activity, now often serves as the final arbiter in patient-provider conflicts, even to the point of dictating clinical decisions. Society, which in a democracy might have been expected to keep its distance from the individual patient's situation, has entered the hospital room because of fears that an individual patient, his or her family, or a provider may overstep the bounds of liberty and exercise license instead. For physicians, nurses, and other care givers, the once-simple charge of doing everything possible for the patient becomes an ethical nightmare when "everything possible" includes treatments, procedures, and decisions that may not, in fact, be in the patient's best interest. When the patient is incapable of rendering a judgment in such a situation because of unconsciousness or other impairment, determining what constitutes appropriate care becomes as much a guessing game as a clinical process.

It becomes even more important, then, to examine the footprints of those hospitals and patients that have gone before, whether they left us wisdom or foolishness from which to learn. In this section, George J. Annas, J.D., M.P.H., offers an impassioned defense of the patient's right to terminate treatment. This is based on the case of William Bartling, a patient who eventually was found to have been within his rights in requesting the termination of life support, despite the opposition of the hospital involved. Sharon H. Imbus, R.N., and Bruce E. Zawacki, M.D., in an article viewed as heretical by many at the time of its publication and now seen as a classic contribution to the debate, share the results of a program that offered autonomy to severely burned patients, long before it was in fashion to provide such options. Mitchell T. Rabkin, M.D., and his coauthors, in another article published before its time, discuss how a hospital can properly configure orders not to resuscitate a patient.

Confronting a more recent dilemma—the provision or withdrawal of food and water from an incompetent patient—Joanne Lynn, M.D., and James F. Childress, Ph.D., examine the special social meaning of nutrients, as opposed to other forms of sustaining life, and offer limited counsel on their use. Finally, Christine K. Cassel, M.D., and Andrew L. Jameton, Ph.D., bring us full circle by challenging the nature and purpose of health care. They ask, in effect, who decides what makes a patient worthy of care. By questioning the medical profession's unwillingness to confront the patient who cannot be "cured," as well as the values that drive medicine itself, they open a window to the future of health care and to the patients who will offer the next generation of ethical dilemmas and possible solutions.

Prisoner in the ICU: The Tragedy of William Bartling

George J. Annas, J.D., M.P.H., Boston University Schools of Medicine and Public Health, Boston

In June 1984, a California court sentenced William Bartling to spend the rest of his life in an intensive care unit. His crime seems to have been that he suffered from fatal diseases instead of "terminal" ones, and that his desire to live seemed at odds with his desire to have the mechanical ventilator that sustained his life removed. The case is important to all who are concerned with respecting the autonomy of patients in hospitals.

The case illustrates how fear of liability can cause a hospital to alter its traditional role of offering services to willing patients, into one of forcing treatment on unwilling patients. It also illustrates how physicians, hospital administrators, and even judges can see themselves as responsible for the actions of a competent patient, and how their ambivalence about the patient's decision can cause them to compromise or abdicate their social roles to the patient's profound detriment.

At the time of his current admission to the hospital, April 8, 1984, Mr. Bartling was seventy years old, had been in failing health for eight years, and had been admitted to the hospital six times in the previous year. He suffers from at least five potentially fatal diseases and disorders: chronic obstructive pulmonary emphysema, which severely restricts his ability to breathe; diffuse atherosclerotic cardiovascular disease (hardening of the arteries); obstructive arteriosclerosis of the coronary arteries; an abdominal aneurysm; and inoperable adenocarcinoma of the left lung.

His lung cancer was diagnosed by biopsy. During this arguably unnecessary procedure Mr. Bartling's lung collapsed, necessitating his prompt transfer to the Medical Intensive Care Unit, the insertion of a chest tube, and the use of a mechanical ventilator to sustain his breathing. The ventilator caused Mr. Bartling significant discomfort, distress, and pain; he repeatedly asked to have it removed, and on many occasions removed it himself. After a time, his hands were tied down to the sides of his bed by cloth cuffs to prevent further attempts to remove the ventilator.

Mr. Barling's attorney, Richard Scott, made arrangements with the hospital and doctors to have Mr. Bartling's wishes honored. His physician, according to Mr. Scott, had no objections to

Reprinted with permission from the author and *The Hastings Center Report* 1984 Dec. 14(6):28–29.
Professor Annas worked with Attorney Richard Scott on the Bartling case and prepared the appeals brief with him and Leonard Glantz.

this course of action and agreed to remove the ventilator if the hospital administrator concurred. The hospital administrator reportedly agreed so long as legal counsel for the hospital agreed also. Legal counsel did not.

Instead of doing what almost all hospitals do in such a situation—go to court to get a declaration of rights and immunity—the hospital took the position that it could not countenance the removal of Mr. Bartling's ventilator because he was neither "terminally ill" nor in a persistent vegetative state nor "brain dead." At this point the hospital took an adversarial position in regard to its patient; instead of seeking legal means to follow the patient's wishes, it sought to use the law to oppose them. Mr. Scott sought judicial relief.

The evening prior to the judicial hearing, Mr. Bartling's deposition was taken and videotaped in his intensive care room. In addition to the lawyers for each side, present in an adjoining room were Mike Wallace and his *60 Minutes* crew. The story they were filming was aired on September 23, 1984. Watchers of that telecast saw the entire deposition. Mr. Bartling's attorney asked him three questions (the ventilator was attached by tracheotomy so Mr. Bartling could only mouth words and shake his head to respond):

> "Do you want to live?" [Indicates yes] "Do you want to continue to live on the ventilator?" [Indicates no] "Do you understand that if the ventilator is discontinued or taken away, you might die?" [Indicates yes]

Brief cross-examination dwelt primarily on whether Mr. Bartling was satisfied with the nursing care. He was.

The hearing was held the next morning, June 22, before Los Angeles Superior Court judge Lawrence Waddington.[1] The judge opened the hearing by expressing his "tentative inclination." He characterized Mr. Bartling's prognosis for recovery as "guarded and cautious, but optimistic"; assumed "he is competent in the legal sense"; and viewed Bartling's request as one for a "mandatory injunction," that is, requiring the affirmative act of ending treatment. He noted that such injunctions were disfavored under California law, and said he could find no case from any jurisdiction where a person applying for injunctive relief was not terminally ill or "in a comatose, vegative or brain-dead state." On this basis he concluded that relief should not be granted.

Mr. Scott responded by noting several non-California cases, such as *Quinlan* and *Saikewicz*,[2] in which courts permitted the withdrawal or withholding of treatment for patients who were not terminal, comatose, or brain-dead. He argued that the key to the case was the patient's competence. If Mr. Bartling was legally competent (and there was no dispute on this point), his wishes had to be respected; the patient in charge of his own body is the "status quo," and that the court had an obligation to restore that: "It is the patient's decision. The doctors can recommend, but the patient must decide."

The judge then asked a number of questions, including one on competence, which led to this response: "He understands the nature and consequences of the act he proposes . . . He absolutely understands that if this ventilator is disconnected, there is a high chance that he would die. I asked him that. He nodded affirmatively . . ."

Finally, when it was clear that the judge would not order any physician to withdraw the ventilator, Mr. Scott asked him to order that Mr. Bartling's hands be untied.

Arguing for the hospital, William Ginsburg attempted to distinguish the previous cases by arguing that unlike them:

> Bartling eats ice cream. He watches L.A. Express games and Angels games. He communicates with nurses. And as Mr. Scott quite correctly states, he is very much with us . . .

But his most important comments were on the issue of competence. Although Mr. Ginsburg did not dispute Mr. Bartling's competence, he characterized his actions as indicating "ambivalence." Specifically, he contrasted "I don't want to die" with "I don't want to live on the respirator," arguing that these positions are inconsistent, and evidence of ambivalence. In his words, "I don't think he really fully spiritually or emotionally understands what it is he is talking about . . . There is a strong possibility that this man can be restored to useful life."

Mr. Scott responded that there was no ambivalence or vacillation:

> He would prefer to live, but he does not prefer to live with that illness and with the necessity of his every breath being sustained by a ventilator, by his trachea being suctioned every two hours around

the clock, confined to an ICU bed for the rest of his life, watching television and eating ice cream.

As for depression, Mr. Scott argued it was real and situational: his serious illnesses, his restraints in the ICU, the constant surveillance, and connection to a respirator all "give him very little cause to be cheerful." The judge was not persuaded, and so did not change his tentative decision, nor would he order that Mr. Bartling's hands be untied.

This is a good example of a case that should never have gone to court, and may even be an example of a case in which a functioning ethics committee could have proven helpful and decisive. For some reason the physician felt he could not act without the approval of the hospital administrator, and the hospital administrator felt, in turn, he could not act without the approval of his attorney. And the attorney, apparently, did not understand either the question put to him by the hospital or the law of California. While we may never know the whole story, since the physicians involved are not talking, it appears that fear of criminal liability for either homicide or assisting suicide led all of the actors involved to defer to others rather than defer to the patient.

According to briefs they filed with the trial court, for example, the hospital attorneys believed treatment refusal by a competent nonterminal individual was suicide if death would result, and potential murder for the physicians involved. These beliefs apparently were fostered by inability to distinguish *Bouvia*[3] or to understand *Barber*.[4] At the hearing Mr. Ginsburg insisted: "The issue of suicide has been raised in the *Bouvia* case . . . And if that wasn't enough, the issue of homicide, murder, was raised in the *Barber* case . . ." The analytical issue in the *Bartling* case is the inability to equate the morality and legality of stopping an ongoing activity with that of not starting the same activity.

Counsel for the hospital also had the non-California cases backwards and was able to at least confuse the judge about their relevance. Far from restricting the right to refuse treatment to comatose, totally incompetent, and brain-dead individuals, cases like *Quinlan* do the opposite: they hold that *even* comatose and incompetent patients must have a mechanism to refuse treatment *because* if they were competent, they would have that right, and to deny it to them simply because they could no longer personally exercise

it would devalue their lives. Likewise, although the California Natural Death Act limits its application to the terminally ill, this has never been a common law or constitutional limitation on the right to refuse treatment.[5] This argument, along with the "eating ice cream" argument, uses the fact that Mr. Bartling knows about his situation, and consciously suffers pain and despair, against him. We can only do this when we are more concerned with our own suffering than that of the patient.

Consistent with this view, the trial judge redefined the case as one in which *he* was being asked to order a physician to terminate Mr. Bartling's wanted life, not his unwanted treatment. Instead of seeing his role as protector of the liberty of an individual who was being held and treated against his will, the judge seemed to see himself as making a medical decision. Medically, the judge determined that Mr. Bartling's prognosis was "Optimistic" and that he was evidencing "ambivalence." The judge seems also to have redefined the legal issue of competence in the case into a medical one so that he would not have to take personal responsibility for a decision that might result in Mr. Bartling's death.

This case is a personal tragedy for William and Ruth Bartling; a dismal failure for physicians trying to administer humane care; and a disgrace for the judiciary. For the lawyers it is a throwback to the post-*Saikewicz* days in Massachusetts when lawyers instructed physicians that they could not write DNR orders or stop treating any patient unless court approval was sought and obtained. Such advice was legally inaccurate and resulted in immeasurable human suffering.

A similar situation exists in California today in a post-*Barber* era. Some physicians are convinced, although *Barber* holds exactly the opposite, that termination of treatment on a competent adult with that person's informed consent could be aiding suicide or murder. This position is indefensible as a matter of law, and attorneys who give their health care provider clients such advice should be held accountable for its foreseeable consequences on the lives of the patients of those clients. Unless lawyers are at risk for negligent, uninformed advice to doctors and hospitals, their incentive will often be to delay and take cases to court. Their clients will pay a high price in terms of transforming their social roles from serving patients to treating them against their wills; and patients will pay the ultimate price:

they will be forced by ambivalent judges "to bear the unbearable and tolerate the intolerable."[6]

NOTE: *Mr. Bartling died on November 6, while attached to the ventilator.*

References

1. Quotations in this article on the hearing are from the Transcript, *Bartling v. Glendale Adventist Medical Center*, Case No. C 500 735, June 22, 1984, Superior Court, Los Angeles, CA (Dept. 86, Waddington, J.).

2. George J. Annas, "Reconciling *Quinlan* and *Saikewicz*: Decision-making for the Incompetent Patient," *American Journal of Law and Medicine 3* (1979), 367.

3. George J. Annas, "When Suicide Prevention Becomes Brutality: The Case of Elizabeth Bouvia," *Hastings Center Report* (April 1984), p. 20.

4. George J. Annas, "Nonfeeding: Lawful Killing in California, Homicide in New Jersey," *Hastings Center Report* (December 1983), p. 19.

5. See George J. Annas and Joan E. Densberger, "Competence to Refuse Medical Treatment: Autonomy vs. Paternalism," *Toledo Law Review 15* (1984), 561.

6. *Foster v. Tourtellotte*, USDC No. CV 81-5046-RMT, Cent. Dist. CA (1981).

Autonomy for Burned Patients When Survival Is Unprecedented

Sharon H. Imbus, R.N., M.Sc., and **Bruce E. Zawacki, M.D.,** both Department of Surgery, Los Angeles County-University of Southern California Medical Center, Los Angeles

No burn is certainly fatal until the patient dies; the most severely burned patient may speak of hope with his last breath. Unable to prophesy, and unwilling to strip the patient of any hope he may cherish, we therefore prefer to diagnose burns as "fatal" or "hopeless" only in retrospect. Every year, however, several patients are admitted to our burn center with injuries so severe that survival is not only unexpected but, to our knowledge, unprecedented. Although difficult to face, the problems that these patients present must be anticipated and not simply ignored.

The surgical literature gives little attention to these patients except for brief phrases allowing an occasional glimpse into a particular surgeon's philosophy.[1-3] The literature on death and dying, voluminous since Kubler-Ross's work,[4] offers rich background but says little about the unique situation of our patients, who, after their injury, often have only a few hours of mental clarity in which to respond to their predicament. Several recent articles about withholding intensive care seem to ignore or incompletely answer the problem of obtaining the patient's informed consent. In some of these discussions, the authors simply assign to the physician what we believe to be the patient's ultimate right to decide whether he will or will not receive a particular form of therapy.[5-7] One suggests, perhaps unconstitutionally, that "certain competent patients" may be excluded from such decision making "when, in the physician's judgment, the patient will probably be unable to cope with it psychologically."[8] Still others, who recognize patient primacy in such decision making, offer no practical suggestion how it is best honored in practice.[9]

Our approach, developed empirically over several years, is based on our conviction that the decision to begin or to withhold maximal therapeutic effort is more of an ethical than a medical judgment. The physician and his colleagues on the burn-care team present to the patient the appropriate medical and statistical facts together with authoritative medical opinion about the available therapeutic alternatives and their consequences. Thus informed, the patient may give or withhold his consent to receive a particular form of therapy, but it is his own decision based on his value system, and it is arrived at before communication and competence are seriously impaired by intubation or altered states of consciousness.

Reprinted, with permission, from *The New England Journal of Medicine* 1977 Aug. 11. 297(6):308–311.

Definitions and Methods

The patient whose management this paper addresses is characterized by some combination of massive burns, severe smoke inhalation or advanced age. Such a patient's condition is designated by "1" on the Bull Mortality Probability Chart[10] and "0" in the National Burn Information Exchange Survival Analysis Diagrams," both indicating nonsurvival from the indexes of age and percentage of body-surface area burned. Furthermore, our staff members cannot, from their own experience, our burn-unit statistics, or references from the literature, recall survival in a similar patient.

To allow the patient maximal clarity of thought in decision making, several points must be communicated to the paramedic teams in the field and to local hospitals who transfer burned patients to our burn center immediately after injury: no administration of morphine or other narcotics before arrival; prompt fluid resuscitation; oxygen administration in treatment of possible carbon monoxide intoxication; avoidance of tracheostomy or endotracheal-tube insertion unless absolutely necessary to preserve the airway and maintain ventilation; and rapid transportation to the burn center.

Upon admission of a patient for whom survival seems in doubt, the burn center's most experienced physician is consulted, day or night, to evaluate the patient. His assessment, combined with a social and family history, is presented to all involved team members. Standard works are rechecked to determine if there has ever been a precedent for survival.

When the diagnosis is confirmed, the physician and other team members enter the room. Family members are not invited into the room to ensure that the decision of the patient is specifically his own. In an attempt to establish a relation with the patient, the attending physician or resident under his guidance tries to assume the role of a compassionate friend who is willing to listen. Hands are often held, and an effort is made to look deeply into the patient's eyes to perceive the unspoken questions that may lie there. Nonverbal cues are watched for closely. The presence of the burn team serves to witness and validate the patient's desires and requests, gives consensus to the gravity of the situation and supports the physician member of the team in this delicate, painful task.

At times, when the question of impending death does not spontaneously arise, suggestions such as "You are seriously ill", "You are sicker than you have ever been" or "Your life is in immediate danger" may be made, always in a caring, gentle way.

Some patients will not respond because of coma or mental incompetency. In those circumstances, the burn team and the family confer, again in a compassionate, concerned relation. All attempts are made to determine and do what the patient would be most likely to want if he were able to communicate.

A few patients will hear but not listen because of a need to deny their predicament. In general, such denials, if persistent, are considered an expression of a strong desire to live, and the patients are treated accordingly with maximal therapeutic effort.

A large majority of patients, however, understand the gravity of their situation and make further inquiries. The very frequent question—"Am I going to die?"—is answered truthfully by the statement, "We cannot predict the future. We can only say that, to our knowledge, no one in the past of your age and with your size of burn has ever survived this injury, either with or without maximal treatment." At this point, those who interpret this diagnosis of a burn without precedent of survival as an indication to avoid heroic measures typically become quite peaceful. Regularly, they then try to live their lives completely and fully to the end, saying things that they must say to those important to them, making proper plans, preparations and apologies and, in general, obtaining what Kavanaugh refers to as "permission to die."[12] These patients receive only ordinary medical measures and sufficient amounts of pain medication to assure comfort after their choice is made explicit. Fluid resuscitation is discontinued, they are admitted to a private room, and visiting hours become unlimited. An experienced nurse and, frequently, a chaplain are in constant attendance, using their expertise to comfort and sustain the patient and his family, chiefly by their continued presence and willingness to listen.

The patients who understand that survival is unprecedented in their case but, nevertheless, choose a maximal therapeutic effort are admitted to the burn intensive-care unit. Fluid resuscitation is continued, and full treatment measures are instituted, as with any other patient in the unit. As with those who choose only ordinary care, however, they may change their minds at any time; their decision is reviewed with them on a daily basis.

In general, when patients are mentally incompetent on admission because of head injury or inhalation injury or some other injury and may reasonably be expected to remain so indefinitely, the socially designated next of kin or other relatives are allowed to speak for the patient.[13] With children who are legally incompetent because of age, however, we have for the past five years been unwilling to declare any burn as being without precedent of survival, chiefly because mortality rates for very large burns in pediatric patients appear to be improving more rapidly than can be reported.

After interviewing the patient or his family, the physician is responsible for recording the salient points and decision in the patient's chart. Accurate documentation serves to clarify communication with other team members and avoids legal ambiguity.

"Postvention," described by Shneidman as "those activities which serve to reduce the aftereffects of a traumatic event in the lives of survivors,"[14] is now being evolved on our unit. Nurses are learning how to help survivors comfort each other and, together with the chaplain and social worker, are arranging for safe transportation of the bereaved to their homes, counseling families on the difficult matters of explaining death to children and explaining such points as legal necessity of an unwanted autopsy. Our hospital chaplain is available to conduct the funeral services if the family does not have its own pastor. He gets in touch with the families on the first anniversary of their loved one's death to answer any unfinished questions that may have been bothering them. The social worker also offers her continuing services to the bereaved.

Results

During 1975 and 1976 there were 748 dispositions from our burn center, excluding readmissions, transfers and nonthermal injuries. Of these patients 126 died—18 children and 108 adults. Of the adults who died, 24, or 22 percent, were diagnosed on admission as having injury without precedent of survival. Twenty-one of these patients or their families chose nonheroic or ordinary medical care. Only three chose full treatment measures, and their desires were fulfilled.

The following case histories illustrate our approach.

Cases 1 and 2

Two sisters, 68 and 70 years of age, and their husbands were searching for a schizophrenic daughter who had disappeared after her discharge from a psychiatric hospital. While their car waited for a stoplight, a nearby construction machine hit a gasoline line. The spraying gas exploded, leveling a city block and igniting the car.

The sisters arrived in our burn center two hours later. The younger sister had 91 percent full-thickness, 92 percent total-body burn, with moderate smoke inhalation; the older had 94.5 percent total-body burn, with moderate smoke inhalation; the older had 94.5 percent full-thickness, 95.5 percent total-body burn, with severe smoke inhalation. The burn team agreed that survival was unprecedented in both cases. Both women were alert and interviewed separately.

The younger sister asked about death directly, looking intently into the physician's eyes. When he answered, she replied matter-of-factly, "Well, I never dreamed that life would end like this, but since we all have to go sometime, I'd like to go quietly and comfortably. I don't know what to do about my daughter . . ."

After she was made comfortable, the nurse obtained a description of the missing daughter and possible whereabouts. The social worker alerted the police to look for her, and telephoned relatives, informing them of the accident as gently as could be conveyed by telephone. The husbands were located at another burn unit. An attempt was made to arrange a final spousal conversation, but both husbands were intubated.

Meanwhile, the older sister doubted whether her injuries were as serious as reported, "I feel so good, wouldn't I be hurting horribly if I were going to die?" The effect of full-thickness burns on nerve endings was explained. The physician reiterated that we wished to do what she thought was best for her. She hedged, "What did my sister say? I'll go along with her decision." Since the patient seemed unsure of her decision, she was offered full therapy in the room with her sister. She then refused the therapy adamantly but denied that she was dying.

The sisters' beds were placed next to each other so that they could see and touch each other easily. They discussed funeral arrangements and then joked, in the next breath, about the damage done to their hair. The hospital chaplain prayed with them. By active listening, he was able to convey to the older that her husband was not to blame for the accident as she had thought. "It's good to go out not cursing him after all our years to-gether," she said. The younger sister died several hours later after her sister lapsed ito a coma; the older died the next day. The daughter was not located.

Case 3

A 58-year-old man was cleaning his kitchen with an aerosol when the fumes were ignited by the stove pilot. He arrived at the hospital one hour later with a 97 per cent full-thickness burn, se-vere smoke inhalation and corneal abrasions. The team consensus that survival was unprecedented was unanimous. When the physicians talked with him, the man replied that he preferred his wife and her mother-in-law to decide for him. His wife and her mother, stunned and horrified by the accident, refused. Further conversation with the patient revealed that he wished to live by any and all means "until God is ready for me." In the burn intensive-care unit he required a tracheostomy and respirator. He continued to communicate, although imperfectly, by "writing" letters in the air. Despite an armamentarium of intensive nursing care, a caridac-out-put monitor, silver nitrate dressings, Swan-Ganz catheter, and intra-venous dopamine, he died three days later in septic shock.

Discussion

Unlike diseases such as uncontrolled cancer, the prognosis of burns without precedent of survival is evident almost immediately at the time of ad-mission, because the extent and severity of burn are easily recognized and rapidly quantifiable, and mortality statistics are more detailed and com-plete than for most other pathologic processes. Although such severe burns are rapid and even violent in onset, the patient is usually alert and mentally competent on admission and may re-main so for hours to a day after the burn—longer if aggressive fluid resuscitation is given. There is no way to predict the length of this lucid interval for a particular patient, but certainly there is lit-tle time for the patient to gain a gradual aware-ness of his condition or for the burn team sud-denly to acquire insight into the ethical issues involved.

The California Natural Death Act requires a 14-day waiting period after a "terminal" condi-tion is diagnosed and the appropriate document is signed and witnessed before a person's wish for nonheroic measures is legally binding. It is not applicable to these patients because death al-most always occurs before the waiting period has lapsed. The lack of specific legal guidelines, how-ever, does not negate the desirability of a planned and efficient approach.

The approach described above evolved slowly and unevenly through experience, interdisciplin-ary conferences and informal debate. Although medical factors were always involved, the final is-sues invariably proved to be primarily ethical and could be stated approximately by the question, "Which is better for this patient, maximal ther-apy or ordinary care, and upon whose value sys-tem should the judgment be based?"

As pointed out by Kubler-Ross, when a pa-tient is severely ill, he is often treated like a per-son with no right to an opinion.[4] Yet it is the pa-tient's life and rights that are at stake. Statistics may describe past experience with a given type of injury receiving maximal therapy or ordinary care; physicians may cite such an experience and are experts in carrying out programs of maximal therapy or ordinary care, but only the patient may choose between them because only he has the right to consent to one or the other.

Just as Lincoln stated that "No man is good enough to govern another man without that oth-er's consent,"[15] so no physician is so skilled that he may treat another without the other's con-sent.[16] If asked, the physician may offer his opin-ion about the choice, but it will be merely his per-sonal, inexpert opinion about whether it is better to accept death or fight to make history as the first survivor in such an injury.

Bioethicists Joseph Fletcher and Paul Ramsey, as interpreted by Robb,[17] urge that *agape* or un-selfish love for the patient and regard for his full stature as a person should be the criterion upon which we base our answers to bioethical ques-tions such as those posed above. When dealing with an alert, competent patient, we need not struggle against distractions and prejudice to imagine what the patient wants; we need only to ask. Who is more likely to be totally and lovingly concerned with the patient's best interest than the patient himself? Whenever in the past we as caregivers tried to decide these matters for the patient, issues such as what was best for the mo-rale of the nursing service, or for the solvency of the hospital, constantly clouded our judgment. It is for this reason that we oppose decision making by select committees convened "[to] explore what the best interest of the patient and his relatives require . . ." without necessarily asking or respecting the opinions of either.[5]

It took many months before we could shed a "we-know-best" defense and actually ask the patient what he wanted on admission when he was most competent to decide. Our approach seems obvious and right to us now; the first few times were agonizing. Our words seemed clumsy and awkward. If we had acted individually, without colleague support, the plan would probably have reverted rapidly to denial, or even worse, to a paternalistic decision making for the patient. Our patients and their families were able to see the human concern behind our first faltering phrases. Their warmth, gratitude and peace confirmed what we later read: that what we say to the patient, the exact words, matters less than how we say it in an atmosphere of honesty, caring and constant human presence.[18]

Weisman wrote, "The pervasive dread in dying seems not only to be the extinction of consciousness, but the fear that the death we die will not be our own. This is the singular distinction between death as a property of life and being put to death,"[19] We believe that on our burn unit, death for these patients has become a property of life. It would be hypocritical to imply that all life-and-death decision making or all "decisions not to resuscitate" are now straightforward and anxiety-free on our burn service. Many patients admitted with head injuries or inhalation injuries are confused or unconscious on admission and never regain competency. Initially competent patients with small but measurable chances of survival still tend to have complications and to become incompetent before we learn what they would want us to do in the event that continued therapy became more a prolongation of death than a prolongation of life. Turning to the family for decision making when death seems imminent for an incompetent patient is rarely satisfactory; guilt-ridden families often find it very difficult to be objective and unselfish in their decision making. The more voiceless and vulnerable the patient, the more easily we have found ourselves slipping into a paternalistic role, using terms such as "hopeless," which we realize now are so obviously prejudicial (literally, judging before the fact). Yet our experience continues to convince us that "truth is the greatest kindness." It seems inevitable that more and earlier communication with the patient will prove to be the most honest and compassionate answer to many of the remaining problems of ethical decision making in the intensive-care unit.

References

1. Jackson D M: The psychological effects of burns. Burns: 1:70–74, 1974

2. Muir I F K, Barclay T L: Burns and Their Treatment. Second edition. Chicago, Year Book Medical Publishers. 1974, p 110

3. Stone H H: The composite burn solution. Contemporary Burn Management. Edited by H C Polk Jr. H H Stone. Boston, Little, Brown, 1971, p 96

4. Kubler-Ross E: On Death and Dying. New York, Macmillan, 1969

5. Critical Care Committee of the Massachusetts General Hospital: Optimum care for hopelessly ill patients. N Engl J Med 295:362–364, 1976

6. Tagge G F, Adler D, Bryan-Brown C W, et al: Relationship of therapy to prognosis in critically ill patients. Crit Care Med 2:61–63, 1974

7. Skillman J J: Intensive Care. Boston, Little, Brown, 1975, p 21

8. Rabkin M T, Gillerman, G, Rice NR: Orders not to resuscitate. N. Engl J Med 295:364–366, 1976

9. Cassem N H: Confronting the decision to let death come. Crit Care Med 2:113–117, 1974

10. Bull J P: Revised analysis of mortality due to burns. Lancet 2:1133–1134, 1971

11. Feller I, Archembeault C: Nursing the Burned Patient. Ann Arbor, Institute for Burn Medicine, 1973, p 10

12. Kavanaugh R E: Facing Death. Los Angeles, Nash, 1972, p 67

13. Brody H: Ethical Decisions in Medicine. Boston, Little, Brown, 1976, p 98

14. Shneidman E: Death of Man. New York, NY Times Book Company, 1973, p 33

15. Lincoln Abraham. In Peoria, Illinois during Lincoln-Douglas debate on Oct. 16, 1854. Quoted in Bartlett J: Familar Quotations. Boston, Little, Brown, 1968, p 635a

16. Ramsey P: The Patient as Person. New Haven, Yale University Press, 1970, p 7

17. Robb J W: The Joseph Fletcher/Paul Ramsey debate in bioethics and the Christian ethical tradition. Religion in Life (in press)

18. Feifel H: Attitudes toward death in some normal and mentally ill populations, The Meaning of Death. Edited by H. Feifel. New York, McGraw-Hill, 1959, p 124.

19. Weisman A D: On Dying and Denying: A psychiatric study of terminality. New York, Behavioral Publications, 1972

Orders Not to Resuscitate

Mitchell T. Rabkin, M.D., Beth Israel Hospital, Boston
Gerald Gillerman, J.D., Widett, Slater & Goldman, Boston
Nancy R. Rice, J.D., Ropes & Gray, Boston

Medical opinions on the inappropriateness of cardiopulmonary resuscitation of certain patients are now openly discussed, as acknowledged by the New Jersey Supreme Court in its recent Quinlan decision. As early as 1974 the AMA proposed that decisions not to resuscitate be formally entered in patients' progress notes and communicated to all attending staff.[1] There has been little open discussion, however, of the process by which a decision not to resuscitate is formulated. Within a single institution, practices may vary among physicians, in part from the lack of a clearly articulated hospital policy.

An apparent need for hospital definitions of the process by which decisions not to resuscitate should be made led to the development of the following statement, which is proposed as a policy statement for hospitals concerned with regulating the process whereby Orders Not to Resuscitate may be cosidered and then implemented. It was developed by us out of discussions held over the past six months in the Law and Ethics Working Group of the Faculty Seminar on the Analysis of Health and Medical Practices, an activity of the Center for the Analysis of Health Practices of the Harvard School of Public Health. We are indebted to the other members of the Working Group for their useful and constructive criticism.

Having witnessed impressive medical developments over the past 25 years, the health-care community is now confronted with complex questions arising from interplay of two such developments, technologic advances and the increased emphasis on the patient's role in decisions cocerning his own health care. There is a growing concern that it may be inappropriate to apply technologic capabilities to the fullest extent in all cases and without limitation. Moreover, increased awareness of the rights of patients to be treated in accordance with their own decisions and expectations means that the use of heroic measures to sustain life can be justified only by adherence to the dictates of both sound medical practice and the patient's right to elect or decline the benefits of medical technology.

Both as a standard of medical care and as a statement of philosophy, it is the general policy of hospitals to act affirmatively to preserve the life of all patients, including persons who suffer from irreversible terminal illness. It is essential

Reprinted, with permission, from *The New England Journal of Medicine* 1976 Aug. 12. 295(7): 364–366.

that all hospital staff understand this policy and act accordingly.

As a matter of policy hospitals also respect the competent patient's informed acceptance or rejection of treatment, including cardiopulmonary resuscitation, and recognize that in certain cases, the unwanted use of heroic measures on a patient irreversibly and irreparably terminally ill might be both medically unsound and so contrary to the patient's wishes or expectations as not to be justified.

To ensure adherence to each of these policies, we have prepared this statement to guide a hospital in the process of decision making regarding the use of cardiopulmonry resuscitation.

Notwithstanding the hospital's pro-life policy, the right of a patient to decline available medical procedures must be respected. For example, if a competent patient who is not irreversibly and irreparably ill issues instructions that under stated circumstances, he is opposed to the use of certain procedures, the following guidelines should be observed. The physician should explore thoroughly with the patient the types of circumstances that might arise, and warn that the consequences of a generalized prohibition may be to allow an unintended termination of life. If after a careful disclosure the patient persists in some form of order declining use of certain medical procedures when otherwise applicable, the physician is legally required to respect such instructions. Such situations are not unknown to hospitals that have treated Jehovah's Witnesses and other persons with fixed opinions unlikely to be affected by unforeseen medical exigencies. If the physician finds the medical program as ordered by the patient so inconsistent with his own medical judgment as to be incompatible with his continuing as the responsible physician, he may attempt to transfer the care of the patient to another physician more sympathetic to the patient's desires.

The specific issue of the appropriateness of cardiopulmonary resuscitation arises frequently with the irreversibly, irreparably ill patient whose death is imminent. We refer to the medical circumstance in which the disease is "irreversible" in the sense that no known therapeutic measures can be effective in reversing the course of illness; the physiologic status of the patient is "irreparable" in the sense that the course of illness has progressed beyond the capacity of existing knowledge and technic to stem the process; and when death is "imminent" in the sense that in the ordinary course of events, death probably will occur within a period not exceeding two weeks.

When it appears that a patient is irreversibly and irreparably ill, and that death is imminent, the question of the appropriateness of cardiopulmonary resuscitation in the event of sudden cessation of vital functions may be considered by the patient's physician, if not already raised by the patient, to avoid an unnecessary abuse of the patient's presumed reliance on the physician and hospital for cotinued life-supporting care. The initial medical judgment on such question should be made by the primarily responsible physician for the patient after discussion with an ad hoc committee consisting not only of the other physicians attending the patient and the nurses and others directly active in the care of the patient, but at least one other senior staff physician not previously involved in the patient's care. The inquiry should focus on whether the patient's death is so certain and so imminent that resuscitation in the event of sudden cessation of vital fuctions would serve no purpose. Although the unanimous opinion of the ad hoc committee in support of the decision of the responsible physician is not necessarily required (for some may be uncertain), a strongly held dissenting view not negated by other staff members should generally dissuade the responsible physician from his or her initial judgment on the appropriteness of resuscitation efforts.

Even if a medical judgment is reached that a patient is faced with such an illness and imminence of death that resuscitation is medically inappropriate, the decision to withhold resuscitation (Orders Not to Resuscitate, "ONTR") will become effective only upon the informed choice of a competent patient or, with an incompetent patient, by strict adherence to the guidelines discussed below, and then only to the extent that all appropriate family members are in agreement with the views of the involved staff. In this context, "appropriate" means at least the family members who would be consulted for permission to perform a post-mortem examination if the patient died.

"Competence" in this context is not to be restricted to the legal and medical tests to determine compretence to stand trial or to form a criminal intent. For the purpose of making an informed choice of medical treatment, "competence" is understood to rest on the test of whether the patient understands the relevant risks and alternatives, and whether the resulting decision reflects a deliberate choice by the patient. Caution should be exercised that a patient does not unwittingly "consent" to an ONTR, as a result of temporary distortion (for example, from pain, medication or metabolic abnormality) in his ability to choose among available alternatives.

It is recognized that it may be inappropriate to introduce the subject of withholding cardiopulmonary resuscitation efforts to certain competent patients when, in the physician's judgment, the patient will probably be unable to cope with it psychologically. In such event, Orders Not to Resuscitate may not be directed because of the absence of an informed choice. Appropriate family members should be so informed, and the physician should explain the course that will thus follow in the event of sudden cessation of the patient's vital functions. This discussion with the family should be noted by the physician in the medical record. If, however, the physician is able to discuss the essential elements of the case with a competent patient without violating the principles of reasonable and humane medical practice, a valid consent may follow.

If the competent patient thus chooses the ONTR alternative, this is his choice, and it may not be overridden by contrary views of family members. Nevertheless, it is important to inform the family members of the patient's decision (with the patient's permission and in accordance with his directions) so that the failure to resuscitate or to take other heroic measures is not unanticipated. In any event, the decision should be documented by the responsible physician and at least one witness. Such decisions shall remain in effect if the patient subsequently becomes incompetent and if the clinical circumstances for Orders Not to Resuscitate otherwise remain in existence.

Minors who are not emancipated by state law will be deemed incompetent to make a decision not to resuscitate. Such persons, however, will be kept informed if such a communication is appropriate, and have the right to reject a decision not to resuscitate, despite their presumed incompetence.

If a patient is incompetent, he should not be denied the benefits of the evaluation process described above. The physician and the ad hoc committee will consider initially whether the conditions of irreversibility, irreparability and imminence of death are satisfied in their opinion. The basis for a final decision for Orders Not to Resuscitate must be concern from the patient's point of view, and not that of some other person who might present what he regards as sufficient reasons for not resuscitating the patient. It is only the clinical interest of the patient that must be considered; consideration of other factors would violate the fundamental policy of the hospital. An additional condition for the issuance of Orders Not to Resuscitate for an incompetent patient is approval of at least the same family members who are required to consent to postmortem examination. Failure to obtain and record family approval of Orders Not to Resuscitate may expose those involved to charges of negligent or unlawful conduct. Thus, the failure to obtain such approval would foreclose further consideration of Orders Not to Resuscitate in cases in which the patient is incompetent.

To prevent any uncertainty or confusion over the status of a patient's treatment, the decision for Orders Not to Resuscitate and its accompanying consent by the competent patient or the appropriate family members should be recorded promptly in the medical chart. In addition to the formal consent, the written and dated record must include the following: a summary of the staff discussion and decision; the disclosures to the patient, which must include the elements of informed consent, the patient's response, the responsible physician's documentation of the patient's competence, the patient's decision to inform appropriate family members and the resulting discussion with them that may then follow. Each hospital must specify what it deems to be the elements of informed consent and the formats in which consent must be witnessed and documented. Whether or not the patient's signature must be required invariably should also be decided; the signature removes ambiguity, but the physical act of signing may be deemed unpalatable by certain patients and therefore unacceptable to them as a necessary or appropriate formalization of the meaningful discussion and their resulting verbal consent.

It is the responsibility of the physician to convey the meaning of the Orders Not to Resuscitate to all medical, nursing and other staff as appropriate, and simultaneously, to insist upon being notified immediately if the patient's condition should change so that the orders seem no longer applicable. If the circumstances described to such a patient do not change, a subsequent resuscitation would constitute treatment without consent.

After the issuing of Orders Not to Resuscitate, the patient's course, including continued evaluation of competence and consent, must be reviewed by the responsible physician at least daily, or at more frequent intervals, if appropriate, and documentation made in the medical chart to determine the continued applicability of such orders. If the patient's condition alters in such a way that the orders are no longer deemed applicable, the Orders Not to Resuscitate must be revoked, and the revocation communicated without delay.

Nothing in the entire procedure leading to Orders Not to Resuscitate, nor the ONTR itself, should indicate to the medical and nursing staff or to the patient and family any intention to diminish the appropriate medical and nursing attention to be received by the patient. It is the responsibility of the physician in charge to be certain that no diminution of necessary and appropriate measures for the patient's care and comfort follows from this decision.

When the incompetent patient is sufficiently alert to appreciate at least some aspects of the care he is receiving (the benefit of doubt must always assign to the patient the likelihood of at least partial alertness or receptivity to verbal stimuli), and especially with a child, whose "incompetence" by legal definition may not be supported by clinical observation, every effort must be made to provide the comfort and reassurance appropriate to the patient's state of consciousness and emotional condition regardless of the designation of incompetence.

In every case in which Orders Not to Resuscitate are issued, the hospital shall make available to the greatest extent practicable resources to provide counseling, reassurance, consolation and other emotional support as appropriate, for the patient's family and for all involved hospital staff, as well as for the patient.

Occasionally, a proposal for Orders Not to Resuscitate may be initiated by family members. It is essential to recognize that a family member's instructions not to resusciate are not to be viewed as the choice of the patient. Thus, the attending physician and the ad hoc committee must not simply concur in the Orders Not to Resuscitate suggested by the family, but such concurrences shall be forthcoming only upon the timing and conditions described above.

Reference

1. Standards for cardiopulmonary resuscitation (CPR) and emergency cardiac care (ECC). V. Medicolegal considerations and recommendations. *Journal of the American Medical Association.* 1974 227(Suppl):864–866.

Must Patients Always Be Given Food and Water?

Joanne Lynn, M.D., Division of Geriatric Medicine, George Washington University Medical Center, Washington, D.C.
James F. Childress, Ph.D., Departments of Religious Studies and Medical Education, University of Virginia, Charlottesville

Many people die from the lack of food or water. For some, this lack is the result of poverty or famine, but for others it is the result of disease or deliberate decision. In the past, malnutrition and dehydration must have accompanied nearly every death that followed an illness of more than a few days. Most dying patients do not eat much on their own, and nothing could be done for them until the first flexible tubing for instilling food or other liquid into the stomach was developed about a hundred years ago. Even then, the procedure was so scarce, so costly in physician and nursing time, and so poorly tolerated that it was used only for patients who clearly could benefit. With the advent of more reliable and efficient procedures in the past few decades, these conditions can be corrected or ameliorated in nearly every patient who would otherwise be malnourished or dehydrated. In fact, intravenous lines and nasogastric tubes have become common images of hospital care.

Providing adequate nutrition and fluids is a high priority for most patients, both because they suffer directly from inadequacies and because these deficiencies hinder their ability to overcomes other diseases. But are there some patients who need not receive these treatments? This question has become a prominent public policy issue in a number of recent cases. In May 1981, in Danville, Illinois, the parents and the physician of newborn conjoined twins with shared abdominal organs decided not to feed these children. Feeding and other treatments were given after court intervention, though a grand jury refused to indict the parents.[1] Later that year, two physicians in Los Angeles discontinued intravenous nutrition to a patient who had severe brain damage after an episode involving loss of oxygen following routine surgery. Murder charges were brought, but the hearing judge dismissed the charges at a preliminary hearing. On appeal, the charges were reinstated and remanded for trial.[2]

In April 1982, a Bloomington, Indiana, infant who had tracheoesophageal fistula and Down syndrome was not treated or fed, and he died after two courts ruled that the decision was proper but before all appeals could be heard.[3] When the federal government then moved to ensure that such infants would be fed in the future,[4] the Surgeon General, Dr. C. Everett Koop, initially stated that there is never adequate reason to deny nutrition and fluids to a newborn infant.

While these cases were before the public, the nephew of Clair Conroy, an elderly incompetent

Reprinted, with permission, from the author and *The Hastings Center Report* 1983 Oct. 13(5):17–21.

217

woman with several serious medical problems, petitioned a New Jersey court for authority to discontinue her nasogastric tube feedings. Although the intermediate appeals court has reversed the ruling,[5] the trial court held that he had this authority since the evidence indicated that the patient would not have wanted such treatment and that its value to her was doubtful.

In all these dramatic cases and in many more that go unnoticed, the decision is made to deliberately withhold food or fluid known to be necessary for the life of the patient. Such decisions are unsettling. There is now widespread consensus that sometimes a patient is best served by not undertaking or continuing certain treatments that would sustain life, especially if these entail substantial suffering.[6] But food and water are so central to an array of human emotions that it is almost impossible to consider them with the same emotional detachment that one might feel toward a respirator or a dialysis machine.

Nevertheless, the question remains: should it ever be permissible to withhold or withdraw food and nutrition? The answer in any real case should acknowledge the psyhological contiguity between feeding and loving and between nutritional satisfaction and emotional satisfaction. Yet this acknowledgment does not resolve the core question.

Some have held that it is intrinsically wrong not to feed another. The philosopher G.E.M. Anscombe contends: "For willful starvation there can be no excuse. The same can't be said quite without qualification about failing to operate or to adopt some courses of treatment."[7] But the moral issues are more complex than Anscombe's comment suggests. Does correcting nutritional deficiencies always improve patients' well-being? What should be our reflective moral response to withholding or withdrawing nutrition? What moral principles are relevant to our reflections? What medical facts about ways of providing nutrition are relevant? And what policies should be adopted by the society, hospitals, and medical and other health care professionals?

In our effort to find answers to these questions, we will concentrate upon the care of patients who are incompetent to make choices for themselves. Patients who are competent to determine the course of their therapy may refuse any and all interventions proposed by others, as long as their refusals do not seriously harm or impose unfair burdens upon others.[8] A competent patient's decision regarding whether or not to accept the provision of food and water by medical means such as tube feeding or intravenous alimentation is unlikely to raise questions of harm or burden to others.

What then should guide those who must decide about nutrition for a patient who cannot decide? As a start, consider the standard by which other medical decisions are made: one should decide as the incompetent person would have if he or she were competent, when that is possible to determine, and advance that person's interests in a more generalized sense when individual preferences cannot be known.

The Medical Procedures

There is no reason to apply a different standard to feeding and hydration. Surely, when one inserts a feeding tube, or creates a gastrostomy opening, or inserts a needle into a vein, one intends to benefit the patient. Ideally, one should provide what the patient believes to be of benefit, but at least the effect should be beneficial in the opinions of surrogates and caregivers.

Thus, the question becomes: is it ever in the patient's interest to become malnourished and dehydrated, rather than to receive treatment? Posing the question so starkly points to our need to know what is entailed in treating these conditions and what benefits the treatments offer.

The medical interventions that provide food and fluids are of two basic types. First, liquids can be delivered by a tube that is inserted into a functioning gastrointestinal tract, most commonly through the nose and esophagus into the stomach or through a surgical incision in the abdominal wall and directly into the stomach. The liquids used can be specially prepared solutions of nutrients or a blenderized version of an ordinary diet. The nasogastric tube is cheap; it may lead to pneumonia and often annoys the patient and family, sometimes even requiring that the patient be restrained to prevent its removal.

Creating a gastrostomy is usually a simple surgical procedure, and, once the wound is healed, care is very simple. Since it is out of sight, it is aesthetically more acceptable and restraints are needed less often. Also, the gastrostomy creates no additional risk of pneumonia. However, while elimination of a nasogastric tube requires only removing the tube, a gastrostomy is fairly permanent, and can be closed only by surgery.

The second type of medical intervention is intravenous feeding and hydration, which also has two major forms. The ordinary hospital or peripheral IV, in which fluid is delivered directly to the bloodstream through a small needle, is useful only for temporary efforts to improve hydration and electrolyte concentrations. One cannot provide a balanced diet through the veins in the limbs: to do that requires a central line, or a special catheter placed into one of the major veins in the chest. The latter procedure is much more risky and vulnerable to infections and technical errors, and it is much more costly than any of the other procedures. Both forms of intravenous nutrition and hydration commonly require restraining the patient, cause minor infections and other ill effects, and are costly, especially since they ordinarily require the patient to be in a hospital.

None of these procedures, then, is ideal: each entails some distress, some medical limitations, and some costs. When may a procedure be foregone that might improve nutrition and hydration for a given patient? Only when the procedure and the resulting improvement in nutrition and hydration do not offer the patient a net benefit over what he or she would otherwise have faced.

Are there such circumstances? We believe that there are; but they are few and limited to the following three kinds of situations: 1. The procedures that would be required are so unlikely to achieve improved nutritional and fluid levels that they could be correctly considered futile; 2. The improvement in nutritional and fluid balance, though achievable, could be of no benefit to the patient; 3. The burdens of receiving the treatment may outweigh the benefit.

When Food and Water May Be Withheld

Futile Treatment

Sometimes even providing "food and water" to a patient becomes a momumental task. Consider a patient with a severe clotting deficiency and a nearly total body burn. Gaining access to the central veins is likely to cause hemorrhage or infection, nasogastric tube placement may be quite painful, and there may be no skin to which to suture the stomach for a gastrostomy tube. Or consider a patient with severe congestive heart failure who develops cancer of the stomach with a fistula that delivers food from the stomach to the colon without passing through the intestine

and being absorbed. Feeding the patient may be possible, but little is absorbed. Intravenous feeding cannot be tolerated because the fluid would be too much for the weakened heart. Or consider the infant with infarction of all but a short segment of bowel. Again, the infant can be fed, but little if anything is absorbed. Intravenous methods can be used, but only for a short time (weeks or months) until their complications, including thrombosis, hemorrhage, infections, and malnutrition, cause death.

In these circumstances, the patient is going to die soon, no matter what is done. The ineffective efforts to provide nutrition and hydration may well directly cause suffering that offers no counterbalancing benefit for the patient. Although the procedures might be tried, especially if the competent patient wanted them or the incompetent patient's surrogate had reason to believe that this incompetent patient would have wanted them, they cannot be considered obligatory. To hold that a patient must be subjected to this predictably futile sort of intervention just because protein balance is negative or the blood serum is concentrated is to lose sight of the moral warrant for medical care and to reduce the patient to an array of measurable variables.

No Possibility of Benefit

Some patients can be reliably diagnosed to have permanently lost consciousness. This unusual group of patients includes those with anencephaly, persistent vegative state, and some preterminal comas. In these cases, it is very difficult to discern how any medical intervention can benefit or harm the patient. These patients cannot and never will be able to experience any of the events occurring in the world or in their bodies. When the diagnosis is exceedingly clear, we sustain their lives vigorously mainly for their loved ones and the community at large.

While these considerations probably indicate that continued artificial feeding is best in most cases, there may be some cases in which the family and the caregivers are convinced that artificial feeding is offensive and unreasonable. In such cases, there seems to be no adequate reason to claim that withholding food and water violates any obligations that these parties or the general society have with regard to permanently unconscious patients. Thus, if the parents of an anencephalic infant or of a patient like Karen Quinlan in a persistent vegetative state feel strongly that no medical procedures should be applied to provide nutrition and hydration, and the caregivers are willing to comply, there should be no barrier in law or public policy to thwart the plan.[9]

Disproportionate Burden

The most difficult cases are those in which normal nutritional status or fluid balance could be restored, but only with a severe burden for the patient. In these cases, the treatment is futile in a broader sense—the patient will not actually benefit from the improved nutrition and hydration. A patient who is competent can decide the relative merits of the treatment being provided, knowing the probable consequences, and weighing the merits of life under various sets of constrained circumstances. But a surrogate decision maker for a patient who is incompetent to decide will have a difficult task. When the situation is irremediably ambiguous, erring on the side of continued life and improved nutrition and hydration seems the less grievous error. But are there situations that would warrant a determination that this patient, whose nutrition and hydration could surely be improved, is not thereby well served?

Though they are rare, we believe there are such cases. The treatments entailed are not benign. Their effects are far short of ideal. Furthermore, many of the patients most likely to have inadequate food and fluid intake are also likely to suffer the most serious side effects of these therapies.

Patients who are allowed to die without artificial hydration and nutrition may well die more comfortably than patients who receive conventional amounts of intravenous hydration.[10] Terminal pulmonry edema, nausea, and mental confusion are more likely when patients have been treated to maintain fluid and nutrition until close to the time of death.

Thus, those patients whose "need" for artificial nutrition and hydration arises only near the time of death may be harmed by its provision. It is not at all clear that they receive any benefit in having a slightly prolonged life, and it does seem reasonable to allow a surrogate to decide that, for this patient at this time, slight prolongation of life is not warranted if it involves measures that will probably increase the patient's suffering as he or she dies.

Even patients who might live much longer might not be well served by artificial means to provide fluid and food. Such patients might include those with fairly severe dementia for whom the restraints required could be a constant source of fear, discomfort, and struggle. For such a patient, sedation to tolerate the feeding mechanisms might preclude any of the pleasant experiences that might otherwise have been available. Thus, a decision not to intervene, except perhaps briefly to ascertain that there are no treatable causes, might allow such a patient to live out a shorter life with fair freedom of movement and freedom from fear, while a decision to maintain artificial nutrition and hydration might consign the patient to end his or her life in unremitting anguish. If this were the case a surrogate decision maker would seem to be well justified in refusing the treatment.

Inappropriate Moral Constraints

Four considerations are frequently proposed as moral contraints on foregoing medical feeding and hydration. We find none of these to dictate that artificial nutrition and hydration must always be provided.

The Obligation to Provide "Ordinary" Care

Debates about appropriate medical treatment are often couched in terms of "ordinary" and "extraordinary" means of treatment. Historically, this distinction emerged in the Roman Catholic tradition to differentiate optional treatment from treatment that was obligatory for medical professionals to offer and for patients to accept.[11] These terms also appear in many secular contexts, such as court decisions and medical codes. The recent debates about ordinary and extraordinary means of treatment have been interminable and often unfruitful, in part because of a lack of clarity about what the terms mean. Do they represent the premises of an argument or the conclusion, and what features of a situation are relevant to the categorization as "ordinary" or "extraordinary"?[12]

Several criteria have been implicit in debates about ordinary and extraordinary means of treatment; some of them may be relevant to determining whether and which treatments are obligatory and which are optional. Treatments have been distinguished according to their simplicity (simple/complex), their naturalness (natural/artificial), their customariness (usual/unusual), their invasiveness (noninvasive/invasive), their chance of success (reasonable chance/futile), their balance of benefits and burdens (pro-portionate/disproportionate), and their expense (inexpensive/costly). Each set of paired terms or phrases in the parentheses suggests a continuum: as the treatment moves from the first of the paired terms to the second, it is said to become less obligatory and more optional.

However, when these various criteria, widely used in discussions about medical treatment, are carefully examined, most of them are not morally relevant in distinguishing optional from obligatory medical treatments. For example, if a rare, complex, artificial, and invasive treatment offers a patient a reasonable chance of nearly painless cure, then one would have to offer a substantial justification not to provide that treatment to an incompetent patient.

What matters, then, in determining whether to provide a treatment to an incompetent patient is not a prior determination that this treatment is "ordinary" per se, but rather a determination that this treatment is likely to provide this patient benefits that are sufficient to make it worthwhile to endure the burdens that accompany the treatment. To this end, some of the considerations listed above are relevant: whether a treatment is likely to succeed is an obvious example. But such considerations taken in isolation are not conclusive. Rather, the surrogate decision maker is obliged to assess the desirability to this patient of each of the options presented, including non-treatment. For most people at most times, this assessment would lead to a clear obligation to provide food and fluids.

But sometimes, as we have indicated, providing food and fluids through medical interventions may fail to benefit and may even harm some patients. Then the treatment cannot be said to be obligatory, no matter how usual and simple its provision may be. If "ordinary" and "extraordinary" are used to convey the conclusion about the obligation to treat, providing nutrition and fluids would have become, in these cases, "extraordinary." Since this phrasing is misleading, it is probably better to use "proportionate" and "disproportionate," as the Vatican now suggests,[13] or "obligatory" and "optional."

Obviously, providing nutrition and hydration may sometimes be necessary to keep patients comfortable while they are dying even though it may temporarily prolong their dying. In such cases, food and fluids constitute warranted palliative care. But in other cases, such as a patient in a deep and irreversible coma, nutrition and hydration do not appear to be needed or helpful, except perhaps to comfort the staff and family.[14] And sometimes the interventions needed for nutrition and hydration are so burdensome that they are harmful and best not utilized.

The Obligation to Continue Treatments Once Started

Once having started a mode of treatment, many caregivers find it very difficult to discontinue it. While this strongly felt difference between the ease of withholding a treatment and the difficulty of withdrawing it provides a psychological explanation of certain actions, it does not justify them. It sometimes even leads to a thoroughly irrational decision process. For example, in caring for a dying, comatose patient, many physicians apparently find it harder to stop a functioning peripheral IV than not to restart one that has infiltrated (that is, has broken through the blood vessel and is leaking fluid into surrounding tissue), especially if the only way to reestablish an IV would be to insert a central line into the heart or to do a cutdown (make an incision to gain access to the deep large blood vessels).[15]

What factors might make withdrawing medical treatment morally worse than withholding it? Withdrawing a treatment seems to be an action, which, when it is likely to end in death, initially seems more serious than an omission that ends in death. However, this view is fraught with errors. Withdrawing is not always an act: failing to put the next infusion into a tube could be correctly described as an omission, for example. Even when withdrawing is an act, it may well be morally correct and even morally obligatory. Discontinuing intravenous lines in a patient now permanently unconscious in accord with the patient's well-informed advance directive would certainly be such a case. Furthermore, the caregiver's obligation to serve the patient's interests through both acts and omissions rules out the exculpation that accompanies omissions in the usual course of social life. An omission that is not warranted by the patient's interests is culpable.

Sometimes initiating a treatment creates expectations in the minds of caregivers, patients, and family that the treatment will be continued indefinitely or until the patient is cured. Such expectations may provide a reason to continue the treatment as a way to keep a promise. However, as with all promises, caregivers could be very careful when initiating a treatment to explain the indications for its discontinuation, and they could modify preconceptions with continuing reevaluation and education during treatment. Though all patients are entitled to expect the continuation of care in the patient's best interests, they are not and should not be entitled to the continuation of a particular mode of care.

Accepting the distinction between withholding and withdrawing medical treatment as morally significant also has a very unfortunate implication: caregivers may become unduly reluctant to begin some treatments precisely because they fear that they will be locked into continuing treatments that are no longer of value to the patient. For example, the physician who had been unwilling to stop the respirator while the infant, Andrew Stinson, died over several months is reportedly "less eager to attach babies to respirators now."[16] But if it were easier to ignore malnutrition and dehydration and to withhold treatments for these problems than to discontinue the same treatments when they have become especially burdensome and insufficiently beneficial for this patient, then the incentives would be perverse. Once a treatment has been tried, it is often much clearer whether it is of value to this patient, and the decision to stop it can be made more reliably.

The same considerations should apply to starting as to stopping a treatment, and whatever assessment warrants withholding should also warrant withdrawing.

The Obligation to Avoid Being the Unambiguous Cause of Death

Many physicians will agree with all that we have said and still refuse to allow a choice to forego food and fluid because such a course seems to be a "death sentence." In this view death seems to be more certain from malnutrition and dehydration than from foregoing other forms of medical therapy. This implies that it is acceptable to act in ways that are likely to cause death, as in not operating on a gangrenous leg, only if there remains a chance that the patient will survive. This is a comforting formulation for caregivers, to be sure, since they can thereby avoid feeling the full weight of the responsibility for the time and manner of a patient's death. However, it is not a persuasive moral argument.

First, in appropriate cases discontinuing certain medical treatments is generally accepted despite the fact that death is as certain as with nonfeeding. Dialysis in a patient without kidney function or transfusions in a patient with severe aplastic anemia are obvious examples. The dying that awaits such patients often is not greatly different from dying of dehydration and malnutrition.

Second, the certainty of a generally undesirable outcome such as death is always relevant to a decision, but it does not foreclose the possibility that this course is better than others available to this patient.[17] Ambiguity and uncertainty are so common in medical decision making that caregivers are tempted to use them in distancing themselves from direct responsibility. However, caregivers are in fact responsible for the time and manner of death for many patients. Their distaste for this fact should not constrain otherwise morally justified decisions.

The Obligation to Provide Symbolically Significant Treatment

One of the most common arguments for always providing nutrition and hydration is that it symbolizes, expresses, or conveys the essence of care and compassion. Some actions not only aim at goals, they also express values. Such expressive actions should not simply be viewed as means to ends; they should also be viewed in light of what they communicate. From this perspective food and water are not only goods that preserve life and provide comfort; they are also symbols of care and compassion. To withhold or withdraw them—to "starve" a patient—can never express or convey care.

Why is providing food and water a central symbol of care and compassion? Feeding is the first response of the community to the needs of newborns and remains a central mode of nurture and comfort. Eating is associated with social interchange and community, and providing food for someone else is a way to create and maintain bonds of sharing and expressing concern. Furthermore, even the relatively low levels of hunger and thirst that most people have experienced are decidedly uncomfortable, and the common image of severe malnutrition or dehydration is one of unremitting agony. Thus, people are rightly eager to provide food and water. Such provision is essential to minimally tolerable existence and a powerful symbol of our concern for each other.

However, *medical* nutrition and hydration, we have argued, may not always provide net benefits to patients. Medical procedures to provide nutrition and hydration are more similar to other medical procedures than to typical human ways of providing nutrition and hydration, for example, a sip of water. It should be possible to evaluate their benefits and burdens, as we evaluate any other medical procedure. Of course, if family, friends, and caregivers feel that such procedures affirm important values even when they do not benefit the patient, their feelings should not be ignored. We do not contend that there is an obligation to withhold or to withdraw such procedures (unless consideration of the patient's advance directives or current best interest unambiguously dictates that conclusion); we only contend that nutrition and hydration may be foregone in some cases.

The symbolic connection between care and nutrition or hydration adds useful caution to decision making. If decision makers worry over withholding or withdrawing medical nutrition and hydration, they may inquire more seriously into the circumstances that putatively justify their decisions. This is generally salutary for health care decision making. The critical inquiry may well yield the sad but justified conclusion that the patient will be served best by not using medical procedures to provide food and fluids.

A Limited Conclusion

Our conclusion—that patients or their surrogates, in close collaboration with their physicians and other caregivers and with careful assessment of the relevant information, can correctly decide to forego the provision of medical treatments intended to correct malnutrition and dehydration in some circumstances—is quite limited. Concentrating on incompetent patients, we have argued that in most cases such patients will be best served by providing nutrition and fluids. Thus, there should be a presumption in favor of providing nutrition and fluids as part of the broader presumption to provide means that prolong life. But this presumption may be rebutted in particular cases.

We do not have enough information to be able to determine with clarity and conviction whether withholding or withdrawing nutrition and hydration was justified in the cases that have occasioned public concern, though it seems likely that the Danville and Bloomington babies should have been fed and that Claire Conroy should not.

It is never sufficient to rule out "starvation" categorically. The question is whether the obligation to act in the patient's best interests was discharged by withholding or withdrawing particular medical treatments. All we have claimed is that nutrition and hydration by medical means need not always be provided. Sometimes they may not be in accord with the patient's wishes or interests. Medical nutrition and hydration do not appear to be distinguishable in any morally relevant way from other life-sustaining medical treatments that may on occasion be withheld or withdrawn.

We are greatful to Haavi Morreim and Steven DalleMura for their helpful comments on an earlier version of this paper. We are also grateful for the instruction provided Dr. Lynn by the staff and patients of The Washington Home and its Hospice.

Notes

1. John A. Robertson, "Dilemma in Danville," *The Hastings Center Report 11* (October 1981), 5–8.

2. T. Rohrlich. "2 Doctors Face Murder Charges in Patient's Death," L. A. *Times*, August 19, 1982, A-1; Jonathan Kirsch, "A Death at Kaiser Hospital," *California 7* (1982), 79ff; Magistrate's findings, *California* v. *Barber and Nejdl*, No. A 925586, Los Angeles Mun. Ct. Cal., (March 9, 1983); Superior Court of California, County of Los Angeles, *California* v. *Barber and Nejdl*, No. A0 25586, tentative decision May 5, 1983.

3. *In re Infant Doe*, No. GU 8204-00 (Cir. Ct. Monroe County, Ind., April 12, 1982), writ of mandamus dismissed sub nom. *State ex rel. Infant Doe v. Baker*, No. 482 S140 (Indiana Supreme Ct. May 27, 1982).

4. Office of the Secretary, Department of Health and Human Services, "Nondiscrimination on the Basis of Handicap," *Federal Register 48* (1983), 9630-32. [Interim final rule modifying 45 C.F.R. #84.61]. See Judge Gerhard Gesell's decision, *American Academy of Pediatrics v. Heckler*, No. 83-0774, U.S. District Court, D.C., April 24, 1983; and also George J. Annas, "Disconnecting the Baby Doe Hotline," *The Hastings Center Report* 13 (June 1983), 14–16.

5. *In re Claire C. Conroy*, Sup Ct NJ (Chancery Div-Essex Co. No. P-19083E) February 2, 1983; *In re Claire C. Conroy*, Sup Ct NJ (Appellate Div. No. 4-2483-82T1) July 8, 1983.

6. The President's Commission for the Study of Ethical Problems in Medicine and Biomedical and Behavioral Research, *Deciding to Forego Life-Sustaining Treatment* (Washington, D.C.: Government Printing Office, 1982).

7. G. E. M. Anscombe, "Ethical Problems in the Management of Some Severely Handicapped Children: Commentary 2," *Journal of Medical Ethics* 7 (1981), 117–124, at 122.

8. See e.g., the President's Commission for the Study of Ethical Problems in Medicine and Biomedical

and Behavioral Research, *Making Health Care Decisions* (Washington, D.C.: Government Printing Office, 1982).

9. President's Commission, *Deciding to Forego Life-Sustaining Treatment*, pp. 171–96.

10. Joyce V. Zerwekh, "The Dehydration Question," *Nursing 83* (January 1983), 47–51, with comments by Judith R. Brown and Marion B. Dolan.

11. James J. McCartney, "The Development of the Doctrine of Ordinary and Extraordinary Means of Preserving Life in Catholic Moral Theology before the Karen Quinlan Case," *Linacre Quarterly 47* (1980), 215ff.

12. President's Commission, *Deciding to Forego Life-Sustaining Treatment*, pp. 82–90. For an argument that fluids and electrolytes can be "extraordinary," see Carson Strong, "Can Fluids and Electrolytes be 'Extraordinary' Treatment?" *Journal of Medical Ethics 7* (1981), 83–85.

13. The Sacred Congregation for the Doctrine of the Faith, *Declaration on Euthanasia*, Vatican City, May 5, 1980.

14. Paul Ramsey contends that "when a man is irreversibly in the process of dying, to feed him and to give him drink, to ease him and keep him comfortable—these are no longer given as means of preserving life. The use of a glucose drip should often be understood in this way. This keeps a patient who cannot swallow from feeling dehydrated and is often the only remaining 'means' by which we can express our present faithfulness to him during his dying." Ramsey, *The Patient as Person* (New Haven: Yale University Press, 1970), pp. 128–29. But Ramsey's suggestion would not apply to a patient in a deep irreversible coma, and he would be willing to disconnect the IV in the Quinlan case; see Ramsey, *Ethics at the Edges of Life: Medical and Legal Intersections* (New Haven: Yale University Press, 1978), p. 275. Bernard Towers describes an appropriate approach to comfort and dignity: "When a patient is conscious to even the smallest degree, and if he appears to be thirsty and to have a swallowing reflex, and if there is no contraindication to oral fluids, his comfort and dignity would surely demand that he be given nourishing liquids, or at least water. If he lapses into coma, good nursing practice has traditionally required sponging out the mouth and moistening the lips. Now, if he lapses into deep coma and is on a dying trajectory, would we then try to 'push' fluids by mouth or nasogastric tube? If we did, dignity would surely suffer. The 'comfort' of the patient would, of course, be unaffected if the coma were deep enough and irreversible." Towers, "Irreversible Coma and Withdrawal of Life Support: Is It Murder If the IV Line is Disconnected?" *Journal of Medical Ethics 8* (1982), 205.

15. See Kenneth C. Micetich, Patricia H. Steinecker, and David C. Thomasma, "Are Intravenous Fluids Morally Required for a Dying Patient?" *Archives of Internal Medicine 143* (May 1983), 975–78.

16. Robert and Peggy Stinson, *The Long Dying of Baby Andrew* (Boston: Little, Brown and Company, 1983), p. 355.

17. A recent article discussed a hypothetical case of maintaining a dying, comatose patient on a respirator while withdrawing IV fluids. The authors contend that this approach is not ironic because withdrawal of the respirator "creates the immediate consequence of death for which we must take responsibility. It represents an extreme form of abandonment." Nevertheless, they were willing to stop IV fluids, knowing that death would occur before long. As the article's survey reported, other physicians would have provided nutrition and fluids. See Micetich, Steinecker, and Thomasma, "Are Intravenous Fluids Morally Required for a Dying Patient?"

Dementia in the Elderly: An Analysis of Medical Responsibility

Christine K. Cassel, M.D., Department of Medicine, University of Chicago, Pritzker School of Medicine, Chicago

Andrew L. Jameton, Ph.D., Department of Medical Jurisprudence and Humanities, University of Nebraska Medical Center, Omaha

Recent attention focused on the health care needs of the elderly includes an increased awareness of the syndrome of chronic dementia, occurring with greater frequency in the aged.[1] Dealing with the complex problems of demented patients causes discomfort in physicians. We believe some of this discomfort is caused by ethical problems underlying the care of demented patients. Yet, it is difficult to pinpoint any single "ethical dilemma." The chronic health problems of the elderly do not often present dramatic crises of decision making where moral imperatives clash. We present a case that provokes the discomfort that some indefinable problem is present. In the discussion, we will clarify the underlying ethical problems.

Mr. P., a 70-year man, was brought to the emergency room of a veterans administration hospital by his wife and daughter after he was found semiconscious on the floor of the bathroom that morning. He had been badly bruised in an automobile accident 3 days earlier but had been seen at another emergency room immediately afterwards and found to have no serious injury nor evidence of neurologic damage. Over the ensuing days he had become more confused, and on the night before admission had collapsed in the bathroom. The morning of admission he had no focal neurologic deficits but was alternately obtunded and agitated. The housestaff were highly suspicious of a subdural hematoma, and decided that a CT scan should be done immediately. If a subdural hematoma was found, he could be admitted directly to the neurosurgical service for evacuation of the clot, eliminating the time it would take for admission to the medical service and subsequent transfer to the neurosurgical service. While awaiting results of the scan, his family revealed a history of gradual onset of dementia over the past few years. Six months before, he had been admitted to the hospital because his confusion had rapidly worsened. Evaluation did not turn up a reversible cause and he was diagnosed as having senile dementia, probably Alzheimer's type. However, during his hospitalization he improved considerably and was able to go home. His memory was poor, but he had been oriented and able to participate in family gatherings.

The housestaff gathered in the CT scan suite.

Reprinted with permission from the author and *Annals of Internal Medicine* 1981 June 94(6):802–807.
When this article was written, Dr. Cassel was at Portland Veterans Administration Medical Center and the University of Oregon Health Sciences Center, Portland, and Dr. Jameton was at the University of California, Health Policy Program, San Francisco.

The patient needed parenteral sedation because he became agitated and would not hold still for the scan. The scan showed only cerebral atrophy. A subdural hematoma was not found. A battery of blood tests, a chest roentgenogram and an ECG showed no abnormalities. The medical team was dismayed because this meant he would probably end up on their service, awaiting placement in a nursing home.

His family hoped that he would recover during this hospitalization as he had during the last. In the hospital he remained alternately lethargic and obstreperous, and usually did not recognize visiting family members. They were told that he might have had a mild concussion that caused decompensation of his borderline mental status, and that he might in time recover from the effects of the concussion enough to go home again. After several weeks, however, it seemed that these were unrealistic hopes and that arrangements would need to be made to place him in a nursing home.

At this point, he knew his name but not where he was or the date and year. He could not dress himself but could feed himself. He was occasionally incontinent. He did not appear to recognize his family. He spoke in obscure sentences, although he seemed to enjoy interacting with staff who took the time to stop and share a few words. He became confused and agitated at night, requiring restraints and routine use of parenteral sedative drugs to keep him from climbing out of bed.

His wife and daughter expressed feelings of guilt about abandoning him although he often appeared not to recognize them. They would not give up the hope that he might improve enough to return home. They called the resident frequently to ask how the patient was doing, and to see if any new information had been found about the cause of his dementia. Because the work-up had already been completed the resident could tell them little except, "There is nothing more we can do." The physicians rarely visited him on their daily rounds, stopping only to renew orders for sedation and restraints.

When this patient was first seen in the emergency room, the medical staff directed a great amount of enthusiasm and energy towards diagnosis and treatment of a suspected subdural hematoma. If the diagnosis had been correct, the course of treatment would have been clear: surgical removal of the blood clot. Surgery can totally reverse the symptoms of deteriorating mental function, and may be life saving. No subtle or difficult ethical decisions would be required in such a case. The differential diagnosis is an interesting problem,[2] requiring substantial technology, and having a finite end-point. The obligation of the physician is clear.

But in the CT scan suite, the tenor of the situation quickly shifted when no subdural hematoma was seen on the scan. The medical housestaff reluctantly accepted this patient and initiated a series of screening tests. They were looking for another treatable cause of his dementia syndrome. Acute deterioration of intellectual function in elderly persons can often be traced to a medical problem such as infection, metabolic disorder, or drug toxicity.[3,4] If mental function was normal before the acute episode then chances are good that the dementia is reversible.[1,3,4]

However, in Mr. P's case, further information from his family suggested that he had a preexisting chronic dementia, not so severe that he was unable to live in a supervised and familiar environment. The worsening of his condition then was seen as somehow inevitable. The car accident may have been just a final insult that worsened his condition. This assessment was supported when all the laboratory test findings were normal. Because the housestaff anticipated a prolonged custodial hospitalization ending in the difficult but familiar problem of nursing home placement, this patient became a "gomer." He had lost his chance to be an "interesting patient."

"Gomer" is one label among many used by health professionals for patients who are disliked or seen as undesirable.[5] A body of literature has begun to appear about these "problem patients."[6,7] Personality conflicts and cultural or life style disparities account for many of the so called "hateful patients"[8,9] or "undesirable patients".[10] Self-destructive or manipulative behavior characterizes many patients who are hateful or undesirable. For example, a patient whose dementia is attributable to self-destructive behavior, such as alcoholism, is more likely to be blamed for his own disability and seen as undesirable. The situation with senile dementia is quite different. Many elderly people suffering from dementia have led useful and productive lives. They cannot be held responsible for being stricken with Alzheimer's disease. They become "undesirable patients" when deterioration of cognitive function changes the possibilities of conventional forms of interaction between doctor and patient. Care of the severely demented is therefore sometimes referred to as "veterinary medicine;" the patient is seen as not fully human.

The outlines of an ethical problem begin to emerge from recognizing that elderly demented patients generally are regarded as uninteresting and problem patients. Physicians' attention is easily drawn away from this group of patients to others with more interesting diseases, and for whom their responsibility is more clearly defined. Yet, being "uninteresting" is not a relevant moral ground for disenfranchising a whole group of people, many of whom have potential for some meaningful participation in their remaining life. Moreover, to ignore patients with chronic dementia, to abandon hope for them, virtually guarantees that they will not improve. No response will be seen if no therapy is offered. This hopelessness then becomes a self-fulfilling prophecy reinforcing the despair of health professionals as well as that of patients, friends, and family, in the face of "irreversible" dementia syndromes.

What is the physician's obligation to such patients? The duty of patient care is perhaps the least controversial obligation. The first section of the American Medical Association "Principles of Medical Ethics" reads: "A physician shall be dedicated to providing competent medical service with compassion and respect for human dignity."[11] The Oath of Hippocrates states: "I will follow that method of treatment which, according to my ability and judgment, I consider for the benefit of my patients."[12] The treatment Mr. P. received and the attitudes reflected by the behavior of the caregivers appear inconsistent with these basic professional principles. Yet, scenarios like that previously described are not unusual.[13]

Two arguments are commonly offered to justify a diminished obligation to patient care in cases like that of Mr. P. We believe that neither argument is convincing.

First, some may be inclined to accept the current low valuation of the aged in our culture. We need not see all stages of life being of equal value (14); thus, limiting resources for these patients and valuing them less is appropriate.

Although the demented aged are held in low esteem, physicians are not justified in imitating this practice. Physicians have a strong tradition of compassion for suffering and care of afflicted persons.[15] The commitment to work with the sick is a commitment to work with those in a disvalued state. If one were to abandon those in a disvalued state, one would have to abandon medical practice altogether. Therefore, disvaluing the demented—or the aged and other "uninteresting" or "hateful" patients—is inconsistent with the basic ethical commitments of the profession. Even when society sets priorities for care through policies and funding, physicians generally have seen their role as advocates for their patients, rather than as administrators of social policy. The tradition of professional medical ethics is much older, more continuous, and more coherent than that of contemporary American culture. Thus, the physician's duty to give care to elderly demented patients remains unless physicians are willing to accept, as a principle of personal conscience, that disvaluing the infirm elderly is a higher principle than their professional responsibility toward their patients.

Second, it may be held that even if our present social and fiscal priorities are regrettable, they have the effect of making it inevitable that physicians do much less for the chronically demented than for other types of patients. Institutional forces are subtle, intricate, and eventually overwhelming. Are we asking physicians, already over-burdened with patient care and a public illusion of medical omnipotence, to change society and its institutions? This is to demand some sort of heroism or saintliness. To devote a full measure of concern to every problem patient is to guarantee burnout and wasted effort.

We admit that the popular image of the physician as especially dedicated, courageous, strong, and humane burdens physicians who feel they must live up to this standard. This message is conveyed to the resident and intern by the heroic levels of labor, energy, and self-abnegation expected during their training. This self-concept can lead physicians to make unrealistic demands on themselves resulting in a high incidence of divorce, drug and alcohol addiction, and suicide.[16] To suggest a supererogatory duty to some physicians will challenge them to undertake it. Others will feel reluctantly forced in the same direction, because in medicine there always seems to be a duty to go beyond duty.[17] Yet, we believe that what at one time may seem heroic can become at a later time conventional and be done with less personal cost. "Heroic" medical interventions and surgery, for example, are now part of the conventional practice of medicine and are relatively easy to accomplish within existing health care institutions. They do not require extraordinary or "saintly" efforts, and are well rewarded both with peer respect and remuneration. If high standards of excellence in the care of demented patients became accepted standards of practice supported by the structures of our health care institutions, physicians would be relieved of the need for supererogatory behavior and personal sacrifice in caring for these patients.

As things stand now, a striking and stable conflict is present between the duty as traditionally expressed and actual practice. Strauss has noted, " . . . there develops a rather amazing pattern of repeated interactional difficulties around these particular kinds of patients." He asks, " . . . why doesn't the staff effectively work out sensible, permanent ways of either preventing or coping better with these recurrent difficulties?"[18] The ethics of the management of patients like Mr. P. are not complex. The real difficulty lies in implementing a clear moral imperative.

Thus at least three major categories of reasons why it is difficult for physicians to take an active interest in the management of chronically demented patients can be identified: the psychological discomfort faced is confronting a demented elderly patient; dominant patterns of medical practice and training; the paucity of positive institutional situations to prevent unnecessary deterioration of the patient's compromised cognitive function.

Psychological Discomfort

The process of aging itself, even without dementia, threatens our illusions of immortality. As has been pointed out many times,[19,20] our culture is strongly oriented towards the values of youth, vigor and physical attractiveness. As a group, physicians value highly for themselves the qualities of intelligence, self-reliance, social mobility, and respect from others. Thus, in addition to the unpleasant prospect of aging, one must confront in these patients symbols of the fearful possibilities of loss of control of one's own mental as well as physical functions, and consequent loss of all those highly prized qualities.

Members of the health professions are not the only ones who shy away from the realities of senescence. Most persons find the experience of visiting an elderly demented relative in a nursing home emotionally trying, even if the home is well-kept and the elderly person is cared for competently and attentively. Such a visit cannot help but raise the spectre of a similar fate for oneself.

The experience often strikes such a deep discomfort that relatives may visit less frequently or stop visiting altogether. Guilt at the feeling of having abandoned the old person intensifies the fear for oneself—the fear of being old, demented, and finally abandoned. This is not to cast blame on persons who have these feelings. These are painful and difficult situations, especially if the old person no longer appears to recognize family members.

Ironically, by ignoring the elderly, our society has made the process of aging even more fearful than it need be. In addition to the problems of physical decline and chronic illness that often accompany the aging process, our image of growing older also includes stereotypes of poverty, loneliness, and boredom, and the loss of a vital role to play in social or professional realms. Although many of these stereotypes are not true for most elderly persons, they are prevalent in our culture, and are shared even by the majority of the population over the age of 65.[21]

If we effectively deny a meaningful role to the elderly in our society, then are we justified in limiting resources expended in their care because they do not have a meaningful role?

Medical Practice and Training

Medical education has been accused of placing an inappropriate emphasis on curative function rather than "management" or "caring" functions, more useful in chronic and terminal disease.[22] Although this emphasis is beginning to change, a tendency is still present among many physicians to prefer pharmacologic and technologic forms of intervention above those that require more investment in human interaction and reorganization of facilities, especially if results are not dramatic.

Because the physician in training learns to perceive patients like Mr. P. as "gomers," interaction with a demented patient lacks the personal satisfaction of the ideal doctor-patient relationship. We cannot elicit a helpful history, answer questions, accept gratitude, or in any of the usual ways experience a satisfying and meaningful therapeutic encounter. The physician may genuinely believe he or she has nothing to offer such a patient and turn management over to the nursing and social work staff. He or she may pay only perfunctory visits until the patient can be placed in a long-term care facility.

The attitude of "therapeutic nihilism" is shown by the treatment of dementia in most medical texts. These chapters are rich with discussions of the differential diagnosis of cognitive dysfunction; histopathologic and neurochemical studies differentiating Alzheimer's and Pick's diseases from multi-infarct dementia and other more rare progressive degenerative brain diseases; and epidemiologic studies seeking etiologic clues. Attention to optimal management of patients who suffer these devastating disabilities is rare except in the nursing literature, which unfortunately is not read by most physicians.

Competence plays an important role in the physician's self image. Because many demented patients will inevitably get worse, physicians see little opportunity to be powerful; instead they may feel helpless. If the physician is not knowledgeable about the management of these problems, this feeling of helplessness is magnified and further compounds the psychological barriers preventing physicians from seeing a case of chronic dementia as an "interesting problem."

Moreover, helpful interventions with demented patients are often technologically simple and require long devotion rather than dramatic and definitive decisions. Their care gives physicians little opportunity for gratifying displays of professional excellence. The profession and the public award less prestige to those skills and specialties involved with direct bedside care, psychological support, and care of the chronically ill than they do to highly technological and scientifically sophisticated interventions.[23] Rigid distinctions between the roles of physicians and nurses, for example, severely limit creative possibilities for therapeutic intervention and contribute to the perception of demented elderly as problem patients. "Custodial" care is not seen as part of the realm of medicine. These patients are perceived as undesirable because devotion to their care has a negative effect on the status of physicians and students who choose to work with them. Poe has suggested (somewhat ironically) the establishment of a new specialty called marantology (from the Greek, "marantos" for "withered") that would include physicians explicitly devoted to the care of the patients nobody else wants.[24]

If the hopelessness was justified, and if it really was the case that nothing could be done by physicians for demented patients, then this attitude might be condoned. However, the notion that nothing can be done is a misconception based on criteria of success that are extravagant. Indeed, many things can be done in the treatment of dementia.

Therapeutic measures cannot cure patients with Alzheimer's and similar diseases, but these measures can improve the level of function and quality of life. Enhancement of functional capacity is an appropriate therapeutic endpoint in many chronic conditions.[25] In fact, management of chronic incurable diseases has become the predominant need of patients seen by internists.[26]

Although no dramatic reversals of cognitive function may occur, some evidence has shown improvements made by pharmacologic, environmental, and even psychological interventions.[27] To be sure, the evidence for therapeutic efficacy of pharmacological agent is controversial, but many examples can be found of other diseases treated with remedies for which no greater proof of efficacy can be demonstrated (adrenocorticotropic hormone for multiple sclerosis and steroids for aspiration pneumonia, for example). In these disorders, we often treat because, "it might help." Certainly chronic dementia is a disorder in which a chance of improvement using drugs of remarkably little risk of toxicity[28] is worth a try. Yet, many physicians scoff at the use of such drugs as dihydrogenated ergot alkaloids, preferring to dedate patients with high doses of medications more likely to do harm.

Problems such as incontinence and nocturnal agitation can be successfully treated by thorough evaluation of their causes and knowledgeable and meticulous attention to care.[29] They are often the result of the unfamiliar and sometimes hostile environment in a hospital, and can be solved by simple human interactions. Mr. P's functional capacity may have improved in a better environment. His occasional incontinence might have been caused by sedation and being restrained in bed with inadequate nursing staff to help him to the bathroom. Unfortunately, most medical training in this country does not address these problems adequately.

Experimental and anecdotal evidence exists that patients with any degree of dementia will either improve or at least deteriorate less rapidly if they are placed in situations where they stay active; are given sensory clues for orientation; are allowed some role in decision making about even minor aspects of the structure of their time and physical environment,[30,31] and are allowed to interact with other people, patients and staff, as much as possible.[32] Improvements in performance on mental status examinations have been reported in demented patients treated with psychotherapy.[33,36]

Highly technological diagnostic interventions may appear to the physician as a high degree of activity, but these may benefit the patient less than simpler means measured in terms of humane support and care. Since the technological and diagnostic techniques are highly developed and the simpler humane and supportive techniques underdeveloped, one could posit the law of diminishing returns to support the hypothesis that progress in the latter category would tend to have a greater net gain for patients than steps taken in the former. If medical students were provided with role models of competent, knowledgeable physicians who perceived the problems of the demented elderly as challenging and interesting, and if the profession acknowledged such expertise with badges of academic recognition comparable to those awarded for advances in esoteric or technological research, medicine could actually be beneficial to a large group of patients sadly and undeservedly identified as "undesirable patients."

Obviously, physicians cannot themselves provide the nursing care, social service assistance, and nutritional and rehabilitative therapies shown to benefit demented elderly patients. However, they can and should recognize the patients' needs and coordinate these labor intensive interventions. Therapists, social workers, and nurses often depend administratively on the active support of physicians for the effective application of their skills. Physicians can also initiate research in interdisciplinary methods of effective palliative treatment of this disorder.

Institutional Obstacles

Institutional structures frustrate positive therapeutic interventions on behalf of demented patients. The interested physician may find it difficult to place patients in a suitable institution. Very few hospitals and nursing homes are set up to provide a therapeutic milieu. More intensive staffing is required, acknowledging time spent in interaction with patients as an important part of the work day.

Patients with dementia often have been observed to have a significantly reduced life expectancy when compared with age matched controls.

The literature provides little information as to why and how the various types of dementia affect the mortality or life span. Dementia, with few exceptions, is probably not the direct cause of death. One may speculate that physical and psychosocial factors may play an important role in the proper prognosis . . . the support systems are often incapable of providing adequate medical and personal care for these patients. Our concept of dementia . . . and the fatalistic attitude and palliative approach that commonly prevail among many laymen and professionals who serve and care for these elderly patients, may also be important factors . . . patients may be overtreated with too many or too large dose of sedatives or psychotropic drugs so that they can be "easily" managed (that) further depress the brain function or jeopardize the cerebral circulation.[37]

Institutionalized patients do not receive the same degree of attention to medical problems that more independent persons receive.[38,39] The occurrence of unevaluated and untreated fever is apparently not unusual in nursing homes.[40] Staff may consider this to be "benign neglect" and feel that more aggressive care of such persons is inappropriate. Institutionalized patients are vulnerable to exploitation, as indicated by the management of some extended care facilities.[41] Overmedication facilitates management of patients whose lethargy decreases their demands for interaction with staff. Profitable contracts between nursing homes and pharmaceutical companies sometimes contribute to this unfortunate practice.[42] Lack of funding in the public sector reduces the availability of institutional care, the staffing of existing institutions, the ability of the public to detect abuses of patients in institutions, and reduces the availability of services to patients living at home.[43] Reduction of family size and urban patterns of employment make management of demented patients in the home difficult. Thus, a heroic effort to improve the functional capacity of a demented person may seem futile in light of the likelihood that he or she will be placed in a nursing home where staffing constraints or negative attitudes prevent continuation of an effective program of care.

The symbolic power of the white coat[44] and the positions of leadership many physicians hold in health care institutions give physicians power to influence public opinion in behalf of the elderly demented patient and to encourage adequate institutional resources to meet their needs. The duty of patient care therefore includes working in social and political spheres for changes in the physical environments and staffing priorities of hospitals and long term care facilities.

Conclusion

In many ways, the problem of Mr. P. is rooted in the concept of medicine. In the suffering of the elderly demented patients and their families, we find one of the most basic and still unresolved ethical questions about the nature of medical practice. One of the tragedies of medicine is to have to witness suffering that one cannot relieve. Suffering has always been an inescapable feature of human existence. Historically, the human response to it has always been to try to give it meaning in philosophic or religious notions of the human condition that emphasize compassion, inner strength, and sense of community.[45] The dramatic successes of medicine in this century have led us to see suffering simply as something to be eliminated: suffering is an evil, and whatever its explanation, the good doctor struggles against it.[46] When the patient's suffering cannot be erased, it is too easy to turn away from that patient and say, "Nothing can be done." Medicine now poses the question again in a new form: How can the new technologies and institutions of medical practice be used to give meaning to suffering caused by disabilities we cannot eliminate? Can we develop effective ways to exercise meaningful compassion towards elderly patients with cognitive impairment?

The tragic dignity in the aging philosopher Immanuel Kant has been described:

Nine days before his death, Immanuel Kant was visited by his physician. Old, ill and nearly blind, he rose from his chair and stood trembling with weakness and muttering unintelligible words. Finally his faithful companion realized that he would not sit down again until the visitor had taken a seat. This he did, and Kant then permitted himself to be helped to his chair and, after having regained some of his strength, said, 'Das Gefuhl fur Humanitat hat mich noch nicht verlassen'—'The sense of humanity has not yet left me.'[47]

We believe that analyzing what physicians should do in the care of demented patients can be helpful in forming a medical ethic that can handle the increasingly prevalent problems of chronic disease. The current status of the demented patient seems to impose on physicians uncomfortable choices. Physicians can look away from the problem, thus becoming accomplices to the neglect of the demented, or attempt to cope with the problem and face internal conflict, frustration, and wasted effort. Where the choices are either heroism or complicity, one has an existential decision to make.[48] One cannot be blamed for a responsible choice of either. It is simply a question of what kind of world one hopes to create.

References

1. National Institute on Aging Task Force. Senility reconsidered: treatment possibilities for mental impairment in the elderly. *JAMA.* 1980;**244**:259–63.

2. Hardison J E. The importance of being interesting. *Am J Med.* 1980;**68**:9–10.

3. Ropper A H. A rational approach to dementia. *Can Med Assoc J.* 1979;**121**:1175–90.

4. Wells C E. Chronic brain disease: an overview. *Am J Psychiatry.* 1978;**135**:1–13.

5. George V. Dundes A. The gomer: a figure of American hospital folk speech. *J Am Folklore.* 1978;**91**:568–81.

6. Malcolm R, Foster H K, Smith C. The problem patient as perceived by family physicians. *J Fam Pract.* 1977;**5**:361–4.

7. Von Mering O, Earley L W. The ambulatory problem patient: a unique teaching resource. *Am J Psychiatry.* 1969;**126**:108–12.

8. Hackett T. Which patients turn you off? It's worth analyzing, *Medical Economics.* 1969;**46(15)**:94–9.

9. Groves J E. Taking care of the hateful patient. *N Engl J Med.* 1978;**298**:883–7.

10. Papper S. The undesirable patient. *J Chronic Dis.* 1970;**22**:777–9.

11. Reinhold R. AMA facing legal pressures adopts less rigid code for doctors. *New York Times.* 1980: July **23**:A–1, col. 4.

12. Reiser S J, Dyck A J, Curran W J. *Ethics in Medicine: Historical Perspectives and Contemporary Concerns.* Cambridge: Massachusetts Institute of Technology Press; 1977:5.

13. Duff R S, Hollingshead AB. *Sickness and Society.* New York: Harper & Row Publishers, Inc.;1968:157.

14. Fletcher J. *Humanhood: Essays in Biomedical Ethics.* Buffalo: Prometheus Books; 1979.

15. Pellegrino E D. *Humanism and the Physician.* Knox-

ville, Tennessee: University of Tennessee Pres; 1979.

16. Bittker T E. Reaching out to the depressed physician. *JAMA*. 1976;**236**:1713–6.

17. Urmson J O. Saints and heroes. In: Feinberg J, ed. *Moral Concepts*. New York: Oxford University Press; 1970:60–73.

18. Strauss A L. *Chronic Illness and The Quality of Life*. St. Louis: The C. V. Mosby Co.; 1975:137.

19. Butler R N. *Why Survive?: Being Old in America*. New York: Harper & Row Publishers, Inc.; 1975:235–6.

20. Collett-Pratt C. Attitudinal predictors of devaluation of old age in a multigenerational sample. *J Gerontol*. 1976;**31**:193–7.

21. Louis Harris and Associates. *The Myth and Reality of Aging in America*. Washington, D.C.: The National Council on Aging; 1975:128–72.

22. *See* Reference 19, p. 175.

23. Fox R C, Swazey J P. *The Courage to Fail: A Social View of Organ Transplants and Dialysis*. Chicago: University of Chicago Press; 1974.

24. Poe W D. Marantology, a needed specialty. *N Engl J Med. 1972*;**286**:102–3.

25. *See* Reference 18, pp. 133–44.

26. Fries J F. Aging, natural death, and the compression of morbidity. *N. Engl J Med. 1980*;**303**:130–5.

27. Shaw J. A literature review of treatment options for mentally disabled old people. *J Gerontological Nursing*. 1979;**5**:36–42.

28. Gaitz C M, Varner R V, Overall J E. Pharmacotherapy for organic brain syndrome in late life. *Arch Gen Psychiatry*. 1977;**34**:839–45.

29. Brocklehurst J C, ed. *Textbook of Geriatric Medicine and Gerontology*. Edinburgh: Churchill Livingstone; 1978.

30. Rodin J, Langer E J. Long-term effects of a control-relevant intervention with the institutionalized aged. *J Pers Soc Psychol*. 1977;**35**:897–902.

31. Schulz R, Hanusa BH. Long-term effects of control and predictability—enhancing interventions: findings and ethical issues. *J Pers Soc Psychol*. 1978;**36**:1194–201.

32. Roshos S R, Terner S. Kline B E. The elderly patient in a therapeutic community. *Compr Psychiatry*. 1979;**20**:359–69.

33. Oberleder M. Crisis therapy in mental breakdown of the aging. *The Gerontologist*. 1970;**10**:111–4.

34. Blank M L. Raising the age barrier to psychotherapy. *Geriatrics*. 1974;**24**(11):14–8.

35. Lewis M I, Butler R N. Life review therapy. *Geriatrics*. 1974;**24**(11):165–73.

36. Harris S L, Snyder B D, Snyder R L, Magrow B. Behavior modification therapy with elderly demented patients: implementation and ethical considerations. *J Chronic Dis*. 1970;**30**:129–34.

37. Wang H S. Prognosis in dementia and related disorders in the aged. In: Katzman R, Terry R D, Bick K L, eds. *Alzheimer's Disease Senile Dementia and Related Disorders*. New York: Raven Press: 1978:312. (Aging; vol. 7).

38. Moss F E, Halamandaris V J. *Too Old Too Sick Too Bad: Nursing Homes in America*. Germantown, Maryland: Aspen Systems Corporation; 1977.

39. United States Senate Subcommittee on Long Term Care. The Special Committee on Aging. *Introductory Report: Nursing Homes Care in the United States: Failure of Public Policy*. Washington. D.C.: U.S. Government Printing Office; 1975.

40. Brown N K, Thompson D J. Nontreatment of fever in extended-care facilities. *N. Engl J Med*. 1979;**300**:1246–50.

41. Mendelson M A. *Tender Loving Greed*. New York: Random House; 1974.

42. Silverman M, Lee P R. *Pills, Profit and Politics*. Berkeley, California: University of California Press; 1974:176.

43. Kane R L, Kane R A. Care of the aged: old problems in need of new solutions. *Science*. 1978;**200**:913–9.

44. Blumhagen D W. The doctor's white coat: the image of the physician in modern America. *Ann Intern Med*. 1979;**91**:111–6.

45. Hawerwas S. Reflections on suffering, death and medicine. *Ethics Sci Med*. 1979;**6**:229–37.

46. Camus A. *The Plague*. New York: Alfred K. Knopf; 1950.

47. Panofsky E. *Meaning of the Visual Arts*. New York: Anchor Press/Doubleday & Co.; 1955:1.

48. Sartre J P. *Existentialism is a Humanism*. New York: Philosophical Library; 1947.

Selected Readings

Articles

Atkinson, G. M. Living and dying with less: An ethic for the 1980s. *Hosp Prog.* 1982 Nov. 62(11):30–34.

Angell, M. Cost containment and the physician. *JAMA.* 1985 Sept. 6. 254(9):1203–1207.

Bayer, R., and others. The care of the terminally ill: morality and economics. *N Eng J Med* 1983 Dec. 15. 309(24):1490–1494.

Bayley, C. Terminating treatment: asking the right questions. *Hosp Prog.* 1980 Sept. 61(9):50–53, 72.

Boyle, J. Should we learn to say no? *JAMA.* 1984 Aug. 10. 252 (6):782–784.

Capron, A. M. An ethical obligation to ensure access to new medical technologies? *J. Health Care Technol.* 1984 Fall. 1(2):103–120.

————. Twenty questions about ethics committees. *Ethics Committee Newsletter.* 1984 June. 1(4):2–9.

Childress, J. Priorities in the allocation of health care resources. *Soundings.* 1979 Fall. 62:561–568.

Forster, J. A communitarian ethical model for public health interventions: an alternative to individual behavior change strategies. *J Public Health Policy.* 1982 June. 3(2):150–163.

Friedman, E. Rationing and the identified life. *Hospitals.* 1984 May 16. 58(10):65–74.

Fuchs, V. The "rationing" of medical care. *N Eng J Med* 1984 Dec. 13. 311(24):1572–1573.

Gutmann, A. For and against equal access to health care. *Milbank Memorial Fund Quarterly.* 1981. 59(4):542–562.

Hampton, J. R. The end of clinical freedom. *Br Med J* 1983. Oct. 29. 287(6401):1237–1238.

Ingelfinger, F. Informed (but uneducated) consent. *N Eng J Med* 1972 Aug. 31. 287(9):465–466.

Jackson, D. L., and Youngner, S. Patient autonomy and "death with dignity"—Some clinical caveats. *N Eng J Med* 1979 Aug. 23. 301(8):404–408.

Levey, S., and Hesse, D. Bottom-line health care? *N Eng J Med* 1985 Mar. 3. 312(10):644–647.

Levine, R. Total artificial heart implantation: Eligibility criteria. *JAMA.* 1984 Sept. 21. 1252:1458.

McCormick, R. A. To save or let die: The dilemma of modern medicine. *JAMA.* 1974 July 8. 229(2):172–176.

Meisel, A. The "exceptions" to the informed consent doctrine: Striking a balance between competing values in medical decisionmaking. *Wis Law Rev.* 1979 Aug., 413–488.

Miller, B. L. Autonomy and the refusal of lifesaving treatment. *Hastings Ctr Rep.* 1981 Aug. 11(4):22–28.

Outka, G. Social justice and equal access to health care. *J Religious Ethics.* 1974 Spring. 2(1):11–32.

Thurow, L. C. Learning to say "no." *N Eng J Med* 1984 Dec. 13. 311(24):1569–1572.

Victoroff, M. Rationing healthcare: An ethical assessment. *HealthSpan.* 1985 Apr. 2(4):3–12.

Weinstein, M., and Stason, W. Allocating resources: The case of hypertension. *Hastings Ctr Rep.* 1977 Oct. 7:24.

Books

Aaron, H. J., and Schwartz, W. B. *The Painful Prescription*. Washington, DC: The Brookings Institution, 1984.

Calabresi, G., and Bobbitt, P. *Tragic Choices*. New York: Norton, 1978.

Cranford, R. E., and Doudera, A. E. *Institutional Ethics Committees and Health Care Decision Making*. Ann Arbor, MI: Health Administration Press, 1984.

Fox, R., and Swazey, J. *The Courage to Fail*. 2nd ed. Chicago: The University of Chicago Press, 1978.

Johnson, A., Siegler, M., and Winslade, W. *Clinical Ethics*. New York: MacMillan Publishing Co., 1982.

Katz, J., and Capron, A. M. *Catastrophic Diseases: Who Decides What?* New York: Russell Sage Foundation, 1975.

Mappes, T. A., and Zembaty, J. S., Editors. *Biomedical Ethics*. New York: McGraw-Hill Book Co., 1981.

Menzel, P. T. *Medical Costs, Moral Choices*. New Haven, CT: Yale University Press, 1983.

Report of the Massachusetts Task Force on Organ Transplantation. Boston: Boston University School of Public Health, 1984. Copies are available from the Massachusettes Department of Public Health, Office of the Commissioner, 150 Tremont St., Boston, MA 02111.

Thomas, L. *The Lives of a Cell*. New York: Viking Press, 1974.

Wong, C. B. *Dilemmas of Dying*. Boston: G. K. Hall Medical Publishers, 1981.

Periodicals

Hastings Center Report. Published six times a year by the Hastings Center, 360 Broadway, Hastings-on-Hudson, NY 10706.

Hospital Ethics. Published quarterly by the American Hospital Association, 840 N. Lake Shore Drive, Chicago, IL 60611.

In Addition, there are many ethics periodicals published by local or regional ethics organizations, such as, *Ethical Currents,* published by the St. Joseph Health System, Orange, CA. Space limitations and the sometimes short publishing lives of these newsletters led us to omit listing them here.